Motor Control and Physical Therapy: Theoretical Framework and Practical Applications

Second Edition
Reprint

Edited by
Patricia C. Montgomery, Ph.D., PT
Barbara H. Connolly, Ed.D., PT

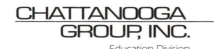

CHATTANOOGA
GROUP, INC.
Education Division

Motor Control and Physical Therapy: Theoretical Framework and Practical Applications

Second Edition
Reprint

Preface

Advances in research in the areas of neurophysiology, biomechanics, motor control, motor learning, motor development, and cognitive training provide physical therapists with new and more effective methods to assess and treat patients with movement disorders. As physical therapy becomes an entry into the health care system for increasing numbers of patients, the physical therapist must become more skilled in diagnosing movement disorders. Additionally, physical therapists are responsible both to patients and to third party payers for measuring and documenting changes in patients' functional abilities as a consequence of treatment interventions. This text attempts to provide "state of the art" information that allows the physical therapy student and the practitioner to apply new concepts in a problem solving approach.

Biographical Sketches

Mary Beth Badke, M.S., PT

Mary Beth Badke is Associate Director and Clinical Assistant Professor of Physical Therapy at the University of Wisconsin Hospital & Clinics, Madison. She received her MS degree from the University of North Carolina, Chapel Hill. She has lectured throughout the U.S. and has published papers dealing with the CNS control of equilibrium and its implications in pathology such as stroke. She is co-editor of the book "Stroke Rehabilitation: Recovery of Motor Control."

Richard P. DiFabio, Ph.D., PT

Dr. DiFabio received his BS degree in physical therapy from the State University of New York at Upstate Medical Center. He earned an MS degree in education from the State University of New York at Cortland and a Ph.D. in therapeutics (physical therapy) from the University of Iowa. Dr. DiFabio holds a joint appointment in the Departments of Otolaryngology and Physical Medicine & Rehabilitation at the University of Minnesota, Minneapolis.

Barbara H. Connolly , Ed.D., PT

Dr. Connolly received her BS degree in physical therapy from the University of Florida and an MEd in special education and an Ed.D. in curriculum and instruction from Memphis State University. She is Associate Professor and Chairman of the Department of Rehabilitation Sciences at the University of Tennessee, Memphis. She holds an academic appointment in physical therapy at the University of Mississippi and serves as a guest lecturer at numerous other programs in physical therapy. Additionally, Dr. Connolly remains active in the clinic through the UT faculty practice.

Carol A. Giuliani, Ph.D., PT

Dr. Giuliani received a BS degree in physical therapy from California State University at Long Beach, and an MS and Ph.D. in kinesiology, with an emphasis in the neural control of movement, from the University of California at Los Angeles. Dr. Giuliani currently is an Assistant Professor in the Division of Physical Therapy at the University of North Carolina at Chapel Hill.

Patricia Leahy, M.S., PT, NCS

Ms. Leahy received a BS degree in physical therapy from the University of Pittsburgh and an MS degree in physical therapy from Temple University. Ms. Leahy has been certified as a Neurologic Clinical Specialist by the American Board of Physical Therapy Specialties. She is an Assistant Professor in the physical therapy department of the Philadelphia College of Pharmacy and Science and is active in the Neurology Section of the American Physical Therapy Association.

Kathye E. Light, Ph.D., PT

Dr. Light received her BS degree in physical therapy from the University of Missouri, Columbia, her MS in physical therapy from the Medical College of Virginia, Virginia Commonwealth University, and her Ph.D. in kinesiological motor control from the University of Texas, Austin. She is presently an Assistant Professor of Physical Therapy at the University of North Carolina at Chapel Hill. Dr. Light's research interests include motor control and learning issues related to neurologic rehabilitation and adult aging.

Sandy Lowrance

Sandy Lowrance is a graphic designer and illustrator who has worked with major institutions and corporations in the United States. She received a Master of Product Design/Visual Design degree from North Carolina State University, and is currently an Associate Professor of graphic design at Memphis State University.

Gin McCollum, Ph.D.

Dr. McCollum received a Ph.D. in theoretical physics from Yeshiva University. She has worked in neuroscience the last twelve years, taking a structuralist-mathematical approach to developing models of movement and the sensory basis for movement. Dr. McCollum is a research scientist at the R.S. Dow Neurological Sciences Institute of Good Samaritan Hospital and Medical Center in Portland, Oregon.

Patricia C. Montgomery, Ph.D., PT

Dr. Montgomery received a BS degree in physical therapy from the University of Oklahoma and an MA in educational psychology and a Ph.D. in child psychology from the University of Minnesota. Dr. Montgomery has a private practice in pediatric physical therapy in the Minneapolis-St. Paul area and holds academic appointments in the physical therapy programs at the University of Minnesota, Minneapolis and Hahnemann University, Philadelphia.

Roberta Newton, Ph.D., PT

Dr. Newton received a BS degree in physical therapy from the Medical College of Virginia, Virginia Commonwealth University and a Ph.D. in neurophysiology from the Medical College of Virginia/VCU. Dr. Newton is an Associate Professor and Director of Advanced Graduate Studies in the Department of Physical Therapy, Temple University, Philadelphia, PA.

Carol A. Oatis, Ph.D., PT

Carol Oatis has a BS in physical therapy from Marquette University and a Ph.D. in anatomy with an emphasis on biomechanics from the University of Pennsylvania. She is an Associate Professor at Beaver College in Glenside, PA, where she teaches applied anatomy and biomechanics. She is also co-founder of and co-principal at the Philadelphia Institute for Physical Therapy, a physical therapist owned facility providing out-patient care as well as research and teaching services. Her present research interests include motion analysis of locomotion particularly modeling pathological gait and the study of elements of normal and abnormal posture.

Mary M. Rodgers, Ph.D., PT

Dr. Rodgers received BS and MS degrees in physical therapy and biomechanics from the University of North Carolina at Chapel Hill, and a Ph.D. in biomechanics from The Pennsylvania State University. Dr. Rodgers is a Research Health Scientist with the Department of Veterans Affairs and holds academic appointments in the Departments of Rehabilitation Medicine and Orthopaedic Surgery at Wright State University School of Medicine, Dayton, OH.

Anne Shumway-Cook, Ph.D., PT

Dr. Shumway-Cook received a BS degree in physical therapy from Indiana University, and a Ph.D. in motor control from the University of Oregon. For the past ten years she has been engaged in research on the physiological basis for postural disorders in the patient with neurologic deficits, and the scientific rationale for rehabilitation strategies. She is currently a private consultant in Seattle.

Ann F. VanSant, Ph.D., PT

Dr. VanSant received a BS degree in physical therapy from Russell Sage College, and an MS in physical therapy from Medical College of Virginia. She received a Ph.D. in motor development from the University of Wisconsin, Madison. Dr. VanSant conducts research in life-span motor development and teaches in the areas of motor development and neurologic physical therapy to entry-level and advanced graduate students in physical therapy at Temple University in Philadelphia.

Table of Contents

— Illustrations by Sandy Lowrance —

Chapter 1
Framework For Assessment And Treatment

Barbara H. Connolly, Ed.D., PT
Patricia C. Montgomery, Ph.D., PT

INTRODUCTION

Physical therapists are members of a dynamic health care profession that is changing constantly as new information becomes available. Advances in research in the areas of neurophysiology, biomechanics, motor control, motor learning, motor development, and cognitive training provide us with new and more effective methods to assess and treat patients with movement disorders. The purpose of this text is to provide physical therapy students and practitioners with practical applications of state of the art information in the above mentioned areas.

A case study format is used to emphasize and illustrate the importance of applying research information in the clinical setting. Students and clinicians need to be diagnosticians of movement disorders and able to apply this state of the art information to patients. Additionally, the case study format allows students, who have little experience in applying theoretical information to practical problems, to use a problem solving approach.

HISTORICAL PERSPECTIVES

For the past 30 years, physical therapists have relied on a number of theories termed "neurophysiologic approaches" to assess and treat patients with neurologically based movement disorders. Most of these approaches are based on a "hierarchial model" of motor control. Within this traditional hierarchial model of motor control, the reflex serves as the basic functional unit of movement. In this model, the cortex is viewed as the highest functioning component of the system and spinal level reflexes as the lowest. Newer models, in particular the "distributed control model," propose a different neural organization of motor control. In this model, the

"controller" varies depending on the task. No longer is the cortex considered the "boss."

Two general models of neural organization that are used to describe motor function are the "open system" and the "closed system." The "open system" model is characterized by single transfer of information without feedback loops (Figure 1). This model is used in the traditional reflexive hierarchial theory of motor control. However, the "closed system" model has multiple feedback loops and supports the concept of distributed control (Figure 2). Additionally, in the closed model, the nervous system is viewed as an active agent with structures that enable the initiation and generation of movement, not merely an agent that reacts to incoming stimuli.

In the field of motor learning, "closed loop" and "open loop" theories are proposed to account for the processes of learning and performing motor tasks. Closed loop theory stresses the use of feedback particularly when learning new tasks. Open loop theory accounts for skills that are well established, performed rapidly, or where feedback is not used due to the speed needed to accomplish the task (i.e., ballistic type movements).

REVIEW OF TRADITIONAL
NEUROPHYSIOLOGIC APPROACHES

Physical therapists use combinations of techniques from a variety of theoretical frameworks in the evaluation and treatment of patients with movement disorders. A majority of the traditional neurophysiologic approaches rely on the assessment of reflexive behavior, i.e., flexor withdrawal, asymmetrical tonic neck reflex, moro response, body right-

FIGURE 1. An open system devoid of feedback. Information travels in only one direction. Neurons 1 and 2 conduct impulses toward Neuron 3, which in turn directs its activity toward the muscle.

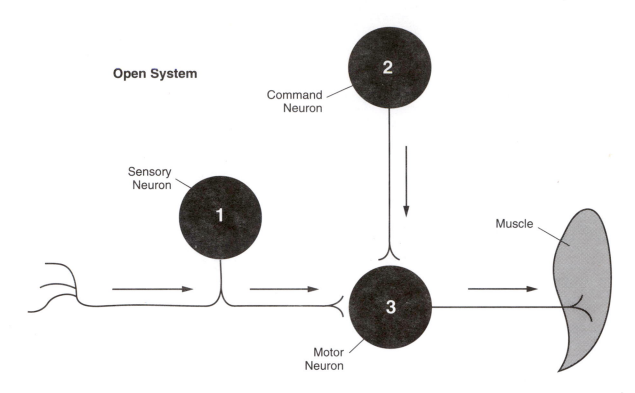

ing, labyrinthine righting, and equilibrium reactions. Descriptions of these reflexes may be found in numerous texts. Emphasis on reflexes has led us to conceptualize the central nervous system (CNS) in a stimulus-response type paradigm or as a passive agent in movement. This has distracted us from attending to other parameters of movement such as initiation, rate, and synergistic organization. Although physical therapy students and clinicians should be familiar with the classic descriptions of these reflexes, it is unclear how reflexes relate to functional movement. We have chosen to emphasize more recent models of motor control in this text.

The most commonly used neurophysiologic approaches are reviewed superficially in the following pages. Refer to the suggested readings at the end of this chapter for further information on the individual approaches.

AYRES - Sensory Integration (SI)

As a young occupational therapist in the early 1950's, A. Jean Ayres Ph.D. realized that functional limitations of many brain damaged adults were due to sensory or perceptual factors rather than to motor problems. She reasoned that understanding how the brain processes sensation, especially vestibular and somatosensory input, would provide the basis for treatment of perceptual dysfunction. Sensory integration is a neurobehavioral theory and the neural model stressed by Dr. Ayres is the CNS's ability to organize and interpret sensory information. Higher level processes of perception

and cognition are considered dependent on brainstem and midbrain processing of sensory input (hierarchial). Ayres devised tests to identify and measure symptoms of sensory dysfunction and began publishing her findings in the mid-1960's. She continued to develop standardized tests until the time of her death in 1988. Through use of these tests, supplemented by clinical observations, she identified several types of disorders in children with learning disabilities including: 1) problems in form and space perception, 2) dyspraxia, 3) tactile defensiveness, 4) auditory-language problems, and 5) vestibular processing disorders and problems in bilateral integration.

Motor dysfunction in sensory integrative theory is addressed primarily from the aspect of motor planning or praxis and SI was not developed to address neuromotor dysfunction as seen in the child with cerebral palsy. Although assessment and treatment principles initially addressed the child with learning disabilities, SI has been incorporated into treatment for patients with varying brain disorders. Motor behavior in treatment is used to assess changes in organization and interpretation of sensory input. Ayres proposed that somatosensory and vestibular functions are ontogenetically and phylogenetically early and are the underpinnings of normal development. Sensory feedback and repetition are important principles of motor learning incorporated into SI theory.

Treatment is administered to meet the sensory needs of the individual, and the sensory environment and sensory requirements of tasks are changed depending on the individual's response to treatment. The "adaptive response" refers to active participation in treatment so sensory information must be organized by the individual in order to complete a task, solve a problem, or plan a movement. Behavioral goals that, as much as possible, are determined by the patient are stressed. Sensory integration is practiced mainly by occupational therapists, but physical therapists also have incorporated SI into treatment regimens for patients with neurologic impairments. Training beyond entry-level preparation is available and consists of professional development courses in theory, test mechanics, and interpretation.

BOBATHS - Neurodevelopmental Treatment (NDT)

Neurodevelopmental treatment is an approach developed by Dr. Karel Bobath, an English physician, and his wife, Berta Bobath, a physiotherapist. Assessment and treatment principles for neuromotor dysfunction were originally proposed in the late 1940's and were based on research done in the 1920's and 1930's with animals and humans. Emphasis has evolved from assessing localized spasticity to evaluating patterns of movement. Dysfunction is envisioned as the result of loss of control from damaged higher CNS centers. The major deficit is in the "normal postural reflex mechanism" with abnormal tone and reflexes interfering with normal movement.

NDT was developed for children with cerebral palsy and adults with acquired hemiplegia, although this approach has been applied to patients with many types of neural dysfunction involving the motor system.

Normal development is the primary model underlying NDT. Principles of motor control are based on the hierarchial reflex model and repetition as a method of motor learning is emphasized primarily in automatic or postural movement. Because emphasis is on postural mechanisms, cognitive aspects of motor control and motor learning are not emphasized. The Bobaths stressed the importance of early intervention in children before abnormal or primitive movement patterns become habitual, leading to muscle asymmetries, contractures, and deformities.

Treatment principles include normalizing abnormal muscle tone (spasticity, flaccidity, rigidity, spasms), inhibiting or integrating primitive postural patterns, and facilitating normal postural reactions. This is done primarily through direct "handling" of the patient through key points (usually proximal) of control, although positioning and family/caregiver education also are stressed. Strengthening is not a principle of NDT and primitive reflexes or patterns and associated reactions are not used to facilitate movement.

In addition to numerous publications, basic training in NDT is taught in continuing education format simultaneously to occupational therapists, physical therapists and speech pathologists, as the Bobaths considered all of these professionals to be concerned with motor aspects of behavior. Instructors are certified by a professional organization, and

FIGURE 2. A closed-loop system with multiple feedback loops. Although Neuron 1 appears to be at the top of the hierarchy, and thus in command of the system, it is apparent on closer analysis that there is no hierarchy in this organizational arrangement of neurons. By inspecting Neurons 1 to 4, it is easy to see that each of these elements could conceivably be under control of at least one other neuron: Neuron 1 receives information from Neurons 2 and 3; Neuron 2 receives information from Neurons 1 and 5; and so on. Only Neuron 5 appears to be outside the sphere of influence of other neurons. Neuron 5 is indirectly affected by the activity in Neuron 4.

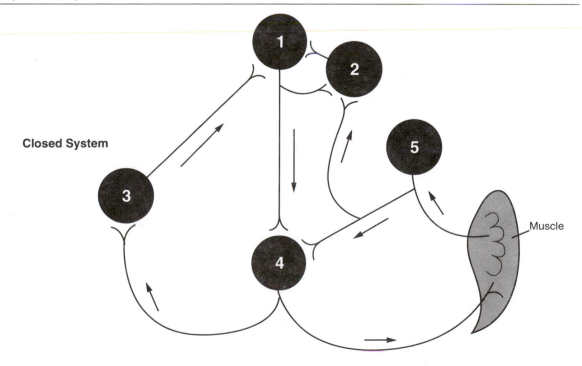

Closed System

Muscle

basic 8 week pediatric courses, 2 - 3 week courses in treatment of adults with hemiplegia, and advanced courses in treatment of infants are offered.

BRUNNSTROM - Movement Therapy in Hemiplegia

The Brunnstrom approach developed by Signe Brunnstrom, a physical therapist, is based on clinical information and neurophysiologic principles that were known during the early 1960's. Brunnstrom identified numerous common characteristics seen in patients with hemiplegia. These common characteristics included the presence of basic limb synergies in both the upper and lower extremities and the order of recovery stages from the time of the initial insult. She stated that, although patients with hemiplegia have common characteristics, individual differences occur since no two patients are exactly alike. In synergistic patterns, these differences are related mainly to the relative strength of the synergy components and not the nature of the synergy.

The evaluation of the recovery stages forms the basis for evaluation of the patient using the Brunnstrom approach. The patient is assessed for the presence of flaccidity (Stage 1), emergence of basic limb synergies (Stage 2), voluntary performance of part or all of the basic limb synergies (Stage 3), mixing and matching of the basic limb synergies (Stage 4), relative independence of basic limb synergies (Stage 5), and isolated, coordinated joint movement (Stage 6). Additionally, the evaluation of sensation (tactile and passive motion sense), pain, passive range of motion, trunk balance, hand function, facial function, presence of selected postural reflexes, and stance/gait are vital to the overall assessment of the patient.

Therapeutic procedures are aimed at promoting voluntary control of the synergies by the patient through the use of sensory input (tactile, proprioceptive, visual, and auditory) and positive reinforcement. Selected postural reflexes such as the asymmetric tonic neck reflex, tonic lumbar reflex, and tonic labyrinthine are used to facilitate voluntary movement. Brunnstrom stressed that training sessions must be planned so that only those tasks which the patient can master, or almost master are demanded. Once the patient is able to move voluntarily through the synergies, the patient is encouraged to learn a number of movement combinations that deviate from the basic synergies and which are more functional. In particular, hand activities are stressed as the patient is able to move out of the basic synergy patterns in the upper extremities.

Brunnstrom advocated that preparation for walking be emphasized early in the treatment approach and that extensive walking be postponed so that a poor gait pattern could be avoided. The preparation for walking included training in trunk balance, modification of motor responses in the legs, and training of alternate responses of antagonistic muscles. In the training for standing and walking, Brunnstrom advocated the use of sensory input and behavioral modification by providing the patient with a knowledge of result of his efforts.

CARR and SHEPHERD - Motor Relearning Approach

The Motor Relearning Approach, developed by Janet Carr and Roberta Shepherd in the 1970's focuses on an understanding of normal movement and how movement is learning or relearned. Carr and Shepherd state that an adult who has experienced a neurologic insult may no longer know how to move and may have to relearn those movements. They further state that those factors that are relevant to the learning of a motor skill are also relevant to the relearning of the skill.

The major factors in the learning or relearning process as identified by Carr and Shepherd include:

- Identification of a goal
- Inhibition of unnecessary activity
- The ability to cope with the effects of gravity and therefore to make balance adjustments while shifting weight
- Appropriate body alignment
- Practice (physical and mental)
- Motivation
- Feedback and knowledge of results

Carr and Shepherd state that the therapist should be aware of the effects of these factors in learning a skill and should assess the impact of problems with any one of these factors on the patient with neurologic deficits.

In this approach, observation is a major part of the assessment procedure. Accordingly, the therapist who understands the subtleties and variations of normal movement should be able to assess with accuracy the patient's problems of movement. Through this critical observation, the therapist should be able to judge the most essential missing or abnormal components of movement and therefore provide treatment to address primary or secondary problems. The assessment includes evaluation of tone through movement, handling, and the effect of tonic reflexes. Additionally, the therapist assesses overall movement and function, hand function, balance (both static and dynamic), and sensation. Although the assessments suggested in the approach are subjective, the authors state that these observations are reliable and provide qualitative information about the patient's function. Other objective quantitative measures should be used as needed. Videotaping the patient is encouraged as a means of assessing function and improvement.

The techniques used in the approach represent a combination of other approaches. However, the authors insist that there can be no routine treatment for patients according to their diagnosis and that the developmental sequence should not be adhered to in adults. Many of the Bobath treatment techniques are suggested for use, such as holding and placing, reflex inhibiting movement patterns, weightbearing/approximation/compression, balance activities on a therapy ball, inhibitive casts, and walking facilitation. Many of the hand activities are based on the Bobath approach. The Rood techniques of brushing, application of ice, pounding, tapping, as well as vibration are incorporated into the treatment. Carr and Shepherd encourage the use of EMG biofeedback as a therapeutic technique to either decrease hypertonus during movement or to aid in the contraction of specific muscles. The use of a mirror for visual feedback is encouraged as a means of self correction and self awareness.

JOHNSTONE - Treatment of CVA

Margaret Johnstone is a Scottish physiotherapist who has worked with patients with neurologic deficits since the time she treated patients with gunshot wounds of the brain in the mid 1940's. The main objective of her treatment approach is to attack spasticity in the patient with a cerebral vascular accident (CVA) 24 hours a day. Treatment is based on reflex inhibition with special attention to the tonic neck reflexes through use of air splints and positioning. The optimal position for the affected upper extremity in the air splint (40 mm HG pressure when fully inflated by mouth) is with shoulder external rotation; elbow, wrist, and finger extension; forearm supination; and thumb abduction. Initial goals are to maintain full wrist extension (avoiding the typical wrist and finger flexion postures of the patient with a CVA) and a pain free shoulder.

During early stages of recovery, the patient is positioned sidelying on the unaffected side with the affected arm in the air splint protracted and supported by a pillow. Attention also is paid to positioning the affected leg in protraction with hip internal rotation, and hip, ankle, and knee flexion. The patient can lie on the affected side if the limbs are positioned properly. Main problems are identified as an imbalance of muscle tone and the presence of unwanted, disabling postures from loss of CNS control from higher centers. Based on a hierarchial, reflex model with sensory as well as motor emphasis, Johnstone's approach also relies on a normal, developmental model following sequences of movements, proximal to distal. The air splint is designed to apply even deep pressure to the soft tissues to address sensory dysfunction. Johnstone outlined principles of early bed and transfer mobility, as well as early mat exercises and more advanced exercises as the patient improves, with emphasis continually on the use of air splints and positioning.

KABAT, KNOTT, VOSS - Proprioceptive
Neuromuscular Facilitation (PNF)

Herman Kabat, MD, has been credited, along with his co-worker, Margaret Knott, physical therapist, for developing the approach initially termed "proprioceptive facilitation." Knott and Dorothy Voss, another physical therapist, later used the term "proprioceptive neuromuscular facilitation" or PNF. PNF was developed initially for use with children with cerebral palsy, but soon was applied to patients with other types of neuromuscular disabilities. Today, PNF is used extensively with patients with orthopedic as well as neurologic problems.

Guidelines for this theory were obtained from studies of animal behavior and learning as well as human development. A developmental framework is evident in such principles as cervicocaudal and proximal to distal progressions and fetal reflexive motor behavior. This suggests that "recapitulation" of motor sequences is important. Sensory elements are incorporated. For example, reversals of movement used in PNF are an orderly sequencing of total tactile, auditory, and visual cues. Manual contacts and tone of voice are used to modulate the patient's efforts to move.

Along with principles of motor development, principles of motor learning using involuntary and voluntary effort with repetition and use of activities are stressed. PNF uses resistance and stretch to facilitate specific motor patterns and rotation is a key element in many patterns. Specific patterns are used with reversing movements to establish an interaction between agonists and antagonists in an attempt to correct imbalances among muscle groups. Diagonal rather than straight plane movements are used primarily and are identified by specific titles, such as D_1 and D_2. Reflexes are stimulated to initiate movement and to promote postural control. These patterns are known as "irradiation patterns." Coordination within patterns of a segment and between segments is stressed. Maximal resistance is used to promote irradiation and the patient's voluntary effort is used whenever possible. Adjunctive physical agents such as heat and cold are employed when appropriate.

General treatment in PNF includes the use of recapitulation of total patterns of developing motor behavior; spiral and diagonal patterns of movement; coupling voluntary movement with postural and righting reflexes; appropriate sensory cues and techniques for facilitating movement and postural responses; maximal resistance for maximal excitation and inhibition; and repetitive activity for conditioning and training. Specific placements of the therapist's hands are an important aspect of the PNF approach as it was originally developed.

ROOD - Rood Approach to Neuromuscular Dysfunction

An approach to treatment of neurologic dysfunction was proposed in the 1950's by Margaret S. Rood, a physical therapist. The approach of Rood to neurologic dysfunction represented her philosophy of treatment which was concerned with the interaction of somatic, autonomic, and psychological factors and their interactions with motor activities. This approach was one of the first that considered motor functions to be inseparable from sensory mechanisms. Therefore, sensory factors and their relationship to motor functions assumed a major role in the analysis of dysfunction and in the application of treatment. Specifically, Rood used sensory stimuli by stroking or brushing at a given speed and for a given duration for activation of a phasic muscle response; applying cold for visceral stimulation and somatic relaxation; and applying pressure and stretch for postural muscle activation. Over the years, the types of stimuli used have been modified by both Rood and other practitioners and brushing is no longer used in treatment.

In the Rood approach, muscle groups are analyzed according to the types of work they perform and their responses to specific stimuli. "Light work" refers to movement with reciprocal inhibition of antagonists. This may occur in voluntary movement or autonomic nervous system action. "Heavy work" is defined as the holding or cocontraction of muscles which are antagonists in normal motion and which are used to provide a stable support of a joint in a fixed position. Some muscles perform both light and heavy work functions. Using these concepts of light and heavy work, Rood outlined the normal developmental sequence by using the following order of activation of muscles groups:

1. Reciprocal innervation — reflex activation for movement patterns using reciprocal innervation of proximal joints in the developmental sequence until voluntary movement

FIGURE 3. The skeletal function sequence according to Rood.

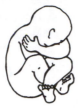

1. WITHDRAWAL–SUPINE
Heavy work of trunk, neck, proximal regions of extremities; motion occurs toward T10; reciprocal innervation pattern.

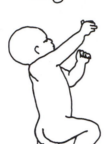

2. ROLL OVER
Flexion of upper and lower extremities on the same side.

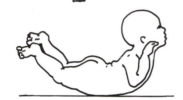

3. PIVOT PRONE
Bilateral holding of proximal extensors in shortened range; reciprocal innervation pattern.

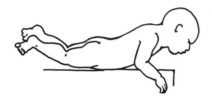

4. COCONTRACTION NECK
Cocontraction of neck extensors and flexors; thoracic extension.

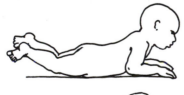

5. ON ELBOWS
Scapular cocontraction; glenohumeral joint cocontraction; pushing backward.

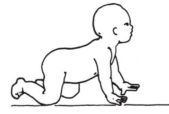

6. ALL FOURS
Weight shifting backward-forward, side to side, alternate arm and leg; creeping.

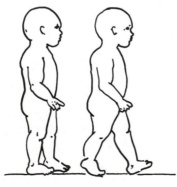

7. STANDING
Static
Shifting weight

8. WALKING
Stance
Push off
Pick up
Heel strike

(Redrawn from Rood.)

without the reflex is achieved

2. Coinnervation — cocontraction of antagonists and agonists working together to stabilize the body beginning at the head and neck and working downward

3. Heavy work — movement superimposed on cocontraction

4. Skill — skilled work with emphasis on distal portions of the body segment which requires control from the highest cortical level.

In addition to using the concepts of light and heavy work in the developmental sequence, the Rood approach identified two major sequences in motor development which are distinctly different, but inseparable due to their interaction. The two sequences are those of skeletal functions (Figure 3) and vital functions. The skeletal functions include activities of the head, neck, trunk, and extremities while the vital functions include vegetative, respiratory, and speech activities.

The developmental sequence, both skeletal and vital, can be used to analyze the stages during which acquisition of the four levels of control (reciprocal innervation, coinnervation, heavy work, and skill) occur. Additionally, stimulation of the sensory receptors is done in the sequence of normal development from the most primitive reflexes to the skill level.

The purpose of treatment is to restore that component in the sequence in the manner in which it is normally acquired. Therefore, the Rood approach to treatment is proposed to be applicable to any type of neurologic dysfunction at any age.

ALTERNATIVE THEORETICAL FRAMEWORKS

Research with animals and humans disseminated in recent years regarding motor control, motor development, and motor learning, has prompted physical therapists to revise our theoretical frameworks for assessing and treating patients with movement disorders. In subsequent chapters in this text, the current concepts are presented in detail to enable physical therapists to revise or develop their own theoretical frameworks. However, it is important that we not "throw out the baby with the bathwater." Theorists of the past 40 - 50 years have provided us with useful theoretical frameworks, a wealth of information regarding normal and pathologic sensory/perceptual and motor functions, and many effective treatment techniques. Whether we opt to use an entirely new theoretical model or to delete portions, revise, or add key elements to our current model, ultimately we will retain principles and treatment techniques that are validated through research.

At the II STEP Conference held in July 1990, evidence was presented that we are on the threshold of major research endeavors in motor control, motor learning, and motor development. As research validates or refutes our currently held tenets, we must be ready to revise our theoretical models and not cling emotionally to what we were taught as students or clinicians. Theoretical frameworks are not "good" or "bad"; they are only "useful" or "not useful." To provide effective assessment and treatment, we need the most "useful" model we can formulate and that model will be in a constant state of revision.

FUNCTIONAL OUTCOMES

An assessment of effective outcomes also must change if we change our theoretical models. No longer can effectiveness of outcome be measured in terms of decreasing spasticity or inhibiting specific reflexes. Outcomes that are effective must be tied to age appropriate functionality. The use of functional behavioral objectives that are well defined and that can be observed and measured must be used to assess effectiveness of physical therapy intervention. A continuum of assessment, treatment, and reassessment is illustrated in Figure 4.

Establishing Functional Objectives

Some physical therapy goals are based on traditional neurophysiologic facilitation techniques and are difficult to document objectively. Examples are decreasing muscle tone or decreasing the influence of primitive reflexes. In these instances, it is preferable to describe functional problems hypothesized to be associated with these factors to determine therapeutic goals and functional objectives. Other goals of physical therapy, such as increasing strength, are easy to quantify. An example would be the patient achieving increased repetitions of specific exercises. The goals and objective documentation of increased strength are not particularly valuable, however, unless they relate to improved function. In this instance, two part objectives are indicated: one related to strength and the second to improved function in which weakness is hypothesized to play a role. If physical therapy intervention improves strength, endurance, flexibility, or some other variable, but does not improve the individual's ability to function, it can be argued that the intervention is of little value to the patient. In a time of soaring health care costs and shortages of physical therapy services, only services that produce functional improvement or maintain levels of function should be provided.

Several examples of physical therapy goals with associated functional problems and objectives for patients with neurologic disorders are provided to assist the physical therapy student who has had little experience in the process of program development. In the process of determining goals and objectives, it is logical to start by defining the patient's functional problems, then determining goals of physical therapy intervention and functional objectives that will measure change in behavior.

EXAMPLES: FUNCTIONAL PROBLEMS, THERAPEUTIC GOALS, AND FUNCTIONAL OBJECTIVES

Functional Problem: decreased strength of the gastrocnemius muscle is hypothesized to decrease propulsion needed during gait
Therapeutic Goal: to increase strength of calf muscles
Functional Objective: Following treatment, the patient will be able to achieve a tip toe position 10 times and demonstrate improved push - off during gait (using chalk on the ball of the foot to document changes in the gait pattern)

Functional Problem: decreased strength of ankle dorsiflexors is hypothesized to impede ability to use an ankle strategy during balancing in stance and to decrease toe clearance during the swing phase of gait

Therapeutic Goal: to increase strength of ankle dorsiflexors

Functional Objective: Following treatment, the patient will perform 3 sets of 10 repetitions of resistive ankle dorsiflexion exercises with red thera-band and will clear the toe during gait 100% of the time

Functional Problems: diminished strength in the hip and knee extensors is hypothesized to interfere with the ability to rise from sitting at a bench to standing and to prevent the patient from walking up stairs

Therapeutic Goal: to increase strength in hip and knee extensors

Functional Objectives: Following treatment, the patient will be able to rise from sitting at a bench to standing independently 3 times and walk up 10 stairs holding onto a railing

Functional Problem: decreased endurance is hypothesized to limit the patient's ability to be a household ambulator

Therapeutic Goal: to increase endurance

Functional Objective: Following treatment, the patient will be able to walk 100 yards using a cane without fatiguing

Functional Problem: decreased endurance is hypothesized to limit the patient's ability to stand to perform ADLs

Therapeutic Goal: to increase endurance

Functional Objective: Following treatment, the patient will be able to stand at the kitchen sink with her walker and wash and wipe dishes without fatiguing

Functional Problem: during gait, decreased range of motion (ROM) in ankle dorsiflexion is hypothesized to interfere with toe clearance

Therapeutic Goal: increase ROM of ankle dorsiflexors

Functional Objectives: Following treatment, the patient will demonstrate an increase of 10 degrees of active dorsiflexion and will clear the toe during gait, 100% of the time

Functional Problem: decreased ROM of the shoulder into forward flexion is hypothesized to interfere with the ability to perform ADLs

Therapeutic Goal: to increase ROM of shoulder

Functional Objectives: Following treatment, the patient will be able to comb his hair with the affected arm and lift large objects using two hands from an overhead shelf

Functional Problem: decreased trunk mobility is hypothesized to interfere with a reciprocal arm swing during gait

Therapeutic Goal: to increase trunk mobility/flexibility

Functional Objectives: Following treatment, the patient will be able to rotate his trunk while sitting to obtain an object placed behind him and demonstrate a reciprocal arm swing during gait, 50% of the time

Functional Problem: patient does not appear to remember instructions

Therapeutic Goal: to improve short term memory

Functional Objectives: Following treatment, the patient will

FIGURE 4.

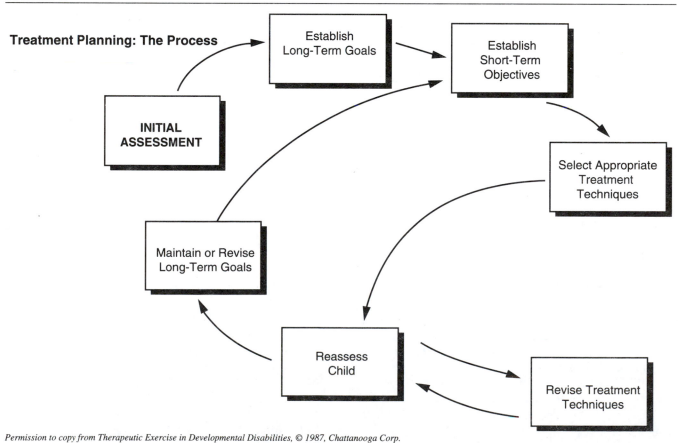

Treatment Planning: The Process

Establish Long-Term Goals

Establish Short-Term Objectives

INITIAL ASSESSMENT

Select Appropriate Treatment Techniques

Maintain or Revise Long-Term Goals

Reassess Child

Revise Treatment Techniques

perform a 3 step command of motor tasks, 2 of 3 trials and will remember the sequence needed for putting on his own socks and shoes

Functional Problem: patient forgets how to get from one place to another
Therapeutic Goal: to improve spatial orientation and memory for places
Functional Objective: Following treatment, the patient will be able to find his way from his room to the physical therapy department independently

Functional Problem: patient cannot identify objects with hemiplegic hand
Therapeutic Goal: to improve tactile processing
Functional Objectives: Following treatment, the patient will match circle, square, and triangle explored tactilly with hemiplegic hand to same 3 dimensional object explored with opposite hand; and will be able to find familiar objects in a dresser drawer, 2 of 3 trials

Functional Problem: patient is hypersensitive to tactile stimuli in the hand and avoids exploration using that hand
Therapeutic Goal: to improve tactile processing
Functional Objectives: Following treatment, the patient will use the involved hand to search for objects hidden in sand and will be able to use the hand to do bilateral tasks such as washing dishes

Functional Problem: patient with hemiplegia disregards left side of the body during ADLs
Therapeutic Goal: to decrease sensory disregard
Functional Objective: Following treatment, the patient will shave both sides of the face with only one verbal reminder

Functional Problem: patient loses balance in situations where there are a number of people moving simultaneously
Therapeutic Goal: to decrease reliance on vision for balance
Functional Objective: Following treatment, the patient will maintain balance using a cane when walking through a crowded shopping mall

Functional Problem: patient leans to one side and appears to have poor appreciation of his position in space
Therapeutic Goal: to improve proprioceptive awareness and perception of the vertical
Functional Objective: Following treatment, the patient will maintain a symmetrical sitting posture for 5 minutes with no more than 3 reminders

Functional Problem: patient has a right visual field deficit and disregards the right side of visual space
Therapeutic Goal: to improve visual scanning and perception
Functional Objective: Following treatment, the patient will orient spontaneously to a television set placed to his right, 2 of 3 trials

Functional Problem: patient demonstrates akinesia
Therapeutic Goal: to improve speed of initiation of movement
Functional Objectives: Following treatment, the patient will be able to move from sitting in a chair to answer a telephone

within 6 rings; will be able to catch a volleyball thrown to him slowly, 3 of 5 trials; and will be able to move on and off an escalator safely

Functional Problems: patient demonstrates bradykinesia and cannot vary speed of movement
Therapeutic Goal: to improve speed of movement
Functional Objectives: Following treatment, the patient will be able to walk safely across a street in the time allowed by a green light and will be able to move into and out of an elevator safely

Functional Problem: patient has a tendency to fall during loss of balance in standing
Therapeutic Goal: to improve balance
Functional Objectives: Following treatment, the patient will maintain independent standing balance for 5 minutes, initiate a step to regain balance when losing balance in upright; and will be able to walk on uneven surfaces, such as grass and gravel without losing balance

Functional Problem: patient does not appear to have posture set before moving and often loses his balance
Therapeutic Goal: to improve synergistic organization of posture and active movement
Functional Objective: Following treatment, the patient will be able to lift a 3 pound object off a desk without falling forward

Functional Problem: patient cannot combine shoulder flexion with elbow extension to reach for objects above the head
Therapeutic Goal: to improve synergistic organization within upper extremity
Functional Objective: Following treatment, the patient will be able to reach overhead to obtain objects from a shelf, 3 of 5 trials

Functional Problem: patient cannot sequence movements to rise from sitting to standing from a chair without arms
Therapeutic Goal: to improve synergistic organization of movement and sequencing of weight shifts
Functional Objective: Following treatment, the patient will be able to rise from sitting to standing from a chair without arms, 1 of 3 attempts

Functional Problem: patient cannot transfer from a wheelchair to a bed and back
Therapeutic Goal: to improve motor planning
Functional Objective: Following treatment, the patient will transfer safely from a wheelchair to a bed with a side rail, 100% of the time

Functional Problem: lack of knee flexion and ankle dorsiflexion are hypothesized to lead to problems with toe clearance in gait
Therapeutic Goal: to improve gait pattern
Functional Objective: Following treatment, the patient will walk 100 yards clearing his toe safely

Functional Problem: inadequate reciprocation of the lower extremities is hypothesized to result in decreased stride length and decreased speed and endurance during gait
Therapeutic Goal: to improve gait pattern

Functional Objective: Following treatment, the patient will demonstrate improved stride length (measured with ink footprints on chart paper) and will be able to walk 50 feet further at a faster rate (timed with stop watch) than noted prior to treatment.

SUMMARY: PROBLEMS, GOALS, AND OBJECTIVES

It should be noted that, in some instances, several factors are hypothesized to contribute to the same functional problem. For example, either weakness in hip and knee extensors or poor synergistic organization of movement, or both, could contribute to difficulty in rising from sitting on a chair without arms to standing. The advantage of focusing on functional objectives is that, if the patient does not improve following treatment, for example to increase strength of hip and knee extensors, then other factors can be considered and emphasized in treatment. If the focus were on improving hip and knee extensor strength alone, this could be accomplished, but the relationship to functional skills would be unclear. Often several goals are worked on simultaneously. An example is poor toe clearance during gait which may be due to weak ankle dorsiflexors, limited range of motion into dorsiflexion, or poor synergistic organization of movement. Following treatment, if the patient has normal active range into dorsiflexion and adequate strength, yet drags the toe during gait, poor synergistic organization may be the most plausible factor contributing to the functional problem.

A controversial treatment issue among physical therapists is the quality of movement displayed by patients with neurologic disorders and the role of physical therapy in improving quality of movement. Quality movement usually is considered to be the ideal or normal pattern of movement. In some instances, the normal pattern is not attainable and the pattern used by the patient is an adequate and desirable compensation for a disordered sensorimotor system. Rather than concentrating on quality or normal movement, the physical therapist should concentrate on improving function. Perhaps the movement pattern that produces the most function and independence should be considered the best pattern. This emphasis on function is evident today in the health care system and is being required increasingly by third party payers to justify physical therapy intervention. Clear descriptions of functional problems and goals of physical therapy intervention are essential for the patient and physical therapist.

SUMMARY

Motor control, motor learning, and motor development are areas of interest to physical therapists who work with patients of various ages with neurologic deficits. This text incorporates theory, specific assessments, treatment techniques, and functional outcomes in a problem solving approach. This text emphasizes the role of the physical therapist as the primary diagnostician of movement disorders. ❑

SUGGESTED READINGS

AYRES

Ayres AJ: Sensory Integration and Learning Disorders. Los Angeles, CA, Western Psychological Services, 1972

Ayres AJ: Sensory Integration and the Child. Los Angeles, CA, Western Psychological Services, 1979

Ayres AJ: Southern California Postrotary Nystagmus Test. Los Angeles, CA, Western Psychological Services, 1975

Ayres AJ: Sensory Integration and Praxis Tests. Los Angeles, CA, Western Psychological Services, 1984

BOBATH

Bobath B: Abnormal Postural Reflex Activity Caused by brain Lesions, ed 3. Rockville, MD, Aspen Publications, 1985

Bobath B: The very early treatment of cerebral palsy. Dev Med Child Neur 9: 373-390, 1967

Bobath B: Treatment of adult hemiplegia. Physiotherapy 63: 310 - 313, 1977

Semans S: The Bobath concept in treatment of neurological disorders. Am J Phys Med 46: 732 - 785, 1967

BRUNNSTROM

Brunnstrom S: Movement Therapy in Hemiplegia: A Neurophysiological Approach. Hagerstown, MD, Harper and Row, Publishers, Inc., 1970

Perry CE: Principles and techniques of the Brunnstrom approach to the treatment of hemiplegia. American Journal of Physical Medicine 46: 789 - 815, 1967

CARR AND SHEPHERD

Carr JH, Shepherd RB: Physiotherapy in Disorders of the Brain. London, England, William Heinemann Medical Books Ltd., 1980

Carr JH, Shepherd RB: A Motor Relearning Program for Stroke. London, England, Aspen Systems, Corp, 1983

JOHNSTONE

Johnstone M: Restoration of Motor Function in the Stroke Patient: A Physiotherapist's Approach, ed 3. New York, NY, Churchill Livingstone, 1987

PNF

Voss DE: Proprioceptive neuromuscular facilitation. American Journal of Physical Medicine 46: 838 - 898, 1967

Voss DE, Ionta MK, Myers BJ: Proprioceptive Neuromuscular Facilitation: Patterns and Techniques ed 3. Philadelphia, PA, Harper and Row, 1985

ROOD

Rood MS: Neurophysiologic Reactions: A Basis for PT. PT Review 34: 444, 1954

Stockmeyer SA: An interpretation of the approach of Rood to the treatment of neuromuscular dysfunction. American Journal of Physical Medicine 46: 789 - 815, 1967

Chapter 2
Motor Control, Motor Learning, and Motor Development

Ann VanSant, Ph.D., PT

INTRODUCTION

As physical therapists we are interested in sciences related to human movement. Our understanding of motor behavior serves as a foundation for our work with individuals with movement disorders. Within the broad area of kinesiology there are varieties of perspectives and approaches to the study of human movement. For example, biomechanists bring to the study of human movement the theory and models of physical mechanics. These theories and models frequently are used by physical therapists to analyze and solve our patients' movement problems. However, biomechanics represents just one approach that can be used to study human movement. Motor control, motor learning, and motor development represent three other areas of kinesiology that have much to offer as foundations for physical therapy. Each of these specialized areas offers a unique perspective that can add to our abilities as physical therapists to analyze and solve our patients' movement problems.

DEFINITIONS OF MOTOR CONTROL, LEARNING, AND DEVELOPMENT

According to Brooks, a neurophysiologist, "motor control is the study of posture and movements that are controlled by central commands and spinal reflexes, and also to the functions of mind and body that govern posture and movement." [1](p. 5) Schmidt, a psychologist and physical educator, defines motor learning as a set of processes associated with practice or experience that leads to relatively permanent changes in the capability for producing skilled action.[2] And finally, the study of motor development, according to Roberton, a physical educator, is "the study of lifespan change in motor behavior." [3]

Motor control, learning, and development represent three distinct approaches to understanding motor behavior. Yet, they have shared ideas and themes in the past and continue to do so. Each is directed ultimately toward understanding motor behavior. For motor control, the question is "how is the control of motor behavior organized?" For motor learning, the question is "how is motor behavior acquired through practice or experience?" And, for motor development, the question is "how does motor behavior change across long periods of time?" The "how" in each of these questions refers to understanding the processes that underlie the motor behavior that we see. One of the differences among these three approaches is the time scale over which the processes are studied. Motor control scientists are interested in operations lasting milliseconds or, at the most, seconds. Motor learning scientists are interested generally in processes that occur across hours, days, and weeks, although for highly practiced skills the processes of learning may extend across months or years. Motor development scientists generally are interested in processes of change that involve time periods ranging from months to decades. The relative span of time that attracts interest has to do with the rate of change in the process studied (Table 1).

Obviously the specialized areas of motor control, learning, and development have as a shared focus the study of motor behavior. Those interested in motor control seek to understand how motor behavior is controlled and organized. Those interested in motor learning study how motor behaviors are acquired through practice and experience. Those interested in motor development examine age related processes of change in specific age groups or across the whole of our human lifespan. The perspectives of each of these special-

TABLE 1. *Motor control, learning, and development: a comparison*

Motor Control	Control and Organization of Processes underlying Motor Behavior	Milliseconds
Motor Learning	Acquisition of Skill through Practice and Experience	Hours, Days, Weeks
Motor Development	Age related processes of Change in Motor Behavior	Months, Years, Decades

ized areas within the study of motor behavior influence and enrich the others and offer to physical therapists alternate perspectives to help solve problems of human movement dysfunction.

MOTOR CONTROL - AN OVERVIEW

The specialized area of motor control as we know it today grew out of the subdisciplines of neurophysiology and cognitive psychology. Early in this century, physiologists studied both motor behavior and the neural processes underlying that behavior. Since that time, and until the very recent past, neurophysiologists tended to concentrate exclusively on understanding microscopic internal neural processes that coordinated and controlled motor behavior of animals. Their studies were carried out in laboratories with anesthetized animals. More recently, technological advances have enabled neuroscientists to study more general processes involved in the control of natural movements of awake animals and human subjects performing motor skills.

Over the last quarter century, cognitive psychologists brought to the study of motor control concepts derived from cybernetics and information processing. Feedback arising from cybernetic theory became a routine element of motor control models and gradually neural function was simulated like a computer, with processes such as motor programs playing a major role.

Physical therapists have a thirty year tradition of studying the neurosciences in order to understand how the nervous system is organized and how it controls motor behavior. The "neurophysiologic approaches" to patient care which originated in the work of Knott and Voss,[4] Rood,[5] the Bobaths,[6] Brunnstrom,[7] and Fay[8] represented a distinct shift from using mechanical concepts alone to solve patient problems, to the use of neuromotor control models (see Chapter 1). The motor control model that was in vogue at the time constituted a hierarchy, with reflexes serving as the foundation for volitional control. This model is still quite common because it helps explain the abnormal motor behavior of individuals with central nervous system (CNS) dysfunction. Simply put, individuals with brain dysfunction demonstrate motor behaviors reflective of the function of intact lower levels of the motor control hierarchy. The model also can be extended to the therapeutic concept of rebuilding control of the motor system. According to the neurophysiologic approaches, control is reestablished by activating the higher levels of control through the use of sensory stimuli and through requests for volitional action.

When the original neurophysiologic approaches to physical therapy were developed, there was widespread study among neurophysiologists of the electrical activity of single neurons and complex sensory receptors, such as the muscle spindle.[9] It was through the study of the muscle spindle and the gamma motor system that feedback loops were examined in detail by neuroscientists. Eventually models of "muscle" control were developed based predominantly on the muscle spindle.[10] The generation of therapists that learned neurophysiologic approaches to patient care as a part of their basic education were presented with models of motor control that incorporated the concept of feedback and the intricate interactions among spinal level neurons for the regulation of posture and movement. While the physiology of the muscle spindle strongly influenced the therapeutic practices incorporated in Rood's[11] approach, as well as those developed in Knott and Voss'[12] proprioceptive neuromuscular facilitation (PNF) approach, Brunnstrom[7] was more hesitant to extract meaning from the flurry of studies of this single receptor system. Similarly, the Bobaths did not attend to details of receptor mechanisms, preferring to focus on more macroscopic elements of motor behavior that can be observed in the individual, such as the spinal and tonic reflexes and righting and equilibrium reactions.[13,14]

As scientific technology advanced, the monitoring of electrical activity at multiple sites within the CNS became possible. This resulted in increasingly complex models of motor control to explain relationships among various elements of the nervous system.[1,15] An interesting tendency within the evolution of these complex models was the move away from assigning specific neural functions to specific nervous system structures (Figures 1 and 2). One of the most important trends in the neurosciences that affects our current perspective of motor control, is the gradual adoption of neural network models to portray complex neural processes. One example of this trend can be seen in modeling of the control of locomotion, where neural networks have been used to portray oscillatory processes that control the alternating phases of gait.[16] The underlying impetus for the adoption of neural network theory is the increasing appreciation for the complexity of neural processes, and the availability of computers to assist in the modeling of network organizations.

FIGURE 1. *A traditional model.*

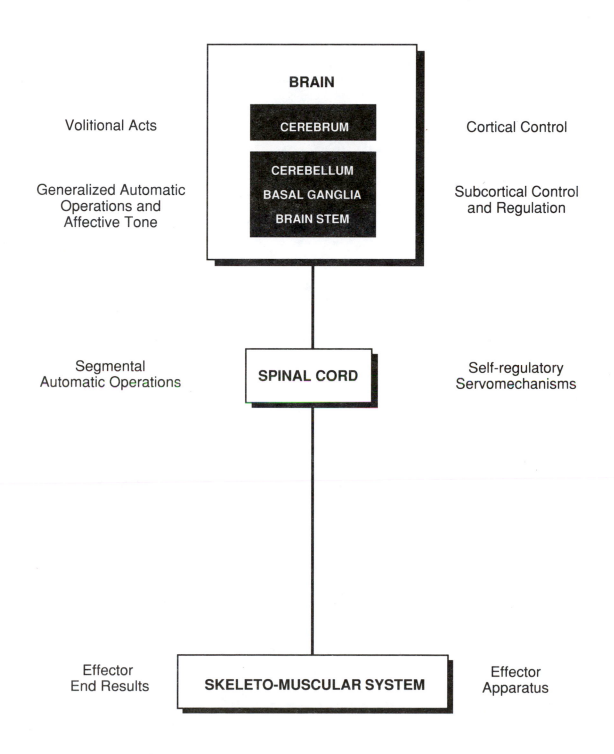

FIGURE 2. A contemporary model taken from Bernstein's work.

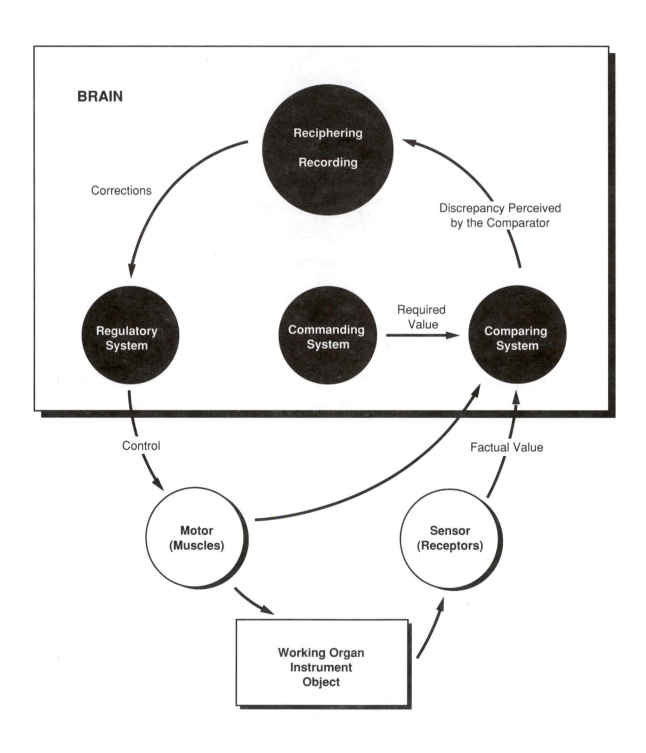

CURRENT ISSUES IN THE STUDY OF MOTOR CONTROL

A general change is taking place in the way theorists view issues related to the control of motor behavior.[17,18] In 1967 the Russian physiologist, Bernstein,[19] published a book in English that has received increasing attention. Bernstein's theoretical stance posed new questions and problems for motor control theorists. Bernstein proposed that a major problem facing the brain is how to control many different joints and muscles of the body. This has become known as the "degrees of freedom" problem. Imbedded within this problem is the recognition of the physical structure of the human body as a control issue. Most models of motor control have not dealt with the physical reality and complexity of the musculoskeletal system. For us, as physical therapists, Bernstein's perspective represents a long overdue integration of principles of physical mechanics which have been used to explain the functions of the musculoskeletal system with concepts of neuromotor control.

The way in which the CNS solves the degrees of freedom problem is proposed to be accomplished through muscle synergies, or coordinative structures.[20] The nervous system simplifies the task of controlling numerous muscles by constraining them to function collectively.[21]

Two lines of thought have emerged to explain these muscle linkages: one emphasizes motor programs; the other emphasizes that muscle synergies are not predetermined like a computer program, rather they arise as a result of complex interactions among individuals and their environments. Motor programs include information that specifies fixed relationships among muscles.[1,2,22,23] Programs are stored in memory and recalled to guide action. Alternately, the CNS creates solutions to demands for action when they are needed. The muscle linkages emerge as a property of the CNS which takes into account the physical context in which the action must be performed and the physical characteristics of the individual.

While the concept of a synergy, or muscles working in patterns is not new to physical therapists, what is new are the processes that underlie muscle linkages. Traditionally, synergies have been viewed as the behavioral manifestation of hard-wired reflexes, present at birth. Synergies are now viewed as programs that are learned and stored in memory,[2] or as emergent properties of the nervous system functioning in the context of a meaningful environment.[24]

Synergies As Motor Programs

A motor program simplifies the degrees of freedom problem by providing a single unit rather than many units to control. Some contemporary models of motor control constitute hierarchies which incorporate motor programs. In these models, the motor program is selected through higher level control processes but carried out by lower levels. This arrangement frees up the higher levels to engage in processes of planning actions. Those who research motor control theory from the perspective of motor programs are interested in determining what elements of the motor program are fixed and what elements are controlled.[1,2]

Currently, a motor program is characterized by an invariant order in which fundamental elements come into action.

Thus, if one were considering a motor program for throwing a ball, the order in which the muscles are fired would be fixed. The relative duration of the various muscular contractions would be fixed, as would the relative force levels among muscles acting in the program.

What can vary in the program, and therefore would need to be controlled, are the absolute level of force and the overall duration of the program. In the throwing task, this means the throw may be light or forceful, or the throw may be carried out slowly or quickly.

The speed and force that can be generated within a specific program are however, limited. For example, if speed is increased in an underarm throwing pattern, the relative timing of various muscles can change and a new program is used as the individual begins to use a "windmill" pattern as a windup for the throw. A similar switch from one pattern to another can be seen when speed of walking increases to a point where a switch to a running pattern occurs. These examples represent shifts from one program to another.

One model that has evolved to explain control within the programming concept is the mass spring model of control. Support for the mass spring model has been provided by Fel'dman, a Russian motor control theorist.[25] He proposed that we control the final position of a limb by specifying the relative stiffness of opposing muscles. Movements end at the point where agonist and antagonist stiffness are balanced across the limb. Non-contractile elastic properties of muscle are a part of the model, and antagonistic muscles are viewed as two opposing springs. Polit and Bizzi, two neuroscientists, found that monkeys, after having learned to perform simple one joint movements involving pointing to targets were able to point correctly with vision occluded and following deafferentation of the limb, regardless of the starting position.[26] It appeared that the monkeys had stored information about muscle tensions at the end position of pointing at the target. This research is supportive of the theory that the motor control system solves the degrees of freedom problem by treating the musculoskeletal system as though it were a mass spring system.

The mass spring model offers a relatively simple explanation of discrete movements to an endpoint. It has been extended to relatively elaborate tasks, such as handwriting. Hollerbach[27] created a system of 4 springs arranged at right angles to each other, with each attached to the same mass or weight. This is like a 4 muscle system attached around a limb segment. If the mass is displaced in any direction, the system oscillates until an equilibrium point is reached. This more complex model of springs in oscillation can produce action similar to handwriting. If the displacement of such a 4 spring system happens to occur in a diagonal direction, the mass oscillates in a circular pattern. By varying the stiffness of the springs, the circular pattern can be altered to make elliptical loops. Attach a pen to the system and the product is much like the letters of cursive writing. Slight alterations to the elliptical loops produce a variety of recognizable letters. Thus, the mass spring model can be extended to explain complex tasks.

Synergies as an Emergent Property of the Nervous System

The notion of emergent properties of a neural network is an outgrowth of application of network models to issues of motor control, particularly to the control of locomotion.[28] By specifically arranging elements, which depict neurons, patterns of neural function can be modeled. If one element in the chain is activated, the others will be activated in a fixed order, mimicking one of the fundamental properties of a synergy or coordinative structure. Not only can fixed patterns result from the function of a network, but sets of neurons can be arranged so that cyclic function can result. Network models

FIGURE 3. This diagram demonstrates the periodic oscillation of the pectoral and dorsal fin of a fish. The relationship between the fins becomes coordinated at the X marked on the diagram. Prior to that time the dorsal fin oscillated at a faster rate than the pectoral fin. The process of entrainment of one oscillating fin to the other resulted in a shared frequency. In this case the dorsal fin has become entrained to the slower rhythm of the pectoral fin, and the movements of the fins are "coordinated."

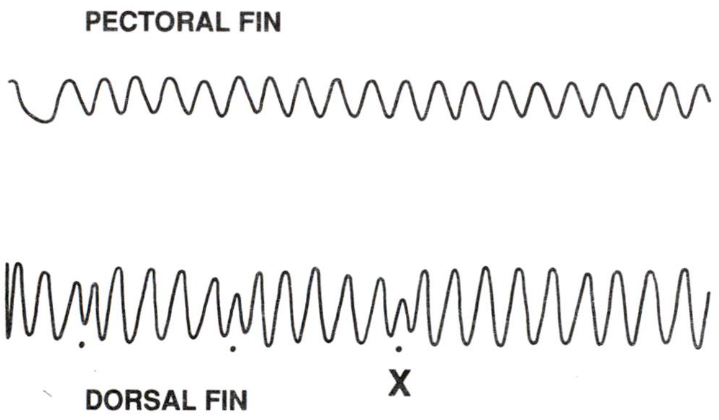

PECTORAL FIN

DORSAL FIN   **X**

Redrawn from von Holst, in Gallistel [1 p. 102]
1. Gallistel CR: The Organization of Action: A New Synthesis. Hillsdale, NJ, Lawrence Erlbaum Associates, Publishers, 1980.

enable depiction and understanding of "emergent properties," by delineating how elements of the system can be combined to produce functions that are not an inherent property of any element of the system.

While networks have their advantages, they also have disadvantages. One particular disadvantage is the tendency for circularly arranged networks to produce resonating oscillatory behavior. This means that they may get progressively carried away during repetitive functions. Damping mechanisms must therefore, be incorporated into network models to control the oscillations. Damps ultimately return oscillators to a point of static equilibrium, when the energy of the system has dissipated.

While oscillatory function is quite common in biological systems,[20] biological oscillations typically do not resonate

uncontrollably. Living organisms have the ability to sustain stable levels of oscillatory function. Thus, the network model breaks down during attempts to explain some fundamental properties of living systems. The problem with network modeling is that it is based in the physics of closed systems in which fuel or energy is not exchanged with the surrounding environment. Ultimately, closed systems are not well suited to modeling the functions of living systems.[29] Biological oscillations appear to be more accurately portrayed by non-linear, or limit cycle oscillators, such as those typical of open systems.

The thermodynamics of open systems is a relatively new area of physics. Yet, the constructs of the newer models of motor control are grounded in principles related to the thermodynamics of open systems (not to be confused with open loop control of movement) and principles of non-linear limit cycle oscillators. One important characteristic of limit cycle oscillators is the property of entrainment of one oscillating function to another, such that they share a common periodicity. Entrainment has been used to explain inter-limb coordination during locomotion.[29] Entrainment underlies the temporally patterned relationship between the limbs during their individual cyclic gait patterns. Figure 3 illustrates the concept of entrainment.

At first glance, the use of oscillators to model motor control appears to be limited to repetitive cyclic tasks, such as various gait patterns. Yet, oscillators may also be used to model discrete non-cyclic behaviors with specific start and end points. The science of thermodynamics of open systems that is leading to formulation of such control models is not just new to us as therapists. The properties of non-linear systems are just beginning to be used to model a host of natural phenomenon, from shoreline formations and tornado development, to the formation of biological structures such as leaves and honeycombs.[30] Why is this new theory preferable to the traditional models? Simply put, complex natural patterns can be reduced to a few simple principles. These principles, when applied in the context of the physical world, lead to new understanding of a vast array of complex natural forms and patterns.

One element of the newer control models is particularly rich for physical therapists. This is the notion that synergies emerge and are constrained by the physical characteristics of the human body and characteristics of the specific environmental context in which actions are performed.[31]

As an example, imagine a child in a huge rocking chair (Figure 4a). If she were to get out of the rocker, there are several options she might use. She could slide off the front of the chair extending her legs and trunk while holding fast to the armrests. Or, she could turn to lie prone on the chair, and get off backwards by lowering her legs to the floor (Figure 4b). One action pattern that she cannot perform from this chair is the common sit-to-stand action pattern that involves flexing forward over feet contacting the floor, followed by extension

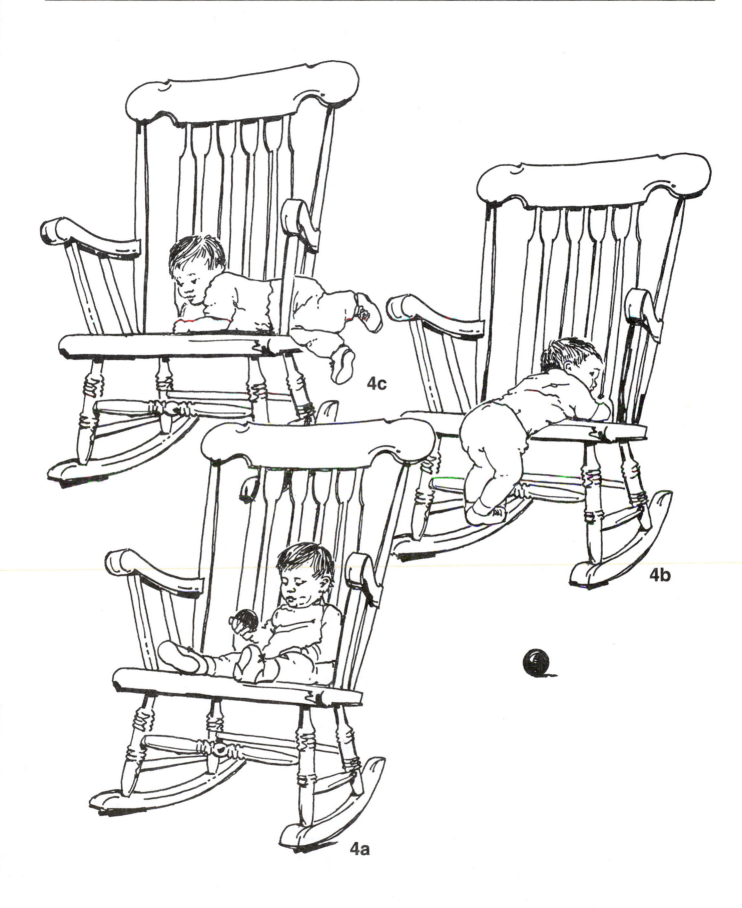

to attain standing. This is because the chair is too big for her to be able to sit and have her feet on the floor. But, the child can perform other actions that relatively larger individuals cannot. She can curl up on her side on the seat of the chair and probably can slide out under the side arms (Figure 4c). Thus, the size of her body and the size of the rocking chair mutually determine the actions possible.

In the examples of throwing and locomotion patterns that were used previously to illustrate different motor programs, when the speed of the individual increased to a critical level, there was an abrupt qualitative shift from one pattern to another. In the programming concept, this shift is regarded as a switch from one program to another. Newer theory, based on principles of the thermodynamics of open systems, would explain this switch as a function of "scaling up" a variable until a qualitatively different organizational pattern emerges from the system. Qualitative change from one action pattern to another is an "emergent property." The laws and principles under which such qualitative change may occur are proposed to be within the thermodynamics of open systems. This newer theoretical framework is termed dynamical action theory.[31]

MOTOR CONTROL THEORY APPLIED TO PHYSICAL THERAPY

The theoretical perspective one adopts affects what aspects of patient function are evaluated and the procedures used to solve clinical problems.[32,33] The classical neurophysiologic approaches to patient care were formulated from the perspective of a motor control hierarchy resting on progressively more complex levels of reflex organization. Therapists evaluated the presence of specific reflexes and reactions that would help indicate the "level of neural function." Therapists facilitated and inhibited reflexes to promote advancement to a higher level of control, ultimately for the purpose of improving the patient's functional competence in daily life.

Functional motor behaviors are of critical importance in the evaluation of patients regardless of the theoretical model adopted to explain motor control. It is important, however, to remember that functional behavior implies that the patient acts in the context of a meaningful environment. Therefore, two basic elements that need to be assessed are functional motor behaviors and the environmental conditions under which they are performed.

A fundamental construct within the newer models of control rest on the notion of coordinative structures, synergy patterns, or muscle linkages. I suggest that the behavioral expression of these linkages within functional tasks should constitute a primary focus of physical therapy evaluation. Specifically, "what postural and movement patterns are part of patients' behavioral repertoire?" can serve as a beginning question for the therapist applying motor control theory in clinical practice.

The movement patterns used to perform fundamental tasks of daily life are beginning to be identified,[34-38] as are postural synergies.[39] However, the descriptions of qualitatively different patterns used to perform the range of tasks of daily life are incomplete.

Another key aspect of a contemporary evaluation scheme is an analysis of the environmental contexts. The environmental conditions under which our patients can function can be systematically explored.[40] Environments can be considered either stable or variable. Stable environments simplify control demands, and they are predictable and allow the individual to perform at a self determined speed. Parallel bars are an example of a stable environment for walking. Stable environments, however, are not all the same. Home and hospital rooms can be stable, in that the elements in the room are fixed and unchanging, yet they differ from one another. We need to concern ourselves with the features of the environments in which our patients ultimately will be required to function. Concern for walking surfaces, the heights of chairs, beds, and so forth are the "variable features" of stable environments.

Variable environments require a greater degree of motor control than do stable environments. This is because the individual must adjust movements to the changing demands of the environment. A busy city street is a good example of a variable environment, as it has a large degree of unpredictability. Yet, even variable environments can have some degree of predictability. We rely on this predictability to ensure our safety. For example, stop lights provide predictable patterns of traffic flow. But there are instances when we must be able to slow, speed up, or stop our movements in order to meet the demands of the environment. Our patients often are not given opportunities to experience variable and unpredictable environments as part of a full course of rehabilitation. Rather, we tend to teach skills in the stable environments of hospitals, rehabilitation centers, and homes. As a result we are unsure, as our patients often are, of their ability to function across the full range of circumstances that are commonly encountered in daily lives.

By viewing the individual and the environment as an interacting unit in the formation of movement patterns, the potential for structuring the environment to bring out specific patterns also becomes apparent as a therapeutic principle. Therapists are familiar with structuring patients' environments to promote general forms of motor behavior. Common examples are arranging the room of a patient with hemiplegia to encourage turning toward the involved side of the body, or positioning a toy so a child will orient and reach to touch it. But we have not fully exploited the idea of the physical environment as a "constraining variable" that would lead to specific motor patterns. Conversely, we need to analyze the environment to determine what actions are possible given the relative size of the patient and objects in the environment.

Several years ago, I was treating a young man recovering from head injury. He consistently postured with his right arm in elbow flexion, and had developed a contracture of approximately 30 degrees. While splinting and casting had been used to prevent further contracture, active extension of this elbow, necessary to maintain functional range of motion, seldom was performed. Traditional techniques of handling and facilitating elbow extension, while effective, were hampered by his limited attention span and motivation to participate in "therapy." Repeatedly asking the patient for elbow straightening or pushing him off balance to evoke protective extension were boring after multiple training sessions. Yet, the young man proved to be quite interested in trying out his abilities in a familiar and meaningful skill. I turned a sliding board into a striking board by having him hold it in a manner similar to the way in which one would hold a baseball bat. A tennis ball was tossed to him, and he swung the sliding board with appropriate timing and directional control to hit the ball. His elbow extended quite naturally, achieving in a matter of seconds what had been an underlying goal of therapy for several months. He performed a task in which he had to straighten his elbow in the context of a meaningful environment. In this example, the environmental conditions were such that the patient had to time his movement to coincide with the arrival of the tennis ball. Had he not been successful, this task could have been simplified by having him use the board to strike a stationary object.

In summary, the newer theories of motor control lead to different assessment and treatment strategies. The types of information gathered in assessment are not the same as those we would gather using our traditional assessment. They go beyond the common view of the environment as the source of reflex stimuli. Rather, the environment is seen as both a constrainer and promotor of meaningful behavior. Motor patterns are more than reflexive responses. They are the elements of behaviors that arise as an emergent properties of a highly complex system that is tuned to function in meaningful environments.

MOTOR LEARNING — AN OVERVIEW

The specialized area of motor learning grew out of the subdiscipline of psychology concerned with processes of learning.[41] In the early part of this century, experimental studies were conducted that explored three main general learning issues: massing versus distributing the practice of tasks, instruction in the whole versus the parts of tasks, and the transfer of learning from one task to another.

By the middle of this century, motor learning had been established as a specialized area of study with problems that differed from those studied by researchers interested in verbal learning. Since that time, cybernetics and information processing science have exerted a major influence on the study of motor learning, as they did on the study of neurophysiology. The contribution of these new sciences to the study of learning includes recognition of the influence of feedback on the motor learning process. Both motor learning theorists and neuroscientists have applied information theory to their areas of study.[1,2] This commonality and technological advances have allowed neuroscientists to study human subjects. Additionally, neuroscientists and motor control scientists from a psychological background now are sharing ideas in interdisciplinary research focused on how skills are acquired and controlled.

Physical therapists, generally, are unfamiliar with traditional motor learning literature. This may be a result of our professional association with medical sciences to the expense of behavioral sciences. The neurophysiologic approaches tended to direct attention away from principles of learning, although there was explicit recognition of the role of learning in the restitution of functional skills.[42,43] "Treatment," however, not "teaching," tended to embody the traditional way of thinking. Regaining motor skills following CNS damage was based predominately on repetitively evoking reflexes to facilitate postures and movements. Practice involved repetition of reflexively facilitated behaviors. Rehabilitative practices involved teaching motor skills, including the breaking of functional activities down into component parts for ease of learning[44] and periods of practice. Much of what therapists learned about teaching motor skills was acquired through practical experiences, rather than through reading literature related to motor learning.

When Adams[45] published a theory of motor learning, much attention and research were generated to investigate his theory. Adams' "closed loop theory," incorporated both ongoing intrinsic feedback arising from the proprioceptive system, as well as extrinsic feedback generated as a consequence of one's actions. The closed loop theory also included two memory constructs as critical components. Schmidt[46] has since proposed an "open loop theory" that incorporates two different memory constructs, the motor schema and the motor program. Schmidt's theory is particularly relevant for skills that are performed either so rapidly or automatically that intrinsic proprioceptive feedback is not used for deliberate control processes.

Over the past 15 years, the theories of motor learning advanced by Adams and Schmidt have forced the attention of those studying motor behavior to theories of motor control. Specifically, the debate of whether movements are controlled centrally or peripherally was a spark that kindled interest in contemporary motor control issues.[47] This debate generated increased understanding of how different types of movements are controlled, and subsequently how different types of movements might be learned. Feedback is essential for learning, but may not be necessary for the performance of well learned tasks.

CURRENT ISSUES IN THE STUDY OF MOTOR LEARNING

Four contemporary issues are presented to demonstrate the importance of motor learning research to physical therapists. These include the difference between motor performance and motor learning, the appropriate use of feedback, practice schedules, and the transfer of learning across tasks and conditions of practice.

Performance And Learning

An issue of importance to physical therapy is the differentiation between performance and learning. Performance can be observed, learning cannot. Motor learning is an internal process that produces a relatively permanent change in the capacity to respond.[43] Although we help our patients learn motor skills, generally, we are more familiar with variables that affect performance than variables that affect learning. Some of the familiar performance variables are those known to evoke temporary reflexive effects, such as muscle stretch, head turning, or the brief application of ice. Learning variables, in contrast, continue to influence performance after they are removed.

Feedback

Extrinsic feedback represents information concerning performance supplied to the learner. Feedback is necessary for learning. The relative frequency with which feedback is supplied to the learner is an area of research that is germane to physical therapists. Current research suggests that contrary to what might be predicted, a relatively low frequency of providing feedback enhances learning.[2,48] This is true despite the fact that performance might suffer under conditions of low frequency feedback. Additionally, Winstein has shown that the "fading" of feedback, or progressively decreasing the rate with which feedback is given, appears to be most effective in promoting learning.[49]

The fading of feedback is contrary to customary practice in physical therapy where more feedback is considered better, particularly if performance is not up to standard. It has been suggested that the reason individuals learn better with less feedback is they do not become as dependent on feedback, rather they engage in processes that enable learning.

Practice Schedules

Among motor learning researchers, the terms "blocked" and "random" practice are used to denote two different practice schedules. Blocked practice refers to consistent practice of one task. Random practice means varying practice among a group of distinctly different tasks. It appears that varying practice among different tasks is more effective in promoting learning than concentrating on a single task.[50] Schmidt has suggested that the recall of tasks inherent in random practice seems to assist with processes that ensure learning.[2]

Transfer of Learning

A final issue that arises from the motor learning research literature that is of great importance to physical therapists concerns the transfer of learning. There are two distinct types of transfer, from one task to another and from one learning condition to another.

Many of our traditional neurophysiologic approaches employ early appearing developmental tasks hypothesized to positively affect the ability to perform higher order tasks. For example, performance in prone extension patterns is considered fundamental to normal performance of standing. Some general ability, such as stability or anti-gravity righting which developed in prone extension, is hypothesized to be essential to normal performance of standing. Research in general motor abilities indicates that transfer from one task to another is very small, if it exists at all.[2]

MOTOR LEARNING THEORY APPLIED TO PHYSICAL THERAPY

Our relative unfamiliarity with motor learning issues is gradually changing. Physical therapists increasingly are aware of the research findings in motor learning, an area of study closely related to the study of motor control. Further, there is an increasing trend for therapists to view their role with patients as a teacher of motor skills. This new perspective is apparent in the recent publications of Carr and Shepherd,[51,52] and Winstein.[48] With the acceptance of the role of teacher comes a concern for the basic principles of motor learning and a reexamination of the traditional guiding hypotheses of physical therapy.

A common experience of therapists is that some traditional treatment procedures affect performance at the time they are applied, but have no lasting effect. The differentiation between variables that affect learning and those that affect performance should lead to more effective use of learning variables.

Understanding that feedback is necessary for learning sheds a new light on therapy sessions. Feedback appears to have held predominantly a motivational role in therapy, being used as an incentive for continued participation in practice sessions. While the idea of withdrawing "hands on" facilitation to promote increased "volitional" participation is a traditional practice, the idea of withdrawing feedback to enhance learning is not. Winstein's finding,[49] that the fading of feedback enhances learning, has great implications for the way we work with our patients in practice settings. In general, we need to allow patients the opportunity to judge and correct their own performance. Accurate and timely feedback that is designed specifically to promote learning should be provided.

Issues related to the transfer of learning are very relevant to therapists. In traditional approaches, much time is devoted to practicing lower order tasks that are considered to positively affect performance of developmentally later appearing tasks. Motor behavior research suggests that this practice is ineffective, to the extent that the tasks are different. Transfer between tasks appears to be dependent on the similarity between the tasks. Further, the similarity seems to rest within the elements that define motor programs. When motor programs differ, transfer of training from one task to another is quite small. Thus, the relative timing and phasing of muscle activity within a motor program is quite specific. Practice of one motor pattern is unlikely to transfer to performance of a different pattern.

How does transfer of training affect our practice as therapists? There are times in therapy when performance of the task is the primary objective, and little concern is directed toward which axial or limb patterns are used to accomplish the task. There are other instances when patients demonstrate a stereotypic set of postural or movement patterns, and the objective of treatment may be directed toward the patient being capable of performing a very specific movement pattern. In this latter example, it is important to state clearly which pattern is the objective of treatment.

In summary, the research findings of motor learning provide useful information for the therapist who accepts the role of a teacher of motor skills. The way we structure practice, provide feedback, and even the way our treatment objectives are stated can be influenced positively by the results of motor learning research.

MOTOR DEVELOPMENT — AN OVERVIEW

The roots of motor development as a specialized area of study can be found in the work of developmental psychologists and physicians early in this century. These individuals described the acquisition of motor skills over extended periods of time. Studies were conducted that examined the relative contributions of maturational and environmental factors to the process of age related change in behavior. The pioneers of motor development were influenced by the motor control and learning theories of their times. For example, McGraw studied the neuromuscular development of infants to look for the onset of cortically mediated volitional control over subcortical reflexive behaviors.[53] She further studied the relative roles of maturational and experiential factors on the motor skill development of a set of twins.[54,55]

The field of motor development has been defined as an area separate from developmental psychology since World War II when psychologists abandoned the study of motor development preferring to focus on the development of cognitive skills.[56] Professionals in physical education, medicine, and health disciplines including physical therapy became more involved in defining and studying the problems associated with age related changes in motor behavior.[57-59] Generally, this second generation of motor developmentalists was interested in development of infants and children, although some adopted a broader perspective involving lifespan changes in motor behavior.

Traditional theories of motor development paralleled traditional concepts of motor control.[59] In fact, the classic hierarchical model of CNS organization, originally proposed as a model of neural evolution,[60] laid the groundwork for developmental theory. Processes of hierarchical integration and progressive differentiation incorporated in Jackson's notion of neural evolution are evident in the work of McGraw.[53] These processes were proposed as fundamental to changes in organismic developmental theories.[61]

For about twenty-five years following World War II, motor development researchers tended to focus on describing the "product" of motor development. These products included performance measures on standardized tests of skill performance, including features such as how far and how fast children of different ages were able to throw or run.[57] Studies during this period carefully described the movement patterns used by children to perform a variety of motor skills.[62] In the 1970s, the influence of the information processing model of motor control began to be seen in the study of the development of motor skills.[63,64] The information processing approach to motor development incorporates a variety of memory structures that are similar to schema and motor programs. Because feedback is an integral part of these models, they are equally well suited for and applied to the study of both motor control and learning processes.

Recently, there has been a resurgence of interest in motor development from within psychology. This seems in large part to be due to the influence of dynamical action theory applied by Kugler, Kelso, and Turvey[65] and Thelen.[66] Their work seems to have given impetus to application of the systems theoretical perspective to infant motor development.[67]

CURRENT ISSUES IN THE STUDY OF MOTOR DEVELOPMENT

The issues in motor development that impact the practice of physical therapy include the concept of motor development

as a life long process; a greater understanding of developmental sequences; new information concerning prenatal development of movement abilities; and the influence of systems theory, particularly dynamical action theory.

Motor Development as a Life Long Process

The concept of lifespan development had its beginnings among developmental psychologists who continued to study their young subjects well into adulthood.[3] The lifespan concept appeared in the motor development literature in the late sixties,[68] and now there are an increasing number of contemporary texts that adopt what is called a life span approach to motor development.[69-72] Roberton[3] has rightfully pointed out, however, that few of these texts have included chapters that cover a single topic across the lifespan. Rather, chapters tend to be devoted to different phases of the lifespan. To a large extent this would seem to result from the paucity of research conducted from a life span perspective. It is easier to gather studies of different phases or age groups and report on them as representative of a particular period within the life span. It is more difficult to integrate the findings of studies of a single function that are carried out under a variety of conditions with representation of age groups.

We are beginning to accumulate a body of literature, generated using a life span developmental perspective, that describes age differences in motor performance of functional tasks. The tasks of rising to standing from the floor,[73-77] rolling from supine to prone,[78-80] rising from a chair,[81] and rising from bed,[78,82,83] have been studied in a variety of age groups. Because the conditions under which the subjects perform have been kept consistent across the age groups, reasonable comparisons can be made across a wide portion of the life span. We are beginning to chart the incidence of the variety of movement patterns used to perform these tasks from early childhood through later adulthood.[84,85] The results of these studies indicate that age differences in movement patterns can be expected across the life span. We have discovered that variability in performance differs with age and with activity level. Currently, the relationship between body dimensions and motor performance in these tasks is under investigation. This line of inquiry is particularly well suited to life span study. Physical growth is a well accepted correlate of childhood motor development. Body dimensions and movement patterns used to perform functional righting tasks demonstrate a variable relationship across the lifespan.[86] The increase in weight that occurs during the middle adult years alters the shape of the body, and may well influence the form of functional movement patterns, long after the physical growth associated with early years is finished.

The patterns of change in movements used to perform functional tasks do not support entirely the traditional concept of developmental progression during childhood to maturity in young adulthood, followed by regression during the middle and later adult years. The variable patterns of movement suggest that patterns of change in motor behavior may be more complex than the simple progression and regression hypotheses would suggest.[59] Much is to be learned from a life span perspective toward motor development. This information will impact our expectations for individuals of different ages who require physical therapy services.

Developmental Sequences

Developmental sequences take many forms. There are sequences of tasks, such as those described by Gesell[87] and Shirley.[88] These sequences outline the order in which a variety of developmental skills are acquired such as rolling before sitting, sitting before creeping and so forth. There are also developmental sequences of body action within performance of a single skill or task. Developmental sequences of body movements within tasks were described by McGraw.[53] She described how the form of body movement changes with age and outlined developmental sequences for several tasks of interest to physical therapists, including rolling, sitting, prone progression, rising to standing, and walking (Figure 5). Finally, there are developmental sequences of movement patterns for body regions.[73,78,81,82]

accomplishments as though it were the singular order for attainment of skills has led to prescriptive use of developmental sequences. Early appearing developmental patterns are construed as essential preparatory steps for later appearing functions. According to Knott and Voss "...a recapitulation of the developmental sequence is a means to the end — the ability to care for one's body, to walk, and to engage in productive work."[12, p 115] It is worth noting that Knott and Voss recognized that recapitulation of developmental tasks is one means to functional competence, not the only means to that end.

Careful reading of the original descriptions of developmental accomplishments,[88,90-93] reveals that they may vary from person to person. This finding raises serious doubts about the prerequisite nature of early appearing tasks for later appearing functions. If one person is able to skip a developmental step, then obviously that step is not universally essential for later functional accomplishments. The extent to

FIGURE 5.   Rolling sequence from supine to prone (redrawn from McGraw).

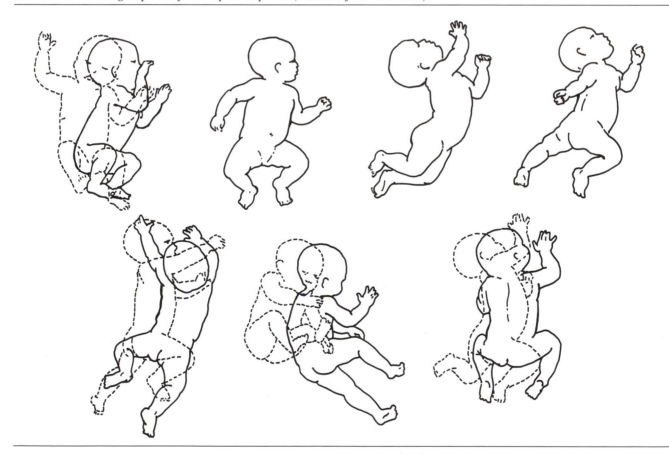

Neurophysiologic approaches to patient care incorporate developmental principles as guides for the progression of patients from states of physical dependency. The predominant pattern of progression was termed "the developmental sequence"[12] or "the skeletal function sequence"[89] and comprises a sequence of motor skills predominantly selected and adapted from the work of McGraw[53] and Gesell.[91] Unfortunately, interpretation of an ordering of developmental

which early tasks lay a foundation for later skills is a matter of conjecture.

Prenatal Development of Movement Abilities

Ultrasonography has allowed a new perspective on fetal development. Rich descriptions of the many varied activities of the human fetus have been made possible by ultrasonography.[94] Most notably, the concept of an active infant has emerged.[95-97] This new concept challenges the older idea that the infant is predominantly passive and dominated by reflexive behaviors evoked by environmental stimuli. As a result, the spontaneous movements of the young infant are no longer ignored and have become the subject of careful study.[98,99] The rhythmical patterns of infancy have been interpreted as suggesting the existence of motor programs[98] and central pattern generators.[99] It is not coincidental that the interpretation of these spontaneous movements has rested on concepts common to motor learning and motor control. As in the past, when reflexes were used to explain behavior, now more contemporary concepts of programs and pattern generators are being used to explain infant behavior.

Systems Theory

Systems theories are influencing our understanding of motor development.[65,100-102] This influence began gradually but has taken on intensity over the past few years. In 1964 Anokhin, a Russian neuroscientist, characterized neural development as a process of systemogenesis[103] in which different regions of the brain develop at different rates in anticipation of the demand for vital functions. Thus, sets of brain structures collectively function to meet the specific circumstances of the individual in an ecologically appropriate context. Importantly, the ecologically appropriate context for infant development involves an interaction with a mother or caregiver. The functions of both mother and infant are matched to assure survival and proper development.

This idea of elements collectively functioning to meet the needs of the individual in concert with environmental demands is seen in Milani-Comparetti's interpretation of fetal movements.[95] He characterized the emerging behavior repertoire of the fetus as directed toward the process of being born and surviving during the early post-natal period. Thrusting and locomotor movements of the fetus were adapted to the process of birth, in which both infant and mother actively participated. Breathing and sucking patterns were developed prenatally to assure extrauterine survival. Thus, behavioral systems were envisioned as ecologically appropriate to the context in which the fetus or infant would function.

There are two systems theories that are currently being used to explain a variety of developmental processes in infancy and childhood. These two theories are termed the perceptual-action theory and the dynamical action theory. Perceptual action theory has roots in the work of the Gibsons[104,105] Perceptual systems are considered critical for any action system. Specifically, motor development is viewed as much a function of perceptual system change as it is a function of motor system change.

Dynamical action theory, another example of systems theory, has been increasingly applied to explain motor development.[65,102,106-110] The idea of increasing the dimension of a variable until a new form of action is produced is at the heart of dynamical action theory. New patterns may emerge, for example by increasing velocity of movement, such as the speed of locomotion.

Changes in the gait pattern from walking to running result from increasing speed. Growth of physical structures can change the motor behavior. If we reconsider the child in the rocking chair, we begin to appreciate the role of physical growth in the emergence of new motor patterns and the potential application of dynamical action theory to the understanding of developmental issues. As one grows, some patterns become impossible, while others are enabled by the changing size of the individual.

MOTOR DEVELOPMENT THEORY APPLIED TO PHYSICAL THERAPY

The issues of life span change in motor behavior, developmental sequences, fetal motor behavior, and systems theory are impacting physical therapy. Because of a new understanding of development as a life long process, the concept of age related change in motor behaviors of individuals across all periods of the life span is beginning to be appreciated. This influences which motor skills and constituent motor patterns are taught to patients. Age appropriate skills and patterns tend to be the focus of therapeutic programs for individuals of all ages.

Careful review of information concerning developmental sequences suggests that they be used less prescriptively. Because there is little information concerning the relationship between early and later appearing behaviors, the use of

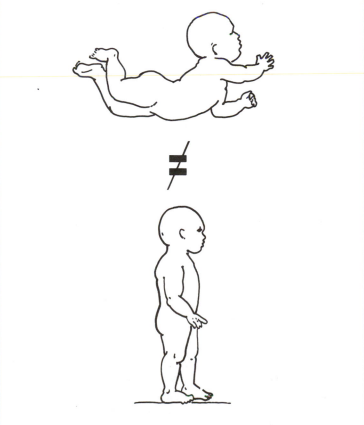

FIGURE 6. *Trunk extension in upright may have different requirements of motor control than extension in prone.*

an early appearing behavior, such as prone extension or creeping, to prepare for a developmentally later appearing function, such as walking, is not well founded (Figure 6). Sequences which describe the skills expected at a particular age do, however, outline the functional accomplishments that are expected of infants and children. Some of these tasks, such as rolling, sitting, rising from supine or sitting to standing, and walking continue as integral elements of physical independence across a wide period of the lifespan.

The new knowledge of developmental sequences of body action and movement patterns is beginning to be applied in physical therapy. At present, the most common interpretation of this information is that age appropriate body actions and movement patterns should be used when instructing patients in performance of functional skills.[73,78,81,82]

Studies of fetal movement have influenced our perception of infants as active agents in their environments. Such active infant concepts are impacting the behaviors we seek to evaluate. The evaluation of self control, as used in the Brazelton neonatal assessment,[111] is more consistent with this active organism concept than is assessment that only focuses on infant reflexes. By recognizing that individuals who come to treatment have a role to play in changing their behavior, we gradually move from a "treatment" model of therapy in which the patient is considered a passive recipient of our procedures to a "teaching" model in which patients are given active roles in producing action, evaluating feedback, and generating corrective action.

The impact of developmental systems theories, particularly dynamical action theory and perceptual action theory, on physical therapy is yet to be realized. It is possible to envision a greater concern for the physical constraints or determinants of motor pattern changes, such as those brought about by physical growth. The short stature of many disabled children may well be a factor in determining which patterns are used to perform motor tasks. The question of whether movement patterns emerge or if they are learned as a part of the developmental process would seem to be a fertile area for debate and research. Such controversy can only lead to a greater understanding of motor control, learning, and development.

SUMMARY

Motor control, learning, and development represent three different approaches to knowledge of motor behavior. The shared ideas and themes of the past continue to be evident today. Motor control theories try to explain how the control of motor behavior is organized. Currently, the concept of muscle synergies or coordinative structures has a central role to play in the organization of motor control. The impact of motor control theories in motor development and learning is strong. The focus on coordinative structures, hierarchical, and systems models of organization prevails in each of these domains of knowledge. Coordinative structures are envisioned by some as motor programs stored in memory and by others as emergent properties of the system. Identification of those variables in a motor program that can be controlled and those which are fixed has implications for the motor learning theorist. By knowing what is controlled, the motor learning

researcher's question "how is motor behavior acquired through practice or experience?" begins to be answered. For the motor development theorist, the question "how does motor behavior change across long periods of time?" is strongly influenced by current concepts of motor control. Systems theory, which had its beginnings as a theory of control, is providing a new understanding of the dynamic relationships in developing individuals among the environment and perceptual, musculoskeletal, and nervous systems. Because all of these systems change across the human lifespan, there are multiple possibilities for explaining life span motor development even in individuals thought to be exhibiting stable behavior. As physical therapists, our understanding of motor behavior is expanded and our approaches to patient care made more versatile by knowledge of theories of motor control, learning, and development. ❏

REFERENCES

1. Brooks VB: The Neural Basis of Motor Control. New York, NY, Oxford University Press, 1986, pp 5, 129-150
2. Schmidt RA: Motor Control and Learning: A Behavioral Emphasis, ed 2. Champaign, IL, Human Kinetics Publishers, 1988, pp 195, 227-298, 346
3. Roberton MA: Motor development: Recognizing our roots, charting our future. Quest 41:213-223, 1989
4. Knott M, Voss DE: Proprioceptive Neuromuscular Facilitation: Patterns and Techniques. New York, NY, Harper and Row, Hoeber Medical Division, 1956
5. Rood MS: Neurophysiological reactions as a basis for physical therapy. Phys Ther Rev 34:444-449, 1954
6. Bobath K, Bobath B: Treatment of cerebral palsy by the inhibition of abnormal reflex action. British Journal of Orthopedics 11:88-89, 1954
7. Brunnstrom S: Associated reactions of the upper extremity in adult patients with hemiplegia. Phys Ther Rev 36:225-236, 1956
8. Fay T: Neuromuscular reflex therapy for spastic disorders. Journal of the Florida Medical Association 44:1234-1240, 1958
9. Matthews PBC: Muscles spindles and their motor control. Physiol Rev 44:219-188, 1964
10. Eldred E: Functional implications of dynamic and static components of the spindle response to stretch. Amer J Phys Med 46:129-140, 1967
11. Stockmeyer SA: An interpretation of the approach of Rood to the treatment of neuromuscular dysfunction. Amer J Phys Med 46:900-956, 1967
12. Knott M, Voss DE: Proprioceptive Neuromuscular Facilitation: Patterns and Techniques, ed 2. New York, NY, Harper & Row, Hoeber Medical Division, 1968
13. Bobath K: The Motor Deficits in Patients with Cerebral Palsy. Clinics in Developmental Medicine, No 23. London, England, William Heinemann, 1966
14. Bobath K: A Neurophysiological Basis for the Treatment of Cerebral Palsy. Clinics in Developmental Medicine, No 75. Philadelphia, PA, JB Lippincott, 1980
15. Hellebrant FE: Motor learning reconsidered: A study of change. In Payton OD, Hirt S, Newton RA (eds): Neurophysiologic Approaches to Therapeutic Exercise. Philadelphia, PA, FA Davis, 1977, pp 33-45
16. Delcomyn F: Neural basis of rhythmic behavior in animals. Science 210:492-498, 1980
17. Greene PH: Problems of organization of motor systems. In Rosen R, Snell RM (eds): Progress in Theoretical Biology, Vol 2, New York, NY, Academic Press, 1972
18. Kugler PN, Kelso JAS, Turvey MT: On the concept of coordinative structures as dissipative structures: I. Theoretical line. In Stelmach GE, Requin J (eds): Tutorials in Motor Behavior. Amsterdam, North Holland, 1980, pp 3-37
19. Bernstein N: The Co-ordination and Regulation of Movements. Oxford: Pergamon Press, 1967
20. Tuller B, Turvey MT, Fitch HL: The Bernstein perspective: II. The concept of muscle linkage or coordinative structure. In Kelso JAS (ed): Human Motor Behavior An Introduction. Hillsdale, NJ, Lawrence Erlbaum, 1982, pp 253-270
21. Gel'fand IM, Gurfinkel VS, Tsetlin ML, Shik ML: Some problems in the analysis of movements. In Gel'fand IM, Gurfinkel VS, Fomin SV, Tsetlin ML (eds): Models of the Structural-Functional Organization of Certain Biological Systems. Cambridge, MA, MIT Press, 1971
22. Schmidt RA: More on motor programs. In Kelso JAS (ed): Human Motor Behavior: An Introduction. Hillsdale, NJ, Lawrence Erlbaum, 1982
23. Keele SW: Movement control in skilled performance. Psychological Bulletin 70:387-403, 1968
24. Kelso JAS, Holt KG, Rubin P, Kugler PN: Patterns of human interlimb coordination emerge from the properties of non-linear, limit cycle oscillatory processes: Theory and data. Journal of Motor Behavior 13:226-261, 1981
25. Fel'dman A: Superposition of motor programs. I. Rhythmic forearm movements in man. Neuroscience 5:81-90, 1980
26. Polit A, Bizzi E: Characteristics of motor programs underlying arm movements in monkey. J Neurophys 42:183-194, 1979
27. Hollerbach JM: An oscillation theory of handwriting. Biological Cybernetics 39:139-156, 1981
28. Davis WJ: Organizational concepts in the central motor networks of invertebrates. In Herman RL, et al (eds): Advances in Behavioral Biology, Vol 18: Neural Control of Locomotion. New York, NY, Plenum Press, 1976, pp 265-292
29. Kelso JAS, Tuller B: A dynamical basis for action systems. In Gazzaniga MS (ed): Handbook of Cognitive Neuroscience. New York, NY, Plenum Press, 1984, pp 321-356
30. Gleick J: Chaos: Making a New Science. New York, NY, Viking, 1987
31. Fitch HL, Tuller B, Turvey MT: The Bernstein perspective: III. Tuning of coordinative structures with special reference to perception. In Kelso JAS (ed): Human Motor Behavior: An Introduction. Hillsdale, NJ, Lawrence Erlbaum, 1982, pp 271-281
32. Rothstein JM, Echternach JL: Hypothesis-oriented algorithm for clinicians: A method for evaluation and treatment planning. Phys Ther 66:1388-1394, 1986
33. VanSant AF: Concepts of neural organization and movement. In Connolly BH, Montgomery PC (eds): Therapeutic Exercise in Developmental Disabilities. Chattanooga, TN, Chattanooga Corporation, 1987, pp 1-8
34. VanSant AF: Rising from a supine position to erect stance: Description of adult movement and a developmental hypothesis. Phys Ther 68:185-192, 1988

35. VanSant AF: Age differences in movement patterns used by children to rise from a supine position to erect stance. Phys Ther 68:1130-1138, 1988
36. Richter RR, VanSant AF, Newton RA: Description of adult rolling movements and hypothesis of developmental sequences. Phys Ther 69:63-71, 1989
37. Sarnacki S: Rising from supine on a bed: A description of adult movement and hypothesis of developmental sequences. Research Platform Presentation. Annual Conference of the American Physical Therapy Association, Anaheim, CA, June 25, 1990
38. Francis ED, VanSant AF: Description of the Sit-to-Stand Motion in Children and Young Adults: Hypothesis of Developmental Sequences. Research Poster Presentation. Joint Congress of the American Physical Therapy Association and the Canadian Physiotherapy Association, Las Vegas, NV, June 16, 1988
39. Nashner LM: Fixed patterns of rapid postural responses among leg muscles during stance. Exp Brain Res 30:13-24, 1977
40. Gentile AM: Skill acquisition. In Carr JH, Shepherd RB, Gordon J, Gentile AM, Held JM: Movement Science: Foundations for Physical Therapy in Rehabilitation. Rockville, MD, Aspen Publishers, Inc., 1987, pp 98-108
41. Kleinman M: The Acquisition of Motor Skill. Princeton, NJ, The Princeton Book Co., 1983, pp 3-29
42. Voss DE: Proprioceptive Neuromuscular Facilitation. Amer J Phys Med 46:838-898, 1967
43. Fischer E: Factors affecting motor learning. Amer J Phys Med 46:511-519, 1967
44. Hoberman M, et al: The use of lead-up functional exercises to supplement mat work. Phys Ther Rev 31:1, 1951
45. Adams JA: A closed-loop theory of motor learning. J Mot Behav 3:111-149, 1971
46. Schmidt RA: A schema theory of discrete motor skill learning. Psychol Rev 82:225-260, 1975
47. Stelmach GE (ed): Motor Control: Issues and Trends. New York, NY, Academic Press, 1976
48. Winstein CJ: Motor learning considerations in stroke rehabilitation. In Duncan PW, Badke MB (eds): Stroke Rehabilitation: The Recovery of Motor Control. Chicago, IL, Yearbook, 1987, pp 109-134
49. Winstein CJ: Relative frequency of information feedback in motor performance and learning. Unpublished doctoral dissertation, University of California, Los Angeles, CA, 1987
50. Shea JB, Zimmy ST: Context effects in memory and learning movement information. In Magill RA (ed), Memory and Control of Action. Amsterdam, North Holland, 1983, pp 345-366
51. Carr JH, Shepherd RB: A motor relearning programme for stroke, ed 2. Rockville, MD, Aspen, 1987
52. Carr JH, Shepherd RB: A motor learning model for rehabilitation. In Carr JH, Shepherd RB, Gordon J, Gentile AM, Held JM: Movement Science: Foundations for Physical Therapy in Rehabilitation. Rockville, MD, Aspen, 1987, pp 31-91
53. McGraw MB: The Neuromuscular Maturation of the Human Infant. New York, NY, Hafner Publishing Co, 1945
54. McGraw MB: Growth; a Study of Johnny and Jimmy. New York, NY, Appleton Century Co, 1935
55. McGraw MB: Later development of children specially trained during infancy; Johnny and Jimmy at school age. Child Dev 10:1-19, 1939
56. Thelen E: The (re)discovery of motor development: Learning new things from an old field. Dev Psych 25:946-949, 1989
57. Clark JE, Whitall J: What is motor development? The lessons of history. Quest 41:183-202, 1989
58. Thomas JR, Thomas KT: What is motor development? Where does it belong? Quest 41:203-212, 1989
59. VanSant, AF: A lifespan concept of motor development. Quest 41:224-234, 1989
60. Jackson JH: Evolution and dissolution of the nervous system. In Taylor J (ed): Selected writings of John Hughlings Jackson. New York, NY, Basic Books, 1958, 45-75
61. Lerner RM: Concepts and theories of human development. Reading MA, Addison-Wesley, 1976
62. Wickstrom RL: Fundamental Motor Patterns, ed 3. Philadelphia, PA, Lea & Febiger, 1983
63. Bruner JS: organization of early skilled action. Child Dev 44:1-11, 1973
64. Connolly KJ: Mechanisms of Motor Skill Development. New York, NY, Academic Press, 1973
65. Kugler PN, Kelso JAS, Turvey MT: On the control and coordination of naturally developing systems. In Kelso JAS, Clark JE (eds): The Development of Movement Control and Coordination. New York, NY, Wiley, 1982, pp 5-78
66. Thelen E: Developmental origins in motor coordination: Leg movements in human infants. Dev Psychobio 18:1-22, 1985
67. Thelen E, Kelso J, Fogel A: Self-organizing systems and infant motor development. Dev Rev 7:39-65, 1987
68. Espenschade A, Eckert H: Motor Development. Columbus, OH, Merrill, 1967
69. Eckert HM: Motor Development, ed 3. Indianapolis, IN, Benchmark Press, 1987
71. Roberton MA: Developmental kinesiology. Journal of Health, Physical Education, and Recreation 43:65-66, 1972

72. Halverson LE, Roberton MA, Harper CJ: Current research in motor development. Journal of Research and Development in Education 6:56-70, 1973
72. Wollacott MJ, Shumway-Cook A: Development of Posture and Gait Across the Life Span. Columbia, SC, University of South Carolina Press, 1989
73. VanSant AF: Rising from a supine position to erect stance: Description of adult movement and a developmental hypothesis. Phys Ther 68:185-192, 1988
73. VanSant AF: Age differences in movement patterns used by children to rise from a supine position to erect stance. Phys Ther 68:1330-1338, 1988
76. VanSant AF, Cromwell S, Deo A, Ford-Smith C, O'Neil J, Wrisley D: Rising to standing from supine: a study of middle adulthood. Phys Ther 68:830, 1988
77. Luehring S: Component movement patterns of two groups of older adults in the task of rising from standing from the floor. Unpublished master's thesis, Virginia Commonwealth University, Richmond, 1989
77. Sabourin P: Rising from supine to standing: A study of adolescents. Unpublished master's thesis, Virginia Commonwealth University, Richmond, 1989
78. Richter RR, VanSant AF, Newton RA: Description of adult rolling movements and hypothesis of developmental sequences. Phys Ther 69:63-71, 1989
80. Lewis AM: Age-related differences in rolling movements in children. Unpublished master's thesis. Virginia Commonwealth University, Richmond, 1987
80. Boucher JS: Age-related differences in adolescent movement patterns during rolling from supine to prone. Unpublished master's thesis, Virginia Commonwealth University, Richmond, 1988
81. Francis ED: Description of the sit-to-stand motion in children and young adults: Hypothesis of developmental sequences. Unpublished master's thesis, Virginia Commonwealth University, Richmond, 1987
82. McCoy JO: Age related differences in the movement patterns of adolescents 11, 14, and 17 years of age rising to standing from supine on the bed. Unpublished master's thesis, Virginia Commonwealth University, Richmond, 1989
83. Ford-Smith C: Age differences in movement patterns used to rise from a bed: A study of middle adulthood. Unpublished master's thesis, Virginia Commonwealth University, Richmond, 1989
84. VanSant AF: A life span perspective of righting tasks. Advances in Motor Development: Current Selected Research. In press, Volume 5, 1991
85. VanSant AF: Assessment of Neuromotor Developmental Status across the Life Span. In Proceedings of Neurology Section Measurement Forum. Alexandria, VA, Neurology Section, American Physical Therapy Association, 1990
86. VanSant AF, Sabourin P, Leuhring S, O'Neil J, Ford-Smith C, Cromwell S, Deo A. Relationships among Age, Gender, Body Dimensions and Movement Patterns in a Righting Task. Poster Presentation, American Physical Therapy Association Annual Conference, Nashville, TN, June, 1989
87. Gesell A, Amatruda CS: Developmental Diagnosis, ed 2. New York, NY, Hoeber, 1947
88. Shirley MM: The First Two Years. A Study of Twenty-Five Babies. Vol. 1: Posture and Locomotor Development. Minneapolis, MN, University of Minnesota, 1931
89. Stockmeyer SA: An interpretation of the approach of Rood to the treatment of neuromuscular dysfunction. Am J Phys Med 46:900-956, 1967
90. Gesell A: Infancy and human growth. New York, NY, Macmillan & Co., 1928
92. Gesell A: The First Five Years of Life. Part I. New York, NY, Harper & Brothers, 1940
93. Gesell A, Ames LB: The ontogenetic organization of prone behavior in human infancy. J Genet Psychol 56:247-263, 1940
93. Shirley MM: The First Two Years: A Study of Twenty-Five Babies. Vol. I. Postural and Locomotor Development. Minneapolis, MN, University of Minnesota Press, 1931
94. Ianniruberto A, Tajani E: Ultrasonographic study of fetal movements. Seminars in Perinatology 5:175-181, 1981
95. Milani-Comparetti A: The neurophysiologic and clinical implications of studies on fetal motor behavior. Sam Perinat 5:183-189, 1981
97. Prechtl HFR: The study of neural development as a perspective of clinical problems. In Connolly KJ, Prechtl HFR (eds): Maturation and Development: Biological and Psychological Perspectives. Clinics in Developmental Medicine, No. 77/78. Philadelphia, PA, JB Lippincott, 1981, pp 198-215
97. Connolly KJ: Maturation and the ontogeny of motor skills. In Connolly KJ, Prechtl HFR (eds): Maturation and Development: Biological and Psychological Perspectives. Clinics in Developmental Medicine, No. 77/78. Philadelphia, PA, JP Lippincott, 1981, pp 216-230
98. Thelen E: Rhythmical stereotypes in normal human infants. Animal Behavior 27:699-715, 1979
99. Kravitz H, Boehm J: Rhythmic habit patterns in infancy: their sequences, age of onset and frequency. Child development 42:399-413, 1971
100. Reed ES: An outline of a theory of action systems. Journal of Motor Behavior 14:98-134, 1982
102. Thelen E, Kelso JAS, Fogel A: Self-organizing systems and infant motor development. Developmental Review 7:39-65, 1987
102. Thelen E: Self organization in developmental processes: Can systems approaches work: In Gunnar M, Thelen E (eds): Systems and development: The Minnesota Symposia on Child Psychology, Vol. 22, Hillsdale, NJ, Lawrence Erlbaum, 1989, pp 77-117
103. Anokhin PK: Systemogenesis as a general regulator of brain development. Prog Brain Res 9:54-86, 1964
104. Gibson JJ: The senses considered as perceptual systems. Boston, MA, Houghton Mifflin, 1966
105. Gibson EJ: The concept of affordances in development: the renascence of functionalism. In Collins WA (ed): The Concept of Development: Minnesota Symposia on Child Psychology, Vol. 15, Hillsdale, NJ, Lawrence Erlbaum, 1982
106. Thelen E: Developmental origins of motor coordination: Leg movements in human infants. Developmental Pyschobiology 18:1-18, 1985
108. Clark JE, Phillips SJ, Petersen R: Developmental stability in jumping. Developmental Psychology 25:1036-1045, 1989
109. Getchell N, Roberton MA: Whole body stiffness as a function of developmental level in children's hopping. Developmental Psychology 25:1020-1028, 1989
110. Goldfield EC: Transition from rocking to crawling: Postural constraints on infant movement. Developmental Psychology 25:1013-1019, 1989
111. Brazelton TB: Neonatal Behavioral Assessment Scale. Clinics in Developmental Medicine, No. 50. Philadelphia, PA, JB Lippincott, 1973

Chapter 3
Neural Systems Underlying Motor Control

Roberta A. Newton, Ph.D., PT

INTRODUCTION

Motor control is the process by which the central nervous system (CNS) receives, integrates, and assimilates sensory information with past experiences for planning and executing appropriate motor and postural responses. How the nervous system produces coordinated and complex motor behavior is of interest to both researchers and clinicians. The purpose of this chapter is to provide an overview of the neural systems underlying motor control. Principles and concepts presented provide part of the foundation for physical therapy assessment and treatment. Changes in assessment and treatment approaches are, in part, reflections of advances in the understanding of the inter-workings of the sensory-motor control system.

What parameters of movement are controlled and how the CNS is organized to produce a variety of movements are not understood fully. Through observation and description of nervous system dysfunction and through research, models have been developed to assist our understanding. These models are based on different perspectives, i.e., neurological, biomechanical, and behavioral. Thus, no singular model of motor control is universally accepted. Models are also based on the type of movement produced, i.e., fast, slow, skilled, voluntary, or postural.

Models may encompass the concept of motor programs. Some motor programs are inherent and contained in neuronal networks, such as the central pattern generators located in the spinal cord.[1] Other motor programs are developed and reside in a shared arrangement with various brain centers.

Which movement characteristics are contained in motor programs is controversial. Some researchers favor a model of a generalized motor program where spatio-temporal sequences of muscles are stored. The specific muscle synergies are supplied at the time of planning the movement. Others consider motor programs as representations of every motor act, thus, the spatio-temporal sequences of specific muscle synergies are stored. This potentially could produce a storage problem in the brain. Which parameters of movement or posture are stored in a motor program may be a reflection of the type of motor or postural behavior. Motor programs are discussed in Chapter 9.

To examine the complex neural system for motor control, various elements will be highlighted. Additionally, an overview of motor control theories will be presented.

SENSORY INFORMATION

Monitoring the internal and external environment is the primary function of sensory receptors. Sensory input denotes the location of the body in space, location of the body parts to one another, and aspects of the environment including temperature, location of objects, and conditions of the support surface. Monitoring is necessary so the organism can detect a potentially harmful environment, resist the forces of gravity to maintain an upright position, or explore and manipulate the environment. The organism relies on a constellation of sensory cues from cutaneous and kinesthetic receptors located in the skin, joints, and muscles, as well as vestibular, visual, auditory, and olfactory information. Motor behavior resulting from sensory information may range from a simple spinal level reflex to a very complex motor pattern based on perception and memory of similar situations.

Sensation is defined as the process by which sensory receptors receive and route information to the spinal level for

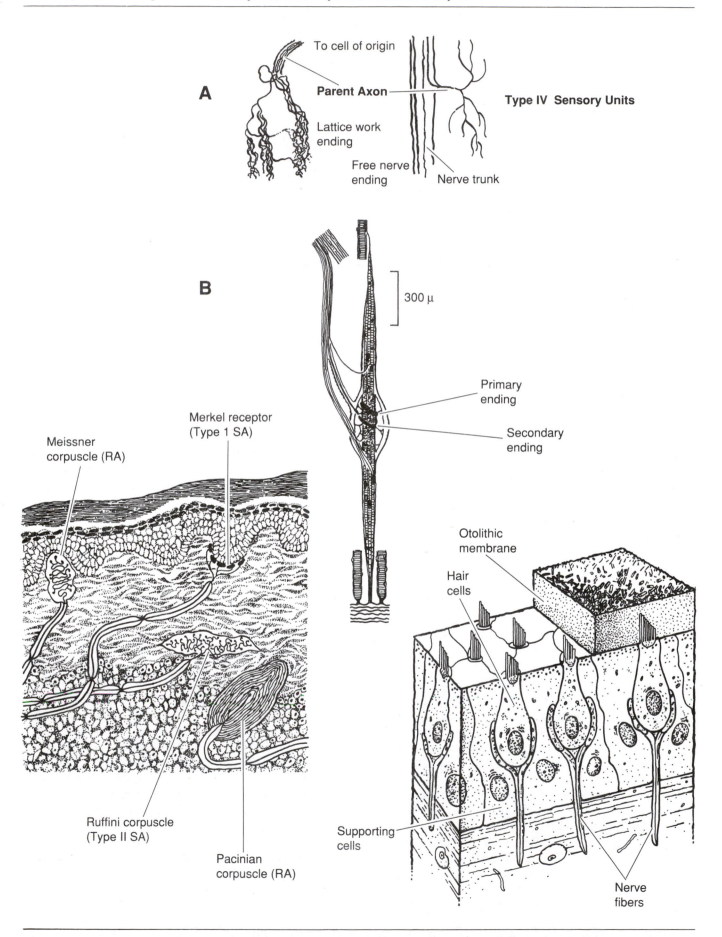

FIGURE 1. *Mechanoreceptors located in skin, muscle and joint.* **A.** *Free nerve endings–type IV joint receptors.* **B.** *Encapsulated endings–cutaneous receptors, muscle spindle, vestibular receptor.*

To cell of origin

Parent Axon

A

Lattice work ending

Free nerve ending

Nerve trunk

Type IV Sensory Units

B

300 μ

Primary ending

Secondary ending

Meissner corpuscle (RA)

Merkel receptor (Type 1 SA)

Otolithic membrane

Hair cells

Ruffini corpuscle (Type II SA)

Pacinian corpuscle (RA)

Supporting cells

Nerve fibers

reflexive autonomic and motor activity, and to higher centers for processing. Perception is the integration of sensory input in conjunction with memory of similar situations. Sensation cannot be changed with repeated experience, whereas, perception is changed with repeated experience.[2]

Sensory information is used in at least in three different modes during motor activity. First, sensory information reflects the location of body parts with respect to one another, and location of the body with respect to space and objects within the environment. This input is used during the planning phase. Second, sensory information can be used to revise motor programs prior to and during the execution of a motor program. This process occurs at the spinal level by altering the excitability level of the internuncial and motoneuronal pool, or at the level of the cerebellum for comparing actual motor behavior to the expected motor response. Third, sensory input from movement may be reduced and stored in motor memory for future use. This use of information is termed knowledge of results.

General Characteristics of Sensory Receptors

Sensory receptors are either free nerve endings or elaborate structures encased in connective tissue capsules (Figure 1). Although receptors tend to be modality specific, responding most efficiently to a single type of sensory stimulus, others are polymodal, responding to several types of stimuli. At the receptor level, sensory information is encoded by a pattern of action potentials. The pattern, or code, is related to the intensity and duration of the stimulus. Sequential activation of receptors indicates direction of the moving stimulus or moving body part. All receptors either partially or completely adapt to a stimulus. With continuous application of a stimulus, the response rate of the receptor will be initially high then, over time, will decrease to a low level or will stop.

The sensory unit is the functional unit of sensation. This entity includes the receptor (or group of receptors) attached to a single afferent neuron. The sensory unit monitors a limited area, the peripheral field. The peripheral field for cutaneous receptors is a specific skin area. For joint receptors, the peripheral field is bounded by a specific joint range and is measured in degrees and direction of movement.

Processing Sensory Information

Although the majority of sensory afferents reach the spinal cord via the dorsal roots, approximately 20% of the unmyelinated pain afferents enter the spinal cord via the ventral root.[3] Sensory input is carried to higher centers via specific ascending pathways as well as routed to various levels of the spinal cord through Lisseaurs tract or short and long propriospinal tracts. Afferent connections at the spinal level influence the internuncial pool, autonomic efferents, and motor efferents.

Cutaneous information reaches higher centers via the dorsal column-lemniscal system or the anterolateral system.

FIGURE 2. Lateral aspect of the cerebrum according to Brodman, with functional localizations.

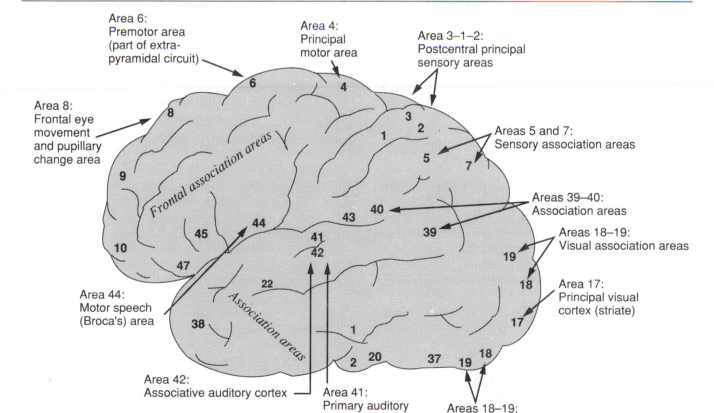

Transmission of information by two distinct pathways is one method for the CNS to distinguish among different sensory modalities. The dorsal column-lemniscal system primarily transmits mechanoreception. This highly organized system produces sparse collateral branching. The result is a high degree of spatial orientation between the perceived stimulus and localization of the stimulus on the body. To increase the discriminatory function of this system, some collateral branching is inhibitory. These inhibitory endings block further spread of the signal, thereby enhancing the contrast of the transmitted signal. This process is called lateral inhibition.

The anterolateral system transmits a broad spectrum of modalities. As this system ascends, collateral branching occurs, therefore this system lacks the discriminatory quality found in the dorsal column-lemniscal system.

In addition to the use of lateral inhibition to enhance the signal, enhancement also occurs though feedback control loops. Corticofugal inhibitory axons impinge on various levels of the neuraxis and are postulated to provide gain control, that is, recurrent inhibition to increase or decrease the threshold level of ascending pathways.

Somatosensory Cortex

Somatic sensory area I lies in the postcentral gyrus of the cerebral cortex (Brodmann areas 3,1,2) (Figure 2). Each side of the cortex receives primarily contralateral sensory input with the exception of the face. Functionally, the region is arranged somatotopically and in vertical columns; each column receives input from a specific sensory modality. Vertical columns in the anterior portion of the postcentral gyrus receive input primarily from proprioceptors, and those in the posterior portion receive input primarily from cutaneous receptors.

Widespread damage to the postcentral gyrus results in deficits in the individual's ability to gauge gradations in weight, pressure, texture of materials, and to judge shapes or forms of objects. Some ability to perceive tactile sensation may return and is believed to be due to crude perception in the thalamus.

Cutaneous Receptors

Cutaneous receptors are classified as mechanoreceptors, thermoreceptors, and pain fibers. Mechanoreceptors monitor the relative position of the stimulus on the surface of the skin as well as assist in determining the rate of movement of body parts relative to one another or to the support surface. Mechanoreceptors provide information relative to exploring and manipulating the environment and determining the texture of the support surface.

Reflexively, cutaneous input is used to provide appropriate facilitation or inhibition of the interneuronal and motoneuronal pools. Only noxious cutaneous stimuli produce reflexive stereotypic movement. The role of tactile input for manipulating the environment, particularly for precise manipulation has been examined by various investigators.[4] Handling small objects between the thumb and finger tips requires refinement of muscle forces, a task which is heavily dependent on cutaneous input. A memory trace for coordinating grip and load forces is constantly updated through tactile input. The automatic adjustment through a closed loop feedback system prevents the object from slipping though the fingers. Because of this automatic feedback loop, a greater portion of the sensory processing can be used for higher level manipulatory or exploratory functions.

Proprioceptors

Muscle, tendon, and joint receptors provide information regarding static position, movement, and sensation pertaining to muscle force. Kinesthesia and proprioception are terms describing these functions, and often are used interchangeably.

The muscle spindle is a complex receptor consisting of two major types of intrafusal muscle fibers, afferent and efferent connections, and a connective tissue covering. The location of the muscle spindle in series with extrafusal muscle fibers permits the receptor to monitor muscle stretch. The muscle spindle is also sensitive to externally applied vibratory stimuli. At the spinal level, this receptor type produces autogenic facilitation of motoneurons. Antagonist muscles receive reciprocal inhibition. Spindle information to higher centers pertains to velocity and length of muscle stretch.

A proprioceptive illusion is created with muscle vibration.[5,6] Vibration activates muscle spindles resulting in reflexive contraction of the muscle, perception of muscle stretch, and distortion of position sense. In individuals with an intact CNS, the apparent conflict can be resolved, however resolution of the conflict may not occur in the patient with CNS dysfunction.

The Golgi tendon organ monitors muscle tension for a group of muscle fibers rather than sampling muscle tension for the entire muscle. Early research suggested that the function of the Golgi tendon organ was to prevent a joint from over exceeding its range. More recently, hypothesized roles of this receptor and the muscle spindle are to regulate muscle stiffness. That is, by monitoring the length and tension of a muscle, these receptors, through feedback loops, influence the amount of muscle tension or stiffness.[7]

Four different types of receptors are considered joint receptors, three true joint receptors and one pain receptor.[8] These receptors signal specific direction and velocity of joint movement as well as static position. Reflexively, they either facilitate or inhibit the internuncial pool. During passive joint movements, receptor input appears to be facilitory. During active movement, joint receptor input appears to facilitate antagonists and inhibit agonists to ensure joint movement in a working range and to provide control when the joint begins to move outside normal physiological range.[9]

The role of joint receptors in kinesthesia has not been fully elucidated. For example an individual's ability to detect passive movements of the fingers and toes is diminished with nerve blockage, however, direction is detected with an increase in the velocity of passive movement. This detection could be reflective of the contribution of muscle receptors.[6] In other studies, intracapsular anesthesia of the knee joint did not affect detection of joint position. Location of anesthesia and the differences in velocity of passive joint movement

FIGURE 3. *The anatomical connections of the basal ganglia.*

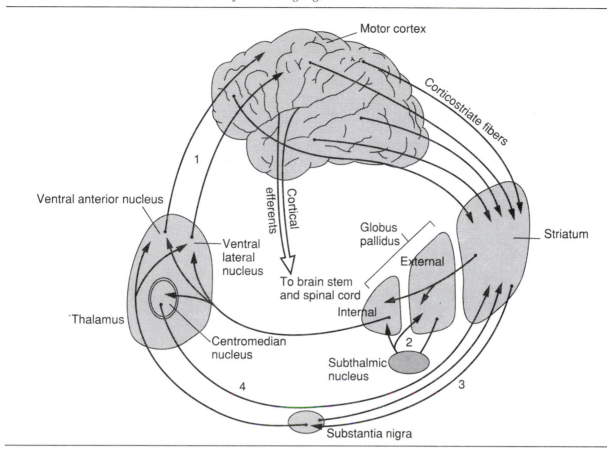

could cause the apparent discrepancies found in the outcomes of these studies.

The role of proprioceptive feedback for development of motor programs, particularly learning a new task, is well documented. Object manipulation is a widely used paradigm for examining this role. Patients with sensory neuropathies are unable to sustain a grip with the affected hand. However, they may be able to drive a car with a manual gear in the absence of peripheral feedback. This example demonstrates that a stored motor program can be executed without peripheral feedback. However, during repetitive manipulation activities performed without visual guidance, motor performance deteriorates due to undetected and uncompensated errors.[10] Although peripheral feedback may not be necessary for execution of stored motor programs, feedback is necessary for the automatic adjustments that accompany movement, particularly adjustments related to load compensation, error detection, and correction. Furthermore, feedback is necessary for learning new motor programs and refining motor output during execution.

Summary

The role of sensory receptors in regulating motor behavior is extensive at both spinal and higher center levels. Depending on the type of movement, the role varies. Rather than examining individual receptors and their role in motor be-havior, future examination should be directed towards functional classifications, i.e., mechanoreception, thermoreception, and nociception.

BASAL GANGLIA

The basal ganglia (BG), by virtue of their interconnections, represent an extremely complex area. Diseases such as Parkinson's disease, hemiballism, and Huntington chorea confirm this center's role in motor control. Movement deficits include abnormalities of righting (labyrinthine and body righting reactions), equilibrium, and initiation and velocity of movement. To consider the basal ganglia's only role to be relative to motor function is too simplistic. More recently, the BG have been demonstrated to be involved in more complex behavior including cognitive functions.

Neuroanatomical Connections

Neuroanatomical connections demonstrate the complexity of this area and the difficulty attributing functions to these nuclei. The three primary nuclei of the BG are the putamen, globus pallidus, and caudate nucleus. Other associated nuclei include the substantia nigra (SN) and subthalamic nucleus. The putamen and caudate nucleus are the primary receiving areas and the globus pallidus is the primary output area. The term, striatum, collectively identifies the putamen and caudate nucleus. Figure 3 demonstrates several circuits involving the BG, cortical, and subcortical centers.

A major circuit arises in the cerebral cortex, projects to the BG via corticostriate pathways, and returns to the cortex via the thalamus. Neurons arise from all areas of the cortex including the primary motor, premotor, and association areas and terminate on neurons in the striatum. The terminations are somatopically organized, with functionally related neurons from different parts of the cerebrum terminating in close proximity. The arrangement of these terminations suggests an integrative role for the BG. Neurons from the striatum terminate upon the globus pallidus and subthalamic nuclei. Neurons transverse to the ventroanterior and ventrolateral thalamus then back to all areas of the cerebral cortex, particularly to prefrontal and premotor areas. This loop is considered a negative feedback loop because of the inhibitory component from the striatum to the globus pallidus.

This major circuit is subdivided into the "complex" ("association") loop and the "motor" loop.[11] The complex loop is identified with frontal association areas of the cortex and uses the caudate nucleus as the major input area. The motor loop originates in the premotor and motor areas of the cortex and uses the putamen as the major input area. Both loops project to different areas of the globus pallidus, substantia nigra, and thalamic nuclei. These loops also recognize and are integrated with the internal circuit between the striatum and substantia nigra. The striatum releases GABA (an inhibitory substance) upon neurons of the SN which, in turn, releases dopamine (an inhibitory substance) at its termination in the striatum. This striatal-SN circuit is a mutual inhibitory pathway. Damage to the SN fibers produces chemical transmitter imbalance within the striatum. Thus cholinergic pathways from the cerebral cortex are totally or partially unchecked when damage occurs to these inhibitory pathways.

Other loops run from the globus pallidus to the subthalamic nucleus and globus pallidus to the centromedian of the thalamus. Other efferent pathways from the BG, not necessarily forming circuits, project to the brain stem and superior colliculus.

Role in Motor Control

The role of this area in motor control has been examined through research and analysis of movement deficits associated with pathologies. Based on recordings of cellular activity in unanesthetized and unrestrained animals performing rapid movements, slow movements, and self paced alternating movements, it can be assumed that the BG are involved with a wide variety of movements. More specifically, these nuclei control specific parameters of movement. Early studies demonstrated that BG cells were active prior to the onset of cortical activity or movement.[12] Movement related cells were also noted to be preferentially active to specific movements or postures.[13] More recently, recordings have been conducted in primates performing pursuit tracking tasks and step tracking tasks. From these studies, researchers concluded these nuclei are not involved in the initiation of a stimulus triggered movement, but are involved with initiation of self generated

or voluntary movement. Moreover, their role includes scaling parameters of movement including velocity, amplitude, and direction.

Parkinson's disease is considered the hallmark of basal ganglia dysfunction and is the first documented example of pathology related to neurotransmitter deficiency.[14] As described by Marsden[15] and Martin,[16] individuals with Parkinson's disease have bradykinesia, tremor at rest, and cog-wheel rigidity. To examine the role of the BG using a disease model such as Parkinsonism, patients need to be observed during early onset. With progression, other cortical and subcortical areas become involved, thereby contaminating observed motor behavior attributed to the BG.

More recently, individuals self exposed to MPTP (1-methly-4-phenyl-1,2,3,4-tetrahydropyridine) developed symptoms similar to Parkinson's disease.[17] This toxin selectively damages dopamine producing neurons of the substantia nigra. The three cardinal symptoms of Parkinson's disease (akinesia, tremor, rigidity) demonstrated in these patients were produced solely by loss of the nigrostriatal projections.[17]

Bradykinesia is a slowing of movement due in part to the inability of the patient to generate sufficient amplitude in the agonists, although the normal triphasic EMG pattern is intact. This finding supports the role of the basal ganglia in a scaling function, particularly in relationship to amplitude or magnitude of the initial burst of EMG activity in the agonists.

Akinesia denotes impaired initiation of movement. To date, the pathophysiologic mechanism for akinesia is not understood completely. Continued, tonic inhibition of thalamic neurons by the internal portion of the globus pallidus is a potential mechanism. Rigidity is believed to be due to loss of the nigrostriatal dopamine system since the symptom is reversed by dopamine agonists. How disruption of this pathway leads to rigidity is still controversial.[18] The pathophysiological basis of tremor is not understood, but may involve either cerebellar-thalamic pathways or pallium-thalamic pathways.

Pursuit tracking paradigms have been used in patients with Parkinson's disease to delineate the BG role in motor control.[19,20] Reaction times to these tasks are increased, with variability attributed to medication. This delay is believed due to the inability to deliver the correct initial motor command to the agonist muscle, as well as the inability to generate appropriate agonist force. These phenomena were demonstrated in standing balance responses to linear perturbation. Horak and Nashner noted the activation of two movement strategies in response to linear perturbation[21] (see Chapter 10). The observed motor behavior could be the result of the inability to select the appropriate motor strategy or the inability to issue a correct initial motor command.

Generally, patients with Parkinson's disease do not achieve high velocity of movements during high amplitude excursions. When tracking targets requiring initial fast movements, patients move slowly to the target using a pause-error correction mode throughout the excursion of the movement, rather than smooth pursuit movement. The faster the speed needed for target pursuit, the greater the impairment. Additionally, slowness and intermittency of movement have been documented with EMG. Alternating activity between agonists and antagonists produces intermittent bursts of activity as the patient follows or approaches the target.[22] Patients demonstrate increasing delay to producing faster movements and a higher error rate than normal when performing tracking tasks. Reduced predictive capabilities and reduced improvement with practice were noticed with step tracking tasks or tracking tasks containing reversals in movement. Patients could learn new motor tasks and learn to predict the course of a target.[23] This is indicative that the patient was able to select a sequence of motor programs necessary to carry out a movement.

In addition, patients with Parkinson's disease have been observed to be dependent on visual input for guidance of limb movements, an indication of impaired kinesthetic mechanisms.[24] DeLong and others noted that the majority of BG cells of non-human primates responded preferentially to joint rotations rather than cutaneous stimulation.[25]

Patients with Parkinson's disease have difficulty performing two simultaneous movements or switching from one motor task to another. "Freezing" in the middle of a motor sequence is not uncommon. Deficits in motor performance of complex movements demonstrate the integral involvement of the basal ganglia in motor control. No single pathophysiologic mechanism can explain movement deficits in Parkinson's disease. It appears that patients perceive the motor task and select and sequence the necessary motor programs, but are unable to execute the motor programs. This is further evidenced by: 1) breakdown of simultaneous tasks into sequential tasks, 2) selection of inaccurate parameters during the initial activation of the agonists, and 3) pause-run mode rather than a smooth running sequence of the motor program.[18]

Postural abnormalities also are evident in Parkinson's disease. The classical flexed posture is due to increased activity of axial and limb musculature. Postural instability is marked by decreased righting and equilibrium reactions. Since postural instability appears later in the course of Parkinson's disease, it may be due to damage in other areas of the brain in concert with progressive damage to the basal ganglia. Anticipatory and compensatory postural reactions, as well as protective reactions, are also compromised.

Role in Cognition

Due to the extensive connections from the cortex to the basal ganglia, the BG are believed to participate in cognition. The caudate nucleus is believed to be the predominate input for cognitive functions. Bilateral lesions to specific areas of the caudate nucleus produce deficits in the animal's ability to perform delayed alternation tasks. These tasks involve a delay between the time instructions are given and when actual motor performance occurs. These deficits are noted when particular areas of the cortex are damaged, specifically those areas having projections to the caudate nucleus.[26]

FIGURE 4. Lobes of the cerebellum.

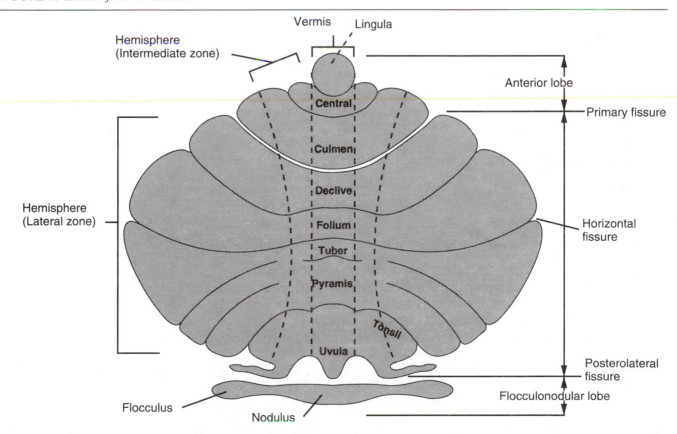

FIGURE 5. Projections of the vestibulocerebellum.

Labels: Vestibular nuclei, Flocculonodular lobe, Medulla, Medial vestibulospinal tracts, Lateral vestibulospinal tract, Spinal cord, Semicircular canals and otolith organs

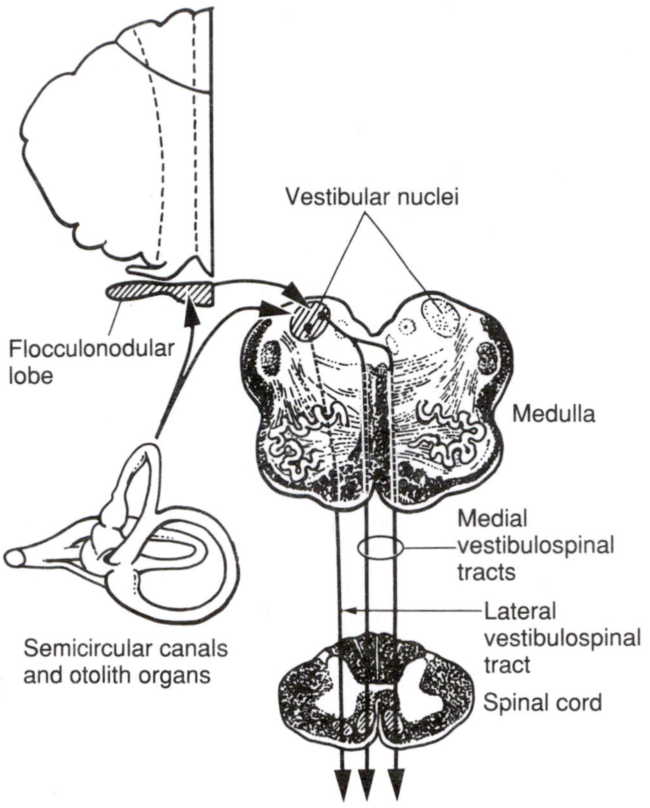

CEREBELLUM

The cerebellum contains half of all the neurons located in the brain, yet constitutes only 10% of the brain weight. This highly organized structure is best analyzed from a three dimensional perspective. The role of the cerebellum in motor control is awesome, ranging from a comparator role to involvement in motor learning.[27]

Deep fissures serve to divide the cerebellum into the anterior, posterior, and flocculonodular lobes (Figure 4). The cerebellum is also divided into three sagittal areas. The vermis is a narrow longitudinal strip located in the midline and separates the left and right cerebellar hemispheres. Each hemisphere is subdivided into an intermediate and lateral zone. Four pairs of deep nuclei associated with this region are the fastigial, dentate, globose, and emboliform nuclei.

Input from the periphery, brain stem, and cerebral cortex terminates either in the cerebellar cortex or deep cerebellar nuclei. The raphe nuclei and locus ceruleus also send projections to the cerebellar cortex. Mossy and climbing fibers transmit all information to the cerebellar cortex. These two excitatory inputs arise from different sources. The mossy fibers originate from the brain stem nuclei and carry information from the spinal cord as well as the cerebral cortex. Mossy fibers terminate on granule cells in the granular layer of the cerebellar cortex. Axons of the granular cells project to the outermost cortical layer, bifurcate, and become known as parallel fibers. By this axonal arrangement, mossy fibers influence a large number of Purkinje cells. Purkinje cells are the sole output neurons from the cerebellar cortex. The second projection system, climbing fibers, originates from the inferior olivary nucleus. These fibers impinge directly on a limited number of Purkinje cells. The mossy fiber-climbing fiber interactive arrangement on the Purkinje cell has been implicated in the cerebellum's role in learning.[27]

The excitatory activity of the mossy and climbing fiber input upon the Purkinje cell is offset by inhibitory interneurons, termed stellate, basket, and Golgi cells. When a group of Purkinje cells are activated, Purkinje cells boarding the active group are inhibited. The function of this lateral or surround inhibition is not clearly understood.

The major output from the cerebellar cortex is to the deep nuclei with some projections to the vestibular nuclei. By virtue of its development, the cerebellum can be considered as three distinctive regions, each with specific efferent projections and each with specific motor functions.

Neuroanatomical Connections And The Role Of Cerebellar Areas In Motor Control

The vestibulocerebellum encompasses the flocculonodular lobe which is termed, the archicerebellum (Figure 4). This area receives input from and projects to the vestibular nuclei and thus is intimately involved with regulation of balance and eye-head movement (Figure 5). Input to this area signals changes in head position and orientation of the head with respect to gravity. Visual information also indicates orientation of the head in space. Output from this area regulates axial muscles used to maintain balance and controls eye movement for coordination of eye-head movement.

Damage to this area is generally due to a medulloblastoma. Patients with this condition may be unable to maintain balance even in a seated position with eyes open, thereby demonstrating lack of postural stabilization. Patients use a wide base of support during stance and gait to compensate for decreased intersegmental stability.[28]

The spinocerebellum (paleocerebellum) runs rostro-caudal to include the vermis and intermediate zones of the cerebellar hemispheres (Figure 4). Sensory information is received from the periphery through the spinocerebellar tracts (hence its name) and from the visual, auditory, and vestibular systems. Input is somatotopically organized, one map lying in the rostral region and the other map in the caudal region. Auditory and visual information are directed more toward the posterior aspect of this region.

Output from the spinocerebellum terminates on different deep cerebellar nuclei, thereby forming two different projection systems (Figure 6). The vermis projects to the fastigial nucleus, which in turn, sends bilateral projections to the lateral vestibular nuclei and the brainstem reticular formation. These latter areas form the medial descending system

FIGURE 6. Projections of the spinocerebellum.

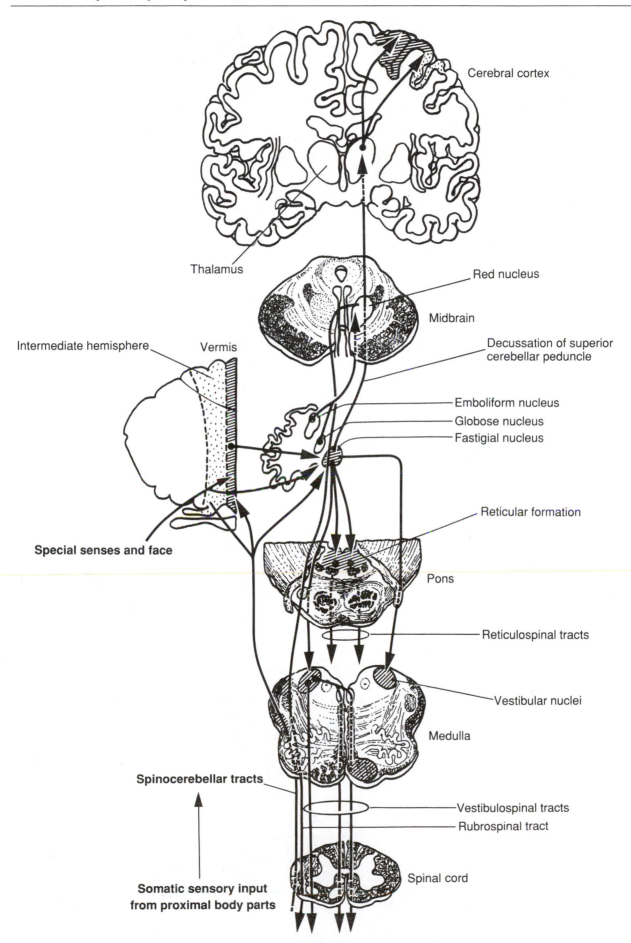

Cerebral cortex

Thalamus

Red nucleus

Midbrain

Intermediate hemisphere

Vermis

Decussation of superior
cerebellar peduncle

Emboliform nucleus

Globose nucleus

Fastigial nucleus

Reticular formation

Special senses and face

Pons

Reticulospinal tracts

Vestibular nuclei

Medulla

Spinocerebellar tracts

Vestibulospinal tracts

Rubrospinal tract

Spinal cord

**Somatic sensory input
from proximal body parts**

FIGURE 7. Projections of the cerebrocerebellum.

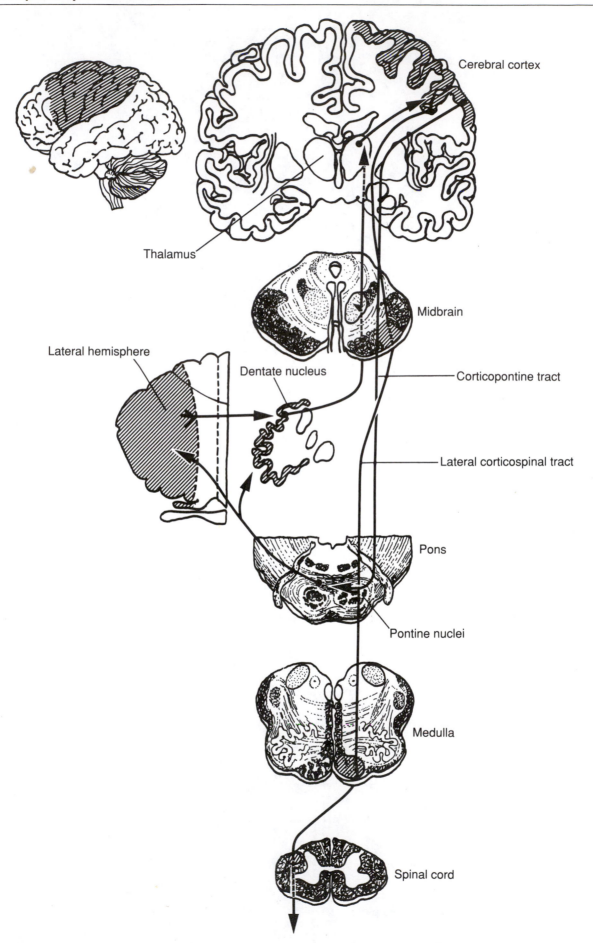

Cerebral cortex

Thalamus

Midbrain

Lateral hemisphere

Dentate nucleus

Corticopontine tract

Lateral corticospinal tract

Pons

Pontine nuclei

Medulla

Spinal cord

that regulates axial and proximal musculature. The fastigial nucleus also sends crossed ascending projections to the motor cortex. The intermediate part of the cerebellar hemispheres impinges upon the emboliform and globose nuclei which project to the red nucleus and cerebral cortex. Thus, the cerebellum influences the lateral descending system, containing, in part, the rubrospinal tract system which affects musculature of the distal portions of the limbs. Projections to the contralateral red nucleus then to limb areas of the motor cortex assist in regulating the corticospinal tract.

Functions of the spinocerebellum include a regulatory role in the execution of movement and regulation of muscle forces to compensate for variations in load encountered during movement. This comparator function is dependent on information received from the cerebral cortex regarding the intended movement and feedback from the periphery regarding the actual movement. A mismatch between the actual and intended movement produces an error signal which is corrected by revising the motor program.

Damage to the spinocerebellum results in an abnormal sequence of muscle contraction. Agonist muscle activity is prolonged and timing of antagonist contraction for limb deceleration is delayed. When deceleration and stop commands are disrupted, movements become inaccurate and tremor occurs, particularly at the end of movement.

Damage usually entails the upper vermal and intermediate part of the anterior lobe, such as that observed in patients with chronic alcoholism. Patients demonstrate extremely large antero- posterior sway paths in standing but rarely exceed sway limits and fall. When tested on sudden tilt of a moveable platform, a relatively normal latency of onset with increased sway amplitude of the compensatory balance response occurs.[29] Patients rely heavily on vision to maintain balance.

The cerebrocerebellum receives widespread input from the cerebral cortex, but does not receive direct input from the periphery. The major inputs arise from the premotor, motor, sensory, and posterior parietal lobes of the cerebrum. This portion of the cerebellum is defined by the lateral parts (zone) of the hemispheres (Figure 4). Because this is the last cerebellar area to evolve, it is also known as the neocerebellum. Phylogenetically, the region increased in size in relation to increases in the size of the cerebral cortex.

Output from this area terminates on neurons in the dentate nucleus, which in turn projects to the ventral lateral nucleus of the thalamus, then to premotor and motor areas of the cerebrum (Figure 7). A feedback loop is evident as fibers of the dentate nucleus project to the red nucleus, then to the inferior olivary nucleus and back to the cerebellum.

Both lesion studies and cell recordings have been used to document contributions of this area to motor control which includes a decrease in control of distal limb musculature. Furthermore, delays in the initiation of movement, hypotonia, and motor incoordination are evident. These deficits can be attributed to the loss of spatio-temporal organization necessary for movement. A delay in initiation has been hypothesized to occur either with loss of the dentate nucleus's participation in commands for initiating movement, or loss of its influence on activation of other centers.[30]

Another possible role for the cerebrocerebellum, along with the premotor cortex, is programming of movement. Thus, this area could serve two purposes, the decision to move, and the initiation of movement.[31,32]

Individuals with tumors or vascular lesions to this region demonstrate some reduction in postural stability, but no abnormal sway characteristics. These individuals may demonstrate a jerky, ataxic path when trying to follow a cursor on a computer screen that represents their center of mass. This observation further confirms the role of this area in spatio-temporal organization necessary for pursuit tasks, either whole limb or whole body.[33]

Role of the Cerebellum in Motor Learning

In the 1970s, the role of the cerebellum in motor learning was based on mathematical models exploring cerebellar circuitry.[34] Further evidence was obtained when researchers noted that the visual fields and the direction of the vestibulo-ocular reflex (VOR) could be reversed by wearing prismatic lenses. Both humans and non-human primates adapted to the reversal, which was considered by some a learning phenomena. Cerebellar damage prevented adaptation. Based on these and other observations, it was postulated that over a period of time climbing fiber inputs modified Purkinje cell response to mossy fiber input. This modification, adaptation, produced the learned changes observed in the VOR.[35]

Changes in Purkinje cell activity occur during learning of skilled motor acts. Neuronal activity was recorded during motor learning tasks in primates, such as altering the task of moving a lever by suddenly adding a new load. As the cerebellum detects mismatch between the intended and actual movement, adjustments occur in the motor program. These adjustments were associated with neuronal activity in the cerebellum.[36] One can question if this is a learning phenomenon or adaptation to a new situation, such as identified in the classical conditioning experiments. Learning represents a permanent change in motor behavior, whereas adaptation represents a temporary change in motor performance. In either case, learning is essential because the individual needs to respond to continuing changes in both the internal and external milieu.

Summary: Parameters Of Motor Control

As stated earlier, the cerebellum's role in motor control extends beyond that just involved with movement. The cerebellum is involved with planning and executing movement as well as serving in a comparater and corrector role. Parameters of the motor control program under cerebellar influence are evident in disease processes. One feature is the loss of smooth coordinated movement (asynergia) which entails a decrease in accurate prediction of force, range, and direction of movement. Many complex movements are broken down into various components which produce a more irregular pattern of alternating movements. The break or stop command also is diminished, causing the limb to overshoot end range and rebound.

Postural adjustments also are regulated by the cerebellum. The extent to which these postural abnormalities are evident depends on the site of damage. Parameters of balance abilities may be near normal, have near normal latency of onset with an increase in sway amplitude, or may be so impaired that the patient is unable to maintain balance even in a seated position.

CEREBRAL CORTEX

Events necessary for purposeful movement include the goal of movement, a strategy for accomplishing the movement, and execution of the motor program via coordinated activity occurring in the different descending pathways.

Motor Cortex

The motor cortex influences alpha motoneurons through both indirect and direct neuronal connections. Since the descending neurons terminate on the same internuncial pool as afferent reflexive connections, the motor cortex participates in motor control though descending pathways as well as regulating spinal level reflexive or oscillatory activity.

The motor cortex tends to be more involved with the production of skilled movement. This area regulates the rate of force development as well as maintaining a steady level of force. Since this area receives and projects to the periphery, these long loop or servo assist loops assist with small load compensations that oppose movement excursion. When the load is large, this loop and other circuits, particularly those associated with the cerebellum, become operational.[37]

The role of the motor cortex for development of the motor program is a shared role with the premotor cortex, the supplementary motor area, the posterior parietal region, and various subcortical centers.

Supplementary Motor Area

This region lies in front of the motor cortex and has a less developed somatotopic map (Figure 2). The major subcortical input is from the basal ganglia. Generally, electrical stimulation in this area produces bilateral movements. This region's role in programming complex movements in humans has been analyzed by cerebral blood flow studies.[38] When individuals compress a spring between the thumb and index finger, an increase in blood flow occurs bilaterally in the motor and sensory cortex, but not in the premotor areas. When the individual performs a more complex movement sequence involving all the fingers, cerebral blood flow in the supplementary motor area significantly increases. A similar increase occurs with mental practice.

Premotor Cortex

This area is located on the lateral surface of the cerebral hemisphere anterior to the motor cortex and under the supplementary motor area (Figure 2). It projects mainly to the brainstem and influences the reticulospinal system, suggesting a regulatory role of proximal and axial muscles, particularly during the early phase of limb movement toward a target.

The premotor area may be involved in response preparation, particularly related to the "go" command. Premotor cortical neurons are activated between the stimulus, "go," and the actual movement. Damage to this area produces a grasp response, the significance of which needs further delineation.

Posterior Parietal Cortex

This region lies posterior to the primary somatic sensory cortex and is interconnected with the premotor area. The posterior parietal cortex is involved intimately with processing sensory information necessary for movement. It provides spatial information necessary for movements that have a target. Damage in this area produces apraxia, which also is seen with damage to the frontal association areas. Neglect of one side of the body or an extremity is noted in patients with damage to this area. This syndrome is believed to be a deficit in the ability to assimilate information from the contralateral side of the body into a body percept. These individuals may have deficits in manipulating objects for exploratory purposes. Cells in the parietal cortex respond to the approach or contact of the desired target and other cells fire in response to hand manipulation.

In summary, the motor systems of the cortex tend to function as modules. Depending on the movement, a different module will be the predominant functioning unit along with subcortical areas. This concept has been termed "distributed processing." It is evident that the motor program does not reside within a single structure, but is an emergent property. That is, the motor program is a function of cortical and subcortical centers assimilating, planning, and coordinating synergies that contain appropriate velocity, direction, and amplitude parameters.

DESCENDING PATHWAYS

Three major descending pathways impinge upon the spinal cord. They are the ventromedial system (VMS), lateral system (LS), and corticospinal system (CS). The VMS is comprised of the vestibulospinal, reticulospinal, tectospinal, and interstitiospinal tracts (Figure 6). These tracts terminate on axial and limb girdle musculature. Due to the high degree of collateralization, the VMS represents the fundamental descending system by which the nervous system regulates movement. This system is involved with regulation of axial musculature for maintenance of intersegmental spinal stabilization for righting and balance. Since the VMS also regulates proximal musculature, this system is involved with integration of body-limb movements and orientation of the body and head with the direction of movement of the organism.

The lateral system arises from the contralateral rubrospinal (Figure 6), rubrobulbar, and ventrolateral pontine tegmentum and terminates on musculature in the distal portions of the limb. This system is involved with independent movements of the shoulder, elbow, and hand, particularly those associated with flexion. The third descending system, the CS system, comprises the corticospinal and corticobulbar pathways (Figure 7). This system terminates at all levels of the spinal cord with some direct synaptic connections on alpha motoneurons. This system is involved with fine finger fractionation and regulatory control over the other two descending systems. Delineation of these two systems and their role in motor control have been obtained primarily through research on non-human primates.[39]

MODELS OF MOTOR CONTROL

Models of motor control have evolved from simple dichotomies to extremely complex interrelationships. Early technology enabled researchers to lesion various areas of the brain and examine remaining motor function. Observed motor and postural patterns were attributed to imbalances between intact and damaged structures. One such model based on ablation studies that, unfortunately, still pervades neurology is that of the extrapyramidal and pyramidal motor system. These two systems were divided into two independent entities: the extrapyramidal system represented by the basal ganglia and the pyramidal system represented by the cortex. This division permitted early neurologists to classify nervous system diseases. Paralysis or spasticity were signs of pyramidal system damage, and rigidity, bradykinesia, or involuntary movements were signs of extrapyramidal system damage. This motor control model should no longer be used for the following reasons. First, by virtue of the extensive interconnections and feedback loops between cortical and subcortical systems, these centers cannot function independently. Second, the basal ganglia, cerebellum, brain stem, and red nucleus, all subcortical structures, play an important role in voluntary movement. And, third, disease or injury does not involve just one area of the brain. For example, Parkinson's disease may initially involve basal ganglia structures, but over time other subcortical and cortical areas become involved. Or, a middle cerebral infarct damages ascending and descending pathways of the cerebrum, and transverse fibers of the basal ganglia. While segregating brain centers was an attempt to understand diseases or damage of the central nervous system, this model has outlived its usefulness and should be viewed from an historic perspective.

Hierarchy is another simplistic model attempting to replicate control of movement. In this model, a commander issues commands and the motor program is carried out by subordinate structures. This model developed by Jackson was based on the evolution and dissolution of the nervous system.[40] Although this model is not useful to study control of extremely complex movements involving feedback or motor learning, it is useful to explain those movements operating in an open loop mode. That is, the motor program is initiated and run without constant feedback. This model is useful in examining quickly executed movements.

A model that is useful for complex movements, for motor learning, and for examination of the role of feedback, is the heterarchy.[41] By virtue of its name, there is no single commander, but rather, depending on the particular type of movement, different systems participate. Since no single commander exists and centers participate in different functions depending on the motor act, the element of redundancy is evident. The concept of the motor program as an emergent property can be supported by this model. That the motor program does not reside in one specific brain center is another concept of the heterarchy. The tripartate model for motor control can be considered a heterarchial model. The basal ganglia, cerebellum, and cortex form the three major centers, and the medial, lateral, and corticospinal descending pathways can be added to this model to form the descending system. As is evident, the different centers serve different functions depending on the type of movement. The concept of emergent properties fits well with this model.

SUMMARY

In order to examine the complexity of neural systems underlying motor control, each element was discussed separately. To fully understand motor control, these elements need to be examined in concert with one another. By understanding neural systems underlying motor control, alternative therapies can be developed to assess and treat the patient with central nervous system damage and the scientific bases underlying these therapies can be better established. ❏

REFERENCES

1. Grillner S: Control of locomotion in bipeds, tetrapods, and fish. In Brookhart JM, VB Mountcastle (eds): Handbook of Physiology. Section I The Nervous System, Vol II Motor Control, part 2, Bethesda MD, American Physiological Society, 1981, pp 1179 - 1236
2. Sage GH: Introduction to Motor Behavior: A Neuropsychological Approach, ed 2. Reading, MA, Addison-Wesley Publishing Co, 1977
3. Yaksh TL, Hammond DL: Peripheral and central substrate involved in rostrad (ascending) transmission of nociceptive information. Pain 13: 1-85, 1982
4. Johansson RS, Westling G: Tactile afferent input influencing motor coordination during precision grip. In Struppler A, Weindl A (eds): Clinical Aspects of Sensory Motor Integration. Berlin, Germany, Springer - Verlag, 1987, pp 3-13
5. Matthews PBC: Where does Sherrington's "muscular" sense originate? Muscles, joints, corollary discharges. Ann Rev Neurosci 5: 189 - 219, 1982
6. Gandevia SC: Neurophysiological mechanisms underlying proprioceptive sensations. In Struppler A, Weindl A (eds): Clinical Aspects of Sensory Motor Integration. Berlin, Germany, Springer - Verlag, 1987, pp 14-24
7. Carew TJ: The control of reflex action. In Kandel ER, Schwartz JH (eds), Principles of Neural Sciences, ed 2. New York, NY, Elsevier Biomedical Press, 1985, pp 457 - 468
8. Newton RA: Joint receptor contributions to reflexive and kinesthetic responses. Phys Ther 62: 22-29, 1982
9. Schaible HG, Schmidt RF, Willis WD: New aspects of the role of articular receptors in motor control. In Struppler A, Weindl A (eds): Clinical Aspects of Sensory Motor Integration. Berlin, Germany, Springer - Verlag, 1987, pp 34-45
10. Marsden CD, Rothwell JC, Day BL: The use of peripheral feedback in the control of movement. In Evarts ED, Wise SP, Bousfield D (eds): The Motor System in Neurobiology. New York, NY, Elsevier Biomedical Press, 1985, pp 215 - 222
11. DeLong MR, Georgopoulos AP, Crutcher MD: Cortico-basal ganglia relations and coding of motor performance. In Massion J, Paillard J, Schultz W, et al (eds): Exp Brain Res Supp 7: 30 - 40, 1983
12. De Long MR: Activity of basal ganglia neurons during movement. Brain Res 40: 127 - 135, 1972
13. DeLong MR, Georgopoulos AP: Motor functions of the basal ganglia. In Brookhart JM, Mountcastle VB (eds): Handbook of Physiology, Section 1. The Nervous System, Volume II. Motor Control, Part 2, Bethesda, MD, American Physiological Society, 1981, pp 1017-1061
14. Hornykiewicz O: Metabolism of brain dopamine in human parkinsonism: Neurochemical and clinical aspects. In Costa E, Cote LJ, Yahr MD (eds): Biochemistry and Pharmacology of the Basal Ganglia. New York, NY, Raven Press, 1966, pp 171-185
15. Marsden CD: The enigma of the basal ganglia and movement. In Evarts ED, Wise SP, Bousfield D (eds): The Motor System in Neurobiology. New York, NY, Elsevier Biomedical Press, 1985, pp 277 - 283
16. Martin JP: The Basal Ganglia and Posture. London, England, Pitman, 1967
17. Ballard PA, Tetrud JW, Langston JW: Permanent human parkinsonism due to 1-methyl-4-phenyl-1,2,3,6-tetrahydropyridine (MPTP): Seven cases. Neurology 35: 949-956, 1985
18. Marsden CD: Basal ganglia and motor dysfunction. In Asbury AK, McKhann GM, McDonald WI (eds): Diseases of the Nervous System, Clinical Neurobiology, London, England, William Heinemann Medical Books, 1986, pp 394 - 400
19. Flowers K: Some frequency response characteristics of Parkinsonism on pursuit tracking. Brain 101:19-34, 1978
20. Flowers K: Lack of prediction in the motor behavior of Parkinsonism. Brain 101:35-52, 1978
21. Horak FB, Nashner LM, Nutt JG: Postural instability in Parkinson's's disease: Motor coordination and sensory organization. Soc Neurosci Abs 10: 634, 1985
22. Hallet M, Shanani BT, Young RR: Analysis of stereotyped voluntary movements at the elbow in patients with Parkinson's disease. J Neurol Neurosurg Psychiatry 40: 1129-1135, 1977
23. Bloxham CA, Mindel TA, Frith CD: Initiation and execution of predictable and unpredictable movements in Parkinson's disease. Brain 107: 371-384, 1984
24. Cooke JD, Brown JD, Brooks VD: Increased dependence on visual information for movement control in patients with Parkinson's disease. Can J Neurol Sci 5:413-415, 1978
25. Crutcher MD, DeLong MD: Single cell studies of the primate putamen. II. Relations to direction of movement and pattern of muscular activity. Exp Brain Res 53:244-258, 1984
26. DeLong MR, Georgopoulos AP: Motor functions of the basal ganglia. In Brookhart JM, Mountcastle VB (eds): Handbook of Physiology, Section 1. The Nervous System, Volume II. Motor Control, Part 2, Bethesda, MD, American Physiological Society, 1981, pp 1017-1061
27. Ito M: The Cerebellum and Neural Control. New York, NY, Raven Press, 1984
28. Dichgans J, Diener HC: Different forms of postural ataxia in patients with cerebellar diseases. In Bles W, Brandt T (eds): Disorders of Posture and Gait. New York, NY, Elsevier Biomedical Press, 1986, pp 207-215
29. Diner HC, Dichgans J, Bacher B, et al: Characteristic alterations of long loop "reflexes" in patients with Friedreich's disease and late atrophy of the cerebellar anterior lobe. J Neurol Neurosurg Psychiat 47: 679-685, 1984
30. Ghez C, Fahn S: The cerebellum. In Kandel ER, Schwartz JH (eds): Principles of Neural Science, ed 2. New York, NY, Elsevier Biomedical Press, 1985, pp 502-522
31. Meyer-Lohmann J, Hore J, Brooks VB: Cerebellar participation in generation of prompt arm movements. J Neurophysiol 40:1038-1050, 1977
32. Brooks VB, Thach WT: Cerebellar control of posture and movement. In Brookhart JM, Mountcastle VB (eds): Handbook of Physiology, Section 1: The Nervous System, Vol II, Motor Control. Bethesda, MD, American Physiological Society, 1981, pp 877-946, 1981
33. Mauritz KH, Dichgans J, Hufschmidt A: Quantitative analysis of stance in late cortical cerebellar atrophy of the anterior lobe and other forms of cerebellar ataxia. Brain 102:461-482, 1979
34. Albus JS: A theory of cerebellar function: Math Biosci 10:25-61, 1971
35. Llinas RR: Electrophysiology of the cerebellar networks. In Brooks VB (ed): Handbook of Physiology, Section 1: The Nervous System, Vol II. Motor Control, Pt.2. Bethesda, MD, American Physiological Society, 1981
36. Thach WT: Correlation of neural discharge with pattern and force of muscular activity, joint position, and direction of intended next movement in motor cortex and cerebellum. J Neurophysiol 41:654-676, 1978
37. Evarts EV: Role of motor cortex in voluntary movement in primates. In Brookhart JM, Mountcastle VB (eds): Handbook of Physiology, Section I: The Nervous System, Vol II, Motor Control. Bethesda, MD, American Physiological Society, 1981, pp 1083-1120
38. Roland PE, Larsen B, Lassen NA, et al: Supplementary motor area and other cortical areas in organization of voluntary movements in man. J Neurophysiol 43: 118-136, 1980
39. Kuypers HGHM: Anatomy of the descending pathways. In Brookhart JM, Mountcastle VB (eds): Handbook of Physiology, Section 1. The Nervous System, Vol II. Motor Control, Part 2, Bethesda, MD, American Physiological Society, 1981, pp 597-666
40. Jackson H: The Croonian lectures on evolution and dissolution of the nervous system. Br Med J. Part 1: 591-593, 1884
41. Davis WJ: Organizational concepts in the central motor networks of invertebrates. In Herman RM, Grillner S, Stein PSG, et al (eds): Neural Control of Locomotion: Advances in Behavioral Biology, v. 18. New York, NY, Plenum Press, 1976, pp 265-292

Chapter 4
Musculoskeletal Considerations In Production and Control of Movement

Mary M. Rodgers, Ph.D., PT

INTRODUCTION

The intent of this chapter is to provide a basic scientific foundation for an understanding of movement which includes consideration of the laws of mechanics as they relate to the description and production of movement, the musculoskeletal structures which produce movement, and specific interactions between the human body and the environment which require movement control. Any study of the production and control of movement requires an interaction of many different systems whose final outcome is biomechanically measurable. In the first section, biomechanical terms and concepts used in the dynamic analysis of motion are introduced. Specific musculoskeletal components and their mechanical characteristics are described in the second section. The final section brings together biomechanical concepts and musculoskeletal structures as they interact in different movements, such as walking.

BASIC BIOMECHANICAL TERMS AND PRINCIPLES

Static analysis simplifies the process of analyzing movement. With large accelerations or masses, however, static analysis would be inaccurate. To more accurately analyze movement of the human body, an understanding of the principles of dynamics is necessary. Dynamics is the study of motion (the relationships between factors causing motion and the motion itself). In statics, bodies are in static equilibrium or in dynamic equilibrium with no great acceleration. In dynamics, bodies are in motion but not in equilibrium.

Dynamics is further subdivided into the areas of kinematics and kinetics. Kinematics is the study of characteristics of motion, or motion descriptors. Kinematics is used to relate displacement, velocity, acceleration and time, without reference to the cause of motion. For example, in the analysis of gait, the pattern of the center of mass of the body, the range of motion of the different segments, and the speed and direction of their motion are all examples of kinematics.

Kinetics is the study of the relationship existing among forces acting on a body, the mass of the body, and the motion of the body. Kinetics is used to predict the motion caused by given forces or to determine the forces required to produce a given motion. Examples of forces which affect the motion of a body are gravity, friction, water and air resistance, muscle contraction, and elastic components. Applying Newton's laws of motion to the characteristics of motion enables the determination of the force characteristics involved in the motion.

The study of dynamics is invaluable in the field of medicine as evidenced by the role biomechanical investigations have played in analysis of gait patterns, development of prosthetics and orthotics, analysis of muscle function in different activities, analysis of the effect of water and air resistance on the moving body, prediction/evaluation of effects of surgical intervention (i.e., tendon transfer), and the analysis of mechanism of injury (i.e., sport injuries).

The analysis of temporal factors is basic to dynamic assessment of human movement. Examples of factors which relate to time include cadence, duration of a movement phase, and the temporal pattern. Cadence is measured by count (strikes per minute) and can be used to determine slow vs fast walking or running. The duration of a movement is important in muscle activity. For example, in a ballistic motion, a larger amount of muscle tension would be required than in a slower motion. Tension requirements may exceed the material strength of the musculotendinous components, causing rupture. In electromyographic studies of the lower extremity muscles during walking, the knowledge that certain muscles are active or inactive is useless unless the time of activity is also known and can be related to the pattern of gait. Changes in position are always connected with changes in time, so that knowledge of timing is essential in kinematic and kinetic analyses of motion.

Kinematics

Dynamic assessment requires an understanding of linear and angular kinematic parameters. This section presents a discussion of these parameters.

Position and displacement. Motion involves a continuous change in position, which in the case of a moving body is called displacement. A change in position may be translatory or linear so that every point of the body is displaced along parallel lines. In translation, a point is moved from one position to another and can be determined as in static analysis. The straight line distance between the two points is the magnitude of the displacement, and the direction must be indicated. Displacement is, therefore, a vector quantity while distance is a scalar quantity (magnitude without direction).

Change in position also may be rotational or axial, causing angular motion. In the body, movement around an axis may occur in a rotational pattern. Motion may be a combination of linear and rotational movement (Figure 1). For example, movements in gait represent a combination of translation (in the general movement of the body) and rotation (as the limbs rotate around many joints to achieve the end result of walking). Human motion can be described as translatory motion which has major contributions from linear, angular, and curvilinear movements. The motion that a body has in translation along a straight course or rotation about a particular axis constitutes one degree of freedom. The joints of the body often have many degrees of freedom, in that they permit motion in more than one plane.

Kinematic analysis has a wide range of applications in physical therapy. Angular displacement is probably the most common kinematic measurement taken for human motion. Because of the structure of the human body as a linked system of rigid segments moving about joint axes, an understanding of the kinematics of the body is often accomplished by analysis of rotational motion. Measurement of joint angles, assessment of deformities, assessment of fracture, planning of osteotomies, and assessment of joint stability are just a few of the medical applications of kinematic analysis.

Velocity. Displacement per unit time gives the rate of displacement or velocity. The average velocity of a body over a time interval is defined as the quotient of the displacement (s) and the time interval (t). Speed or velocity provides an account of both the spatial and temporal elements

FIGURE 1. *Translation and rotation movements during walking. The stick figure is reconstructed from three-dimensional motion analysis. It shows the combination of angular movement of the limbs about the joints and translation of the center of mass (highlighted) which occur during walking.*

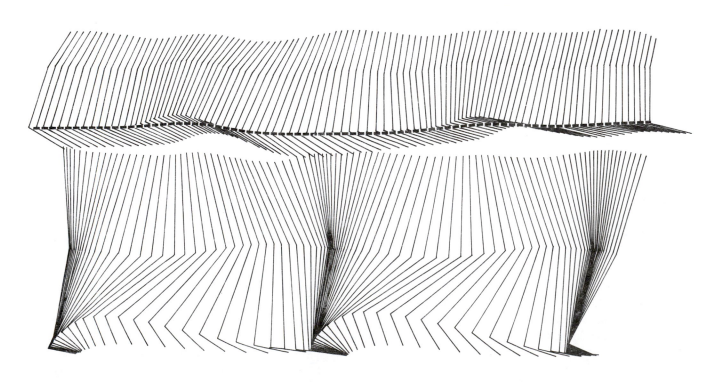

of motion. However, velocity is a vector quantity (includes direction of movement), whereas speed is scalar only (shows magnitude of the velocity vector without regard for change in direction). Average velocity can be used when the velocity is relatively constant. Additionally, average velocity calculated over a short period of time will approach the value for instantaneous velocity (eg. velocity at a specific instant of time or at a certain point on its path).

Linear velocity is the time rate of change of position and displacement. The units are expressed as meters per second (m/s). Graphically, velocity refers to the slope of the position-time graph. A change in the slope of the position line depicts a change in the relationship (or velocity). Angular velocity is the time rate of change of angular positions and is expressed in radians per second (rad/s) or degrees per second.

Acceleration. When an object moves from one location to another, its velocity may not be constant over the entire distance. The magnitude of the velocity may increase or decrease relative to its straight line of displacement, or the direction of velocity may change. These changes in velocity are referred to as acceleration and deceleration (negative acceleration). Since change in velocity takes place over a certain time interval, acceleration is considered the rate of change in velocity.

Linear acceleration is expressed in meters per second squared (m/s^2). If final velocity is greater than initial velocity, the object is accelerating or has positive acceleration. If final velocity is less than initial velocity, the object is decelerating or has negative acceleration. Instantaneous acceleration would be approximated by using small time intervals in the analysis. Angular acceleration (alpha) is the time rate of change of angular velocity. The units for angular acceleration are radians per second squared (rad/s^2) or degrees per second squared.

As an example, suppose a patient is moving her arm through a range of 105 to 135 degrees of shoulder abduction. The angular displacement would be 30 degrees or .52 radians. If the starting position were stationary and the movement occurred in 2 seconds, the average angular velocity of shoulder abduction would be .26 rad/s (15 deg/s). If the patient continues to abduct the arm, and at 2.5 seconds the arm is travelling at a velocity of 1.57 rad/s (90 deg/s), the average angular acceleration would be .63 rad/s (36 deg/s^2).

Relative motion. In many applications of dynamics, the description of a frame of reference is necessary in order to relate motion at different locations. For example, motion of the ankle joint occurs in several different planes. Motion at the knee joint occurs primarily in one plane. The three-dimensional motion of the ankle during locomotion cannot be compared to that of the knee unless the kinematics and kinetics are described in the same planes for each joint. Similarly, the coordinate systems must be defined when analysis involves more than one technique.

If two bodies are moving along the same straight line, the position coordinates can be measured from the same origin. The difference in their positions defines the relative position coordinate of point A to point B and is denoted as $s_{A/B}$. The relative linear velocity between the points is the rate of change of relative displacements ($v_{A/B}$). Similarly, the rela-

tive linear acceleration between the points is the rate of change of relative velocities (aA/B). Relative motion may also be angular, in which case the same relationships are expressed using angular terms.

The applications for relative motion analyses are many. The effects of reconstructive surgery on joint motions can be documented using motion analysis prior to and following surgery. Additionally, basic research involving the effects of total joint kinematics on ligaments uses motion analysis.

Three-dimensional motion. Planar motion is movement in which all points of a rigid body move parallel to a fixed point. This motion has three degrees of freedom, including sliding anteriorly or posteriorly, sliding laterally, and rotating about an axis perpendicular to the translatory axes. The movements of vertebrae in trunk flexion illustrate planar motion as they rotate forward and translate simultaneously.

Plane motion is described by the position of its instantaneous axis of rotation and the motion's rotational magnitude about this axis. In cervical flexion, for example, as a vertebra moves in a plane, there is a point at every instant of motion somewhere within or without the body that does not move. If a line is drawn from that point so that it perpendicularly meets the line of motion, the point of intersection is called the instantaneous axis of rotation (or screw axis) for that motion at that point in time. Most joint movement is primarily rotatory motion, but the axis of motion may change its location and/or its orientation during a complete range of motion.

The term three-dimensional motion implies that an object may move in any direction by combining multidirectional translation and multiaxial rotation. In the human body, most movements are three-dimensional in that they move in more than one plane. The normal range of motion of joints denotes the extremes of rotation and translation of the joint. An articulation may have several degrees of freedom and a limited range of motion. Degrees of freedom refer to the ability to move in planes (number of axes), while the range of motion is dependent on soft tissue restraints, the number of joint axes, the joint architecture, and the size and position of adjacent tissue which may affect motion of a part. For example, the knee joint has one degree of freedom and a large range of motion, while the L5 vertebrae has six degrees of freedom and a limited range of motion. A range of motion can be expressed for each degree of freedom in a joint.

Kinetics

So far, only the movement itself, without regard for the forces which cause the movement, has been discussed. The study of these forces and the resultant energetics is called kinetics. The forces which cause motion can be internal or external. Internal forces may result from muscle activity, ligaments, or from friction in the muscles and joints. External forces may come from the ground or from external loads ,or from active bodies or passive sources (i.e., wind resistance). Since most of these forces are not directly measurable, they can be calculated using readily available kinematic and anthropometric data. Three forces constitute all of the forces acting on the total body system (gravity, ground reaction forces, and muscle/ligament forces).

The force exerted on an object as a result of gravitational pull is referred to as gravitational force. This force may be considered as a single force representing the sum of all the individual weights within the object. For internal force calculations, gravitational forces act downward through the centers of mass of each segment and are equal to the magnitude of the mass times acceleration due to gravity.

The forces that act on the body as a result of interaction with the ground are called ground reaction forces (GRF). Newton's third law implies that GRF are equal and opposite to those that the body is applying to the ground. GRF are external forces which can be measured using a force transducer (force platform). GRF are distributed over an area of the body (i.e., under the foot). For calculation purposes, GRF may be considered to act at a point so that the forces are represented as vectors. Under the foot, the point at which GRF act is referred to as the center of pressure.

Muscle and ligament forces can be calculated in terms of net muscle moments in order to represent the net effect of muscle activity at a joint. In the case of cocontraction at a joint, the analysis yields the net effect of both agonists and antagonists. The analysis includes any frictional effects at the joint or within the muscle. Increased friction reduces the net muscle moment, so that the moments created by the muscle contractile elements are higher than the tendon moments. At the extreme end of range of movement, the passive structures such as ligaments become important in limiting movement. The moments generated by these passive structures then add or subtract from those produced by the muscle.

The previously described forces act on the total body. In analysis of internal forces, body segments must be examined one at a time. Joint reaction forces are the equal and opposite forces that exist between adjacent bones at a joint caused by the weight and inertial forces of the two segments. Bone-on-bone forces are seen across the articulating surfaces and include the effect of muscle activity. In actively contracting muscles, the articulating surfaces are pulled together creating compressive forces. In this situation, the bone-on-bone force equals the compressive force due to muscle, plus the joint reaction forces.[1]

Approaches to analysis of movement

The kinematics of a motion can be used to examine the forces which actually cause the movement to occur. Force and motion may be studied using one of three approaches which are based on Newton's laws of motion. The law of inertia states that if a resultant force acting on a body is 0, the body will remain at rest (if originally at rest) or will move with constant speed in a straight line (if originally in motion). Another law of motion, the law of acceleration, states that if the resultant force acting on a body is not 0, the body will have an acceleration proportional to the magnitude and in the direction of this resultant force. A third law of motion, the law of action/reaction, states that forces of action and reaction between bodies in contact have the same magnitude, same line of action, and opposite sense. These three laws form the basis for kinetic analysis using the acceleration, impulse-momentum, and work-energy approaches.

In the acceleration approach, statics is defined as having acceleration equal to 0, so that the resultant force acting on the body is also 0. In dynamics, the resultant force is not equal to 0, therefore the body will accelerate. Since mass does not change, the force is proportional to the acceleration. Mass is the quantity determining the inertia of the body, therefore a large mass will have a large inertia. Units involved in the acceleration approach include Newtons for force, kilograms for mass, and meters/second^2 for acceleration.

The acceleration approach can be used to convert weight (a force) to mass. For example, the mass of a man who weighs 667.5 N (150 pounds) would be equal to force divided by gravity (9.8 m/s^2) or 68 kg. In another example of the acceleration approach to problem-solving, the resultant force required for a runner weighing 620 N (139 lbs.) to reach an acceleration of 28 m/s^2 would be:

$$F = (620 \text{ N} / 9.8 \text{ m/s}^2) * 28 \text{ m/s}^2$$
$$= 1771 \text{ N}$$

Acceleration is also involved with angular motion. A force acting through a distance from the axis of rotation causes motion since the moment is not balanced as in statics. The law of acceleration, therefore, has several angular analogies or correlates. In angular motion, the mass is represented by the moment of inertia, which relates resistance of a mass to its distance from an axis. In angular terms, the linear formula F = ma becomes: moment or torque equals moment of inertia multiplied by angular acceleration.

If the body is divided into many particles, each has a mass (m) and a perpendicular distance (r) from the axis. The sum of all the particles (mr^2) is the moment of inertia for the entire body. In linear terms, the center of mass represents the place at which the mass of the body is concentrated. In angular motion, this location is designated using the radius of gyration (k). An increase in either mass or distance from the axis will increase resistance of the body to angular acceleration (distance more so than mass since it is a squared term). For example, the k for a below knee prosthesis will influence how easily it swings (or the amount of resistance to movement) even more so than its mass. The placement of a leg cast will also influence resistance to motion more so than the mass of the cast.

If no external torque acts on a closed system, the total angular momentum remains unchanged even when the moment of inertia is changed. This principle is often expressed in athletics. A gymnast, high diver, or free-fall parachutist can regulate speed as the body rotates about its center of gravity by changing postures. If the limbs are tucked, the radius of gyration is shorter than when the limbs are abducted, so that the moment of inertia will be small and the body will spin rapidly about a transverse axis in the coronal plane. This is how the spinning figure skater can increase rotational speed by bringing the arms toward the center of the body. Conversely, the speed of rotation can be decreased by extending the extremities to increase the radius of gyration and increase the moment of inertia.

The following is an example of the acceleration approach to solve a human motion problem. A patient is able to hold the forearm in static equilibrium (Figure 2) using a muscle force of 108 N. How does the muscle force requirement change if the arm is accelerating at 80 rad/s² into elbow flexion? Almost three times as much muscle force is required when the forearm is accelerating compared to a static position. The potential for muscle tears and strains in ballistic types of movements is evident from this example.

A second method used to solve dynamic problems is the impulse-momentum approach. This approach is useful when the force involved in a dynamic problem acts over a period of time, and is essential when a collision is involved.

Impulses are forces developed during impact, the product of force and time. The value of momentum will increase with an increase in force, the application of force over a longer period of time, or a combination of both. The direction of the velocity vector will be that of the resultant force, so that velocity will be increased or decreased depending on the direction of the force. Whether the impact is delivered or received, its force will depend on the relative velocities of the colliding bodies. Thus, a greater impact force occurs when a hip impacts than when an elbow impacts because the trunk has a greater mass. When impact is made by elbow or knee extension (as in throwing or kicking), a greater velocity must be developed.

Applying force for a longer period of time increases the change in momentum. The impulse involved to stop a moving object corresponds directly to the change in momentum of the object so that the force and time of the impulse are inversely related. A longer time taken to stop a moving object will require less force by allowing an increased time for the momentum to change, as when the hand is allowed to go backward when catching a ball, or when a person rolls to decrease the force of a fall. Conversely, an increased force will reduce the duration necessary to stop the object. Postural adjustments just prior to receiving an impact (such as using one's center of gravity, going with the direction of force, and prolonging the duration of impact) can decrease the force of impact. For example, a toppling force can be minimized by receiving impact as close as possible to the center of gravity. Impact force can be decreased by moving in the same direction as the force (i.e., rolling with the punch).

Moment of inertia multiplied by the change in velocity represents the angular momentum of the rotating body. The torque applied to a rotating body is directly proportional to the product of its moment of inertia and angular velocity and inversely to its duration. The angular impulse is defined as the torque times the duration of torque application, which equals the angular momentum. The change in angular momentum of a rotating body depend on the magnitude and direction of the torque, and the duration of the torque applied.

A common example of angular impulse occurs during the gait cycle. Electromyographers have studied the coordinated action of the lower limb muscles. These muscles exert a force over a period of time. The force in this case produces a torque which changes the angular momentum of the limb. The impulse-momentum approach may be applied to rotator cuff lesions which occur during throwing. The velocity involved in the angular momentum of the arm and ball is directed backward, then suddenly the direction of the angular velocity

is changed by the internal rotator muscles as the throwing phase starts. The rapid change in angular momentum may produce immediate muscle or joint damage, or a fracture of the humerus. Angular momentum also plays an important role in exercise. A quick, forceful muscular contraction at the beginning of the movement may produce sufficient impulse to allow the body part and exercise weight to move through

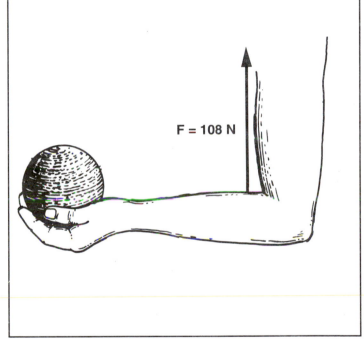

FIGURE 2. *Patient holding a forearm weight. In the static position, the arm and weight are balanced using a muscle force of 108 N. If the arm is accelerating at 80 rad/s2, the force required of the muscle must increase almost three times.*

F = 108 N

the range of motion without further muscle contraction. This minimizes the strengthening effects of the exercise. Momentum of a body part is often used in stretching exercises. If the momentum caused by a large mass or velocity is too great, the tissues may not be capable of supplying sufficient force to stop the movement. The force needed may be greater than the rupture strength of the tissues, and they may tear. Prolonged stretching of low velocity will decrease the chances of injury.

When the forces acting on the system are known as a function of the position of the body, the work-energy approach is the more convenient method to solve for motion. Work is defined as a force overcoming a resistance and moving an object through a distance. Its value is determined by multiplying the force by the displacement of the object. If force is not in the same direction as the displacement, the component of force in the direction of the displacement must be used to determine the work done. The displacement must be along the same line and in the opposite direction to the resisting force of the object. For example, movement perpendicular to the force of gravity will produce no work against gravity. A component of applied force must be parallel to elastic resistance as in a spring or with friction for work to be done.

The unit of measure for work is the newton-meter Nm or Joule. These units should not be confused with torque or moment which have similar units and are also defined as a force times distance. The resultant force producing work is concerned with a displacement and lies along the same line as the distance the object is moved. Conversely, the resultant force producing torque is perpendicular to a lever arm distance. A force producing torque can also produce work, but the correct distance must be used. By converting angular to linear motion, the work done during angular motion can be calculated (torque times angular displacement).

Work is usually considered as a force which lifts an object against gravity, although this is not the only way to perform work. If a resultant force moves a resistance through a distance parallel to the line of action of the force, work is accomplished. For example, a spring, friction, and a balloon all resist force so that work is performed when movement occurs. Work is also performed when acceleration occurs. In Newton's second law, force causes acceleration of an object and the accelerated motion is parallel to the force. Negative work refers to the situation in which a force acts parallel to the movement, but in the opposite direction. When a weight is lowered from a height with the force controlling the descent, negative work is said to occur. A spring which is released gradually or a moving object which is decelerated are two more examples of negative work.

Energy is the ability or capacity to do work. Although other forms of energy exist (i.e., heat, light, nuclear, electrical), our focus is on mechanical energy. Potential energy (PE) is energy by position, due to gravity. Potential energy equals the work done to elevate an object. For example, a 20 kg barbell lifted 1 meter above the floor has a potential energy equal to the force needed to overcome gravity (F) times the height (h) above the floor (PE = F* h = mgh). Therefore, the barbell at this position has 20 kg (9.81 m/s²) (1 m) or 196.2J of potential energy. The units to measure energy are the same as those used to measure work, and the work done equals the potential energy of the object. When work is done to overcome gravity, the PE of the object is increased.

Kinetic energy (KE) of the body is defined as the energy of motion. The work done on an object equals the change in its kinetic energy. Any moving body must possess energy because a force must be exerted to stop it, and it cannot be stopped in zero distance. To start an object moving, force must be exerted over a distance.

The law of conservation of energy states that energy cannot be created or destroyed, but may be transformed from one form to another. This law deals with the transmission, absorption, and dissipation of energy. The sum of potential energy and kinetic energy equals the total energy of the system. The principle of conservation of energy is that as potential energy decreases, the kinetic energy increases.

Conversion of PE to KE in falls relates to mechanisms of injury. The KE at the instant of impact may be determined from the PE of the body before the fall, and the height of the body's center of mass at impact. For example, a 70 kg man who falls on his hip has a center of mass located at 70 cm above the floor. His PE while standing is (70kg * 70cm) equal to 4900 kgcm. Normally the KE at impact is dissipated by bones, ligaments, muscles, and other soft tissues so that the energy absorption is within tolerable limits. According to Frankel and Burstein, if the hip carries most of the impact, a fracture is likely to occur since the femoral neck cannot absorb over 60 kgcm.[2]

The speed of loading a body tissue is related to its energy absorption. Frankel reported that with the slow loading of a bone, a greater load will be needed to fracture it.[3] However, with a rapidly applied load, the bone will break with a high energy explosion, while slow loading produces low energy fractures. Noyes determined that the speed of loading affected the type of tissue damaged.[4] A fast loading produced more ligament failures, whereas a slow rate resulted in more avulsion fractures.

The quantity of work required for a certain task or movement does not address the amount of time needed for the task or movement to take place. For example, the same amount of work is done if a 10 kg weight is lifted 1 meter whether the lifting is performed in one second or one minute. However, the power is different between the two situations. Power is the rate of doing work or the rate at which energy is expended. If the torque and angular velocity are known, the rotational power or development of rotational kinetic energy about an axis can be determined.

MUSCULOSKELETAL COMPONENTS

Because human movement is such a complex phenomenon, a number of simplifying assumptions are necessary for any analysis. For example, the dynamics section of this chapter describes methods of analysis in which the segments being moved are assumed to be rigid and the muscle forces are assumed to be in one direction. These assumptions ignore the complexity of both the bone and muscle structures, but allow the use of basic concepts in the study of human movement. Enoka described a "simple joint system" which is responsible for the production of human movement.[5] The system is composed of five parts: rigid link, synovial joint, muscle, neuron, and sensory receptor. The motor commands and sensory information must interact with the musculoskeletal components in order to produce and control movement. Description of these five components of the simple joint system follows.

Bone

The rigid link component of the simple joint system includes bone, tendon, and ligament. Bone has unique mechanical properties which allow it to provide rigid kinematic links and attachment sites for muscles, thereby facilitating muscle action and body movement. Strength and stiffness are the significant mechanical properties of bone. Bone strength, or the amount of force necessary to break bone, varies according to the angle and direction of force application. For example, Cowin found that a human femur has over twice as much tensile strength along the length of the bone as opposed to tensile strength perpendicular to the bone.[6] Because function has a direct affect on the mechanical characteristics of bone, it is strongest in the direction of most frequent stress. According to Alexander, bones are generally two to five times stronger than the forces they commonly encounter in everyday activities.[7]

The method of load application affects bone strength. For example, mature bone is strongest in compression. Additionally, bone increases in strength and stores more energy with increased speed of loading. The loading applied to bone through muscle activity alters the in vivo stress patterns in bone. Living bone is continually undergoing processes of growth, reinforcement, and resorption which together are referred to by Lanyon and Rubin as remodeling.[8] When the frequency of loading prevents the remodeling necessary to prevent failure, bone fatigues. Bone is laid down when needed and resorbed where not needed (Wolff's law), and remodels in response to mechanical demands. Examples are seen in the bone loss which occurs with space (no gravity) travel and with spinal cord injury (disuse osteoporosis). Conversely, bone hypertrophy is often seen in athletes who are routinely applying high loads to specific bones.

Tendon and Ligament

The tendons and ligaments surrounding the skeletal system are passive elements in the simple joint system in that they do not produce movement, but rather transmit movement. Tendons attach muscle to bone, and ligaments tie bone to bone. The structural organization of these two connecting links varies with the different function performed by each. Tendon and ligament are composed of three types of fibers: collagen, elastic, and reticulin fibers. The behavior of tendon and ligament is related to the structural orientation of these fibers, the properties of the collagen and elastic fibers, and the proportion between the collagen and elastic fibers. The function of tendon is to transmit force from muscle to bone or cartilage, therefore, its strength is needed in tension. The almost completely parallel alignment of the fibers provide tendons with high tension load tolerance (higher than that of ligament). The larger the cross-sectional area of the tendon, the more force it can withstand. Conversely, tendon can be deformed by small compressive and shear forces. Ligaments have a principal purpose of stabilizing joints, and ligament fibers are less consistently parallel than tendon fibers. Since joints may encounter forces which are tensile, compressive, or shear, the arrangement of fibers within a given ligament reflect the primary forces it must resist. They may be aligned in parallel, oblique, or spiral arrangements to accommodate forces in different directions.

The transition between bone and either tendon or ligament is gradual, creating a series of junctions instead of a marked change in structure. The bone-ligament and bone-tendon junctions are most susceptible to injury. However, all parts of the connecting links (ligament, tendon, and bony junctions) are affected by activity. Several investigators have shown that increased use results in increased strength of all parts of the connecting links, and enhances the healing process.[9,10]

Synovial Joint

In the calculations made using rigid body link segments, the segments are assumed to be joined by frictionless pinned joints. Since the synovial joint most closely approximates these assumptions, it will be described as the joint component of the simple joint system. The surfaces of the bones that form the joint are lined with articular cartilage which functions to absorb impacts, to prevent direct wear to the bones, and to modify the shape of the bone to insure better contact between the bones. The cartilage increases its thickness by increasing fluid absorption when a person goes from resting to active states. This increased thickness provides more protection during activity. The articulating surfaces are enclosed in a joint capsule which is covered internally with synovial membrane. The structure of the joint is quite variable, and determines the quality of movement between two adjacent body segments. A joint will have one to three axes, referred to as degrees of freedom.

Muscle

Muscles are able to respond to a stimulus, propagate a wave of excitation, modify length, grow, and regenerate to a limited extent. Of the different types of human muscle, skeletal muscle most closely approximates the role needed in the simple joint system analysis — to provide a force that interacts with those exerted by the environment on the system. Skeletal muscles act across joints to produce rotation of body segments (rigid links) about their joint.

The two most important elements of muscle function are the relationship between the sarcolemma and the sarcoplasmic reticulum and the components of the sarcomere. Sarcolemma is the cell membrane which surrounds each set of myofilaments that comprises a muscle fiber. The sarcolemma provides active and passive selective membrane transport in its function as an excitable membrane. Sarcoplasm is the fluid enclosed inside of the sarcolemma which contains fuel sources, organelles, enzymes, and contractile components (myofilaments bundled into myofibrils). The sarcoplasm also contains a hollow membranous system which is linked to the surface sarcolemma and assists the muscle in conducting commands from the nervous system.

The sarcomere is the basic contractile unit of the muscle which is arranged in series, end to end, to form a myofibril. An interdigitating set of thick and thin contractile proteins, or myofilaments, comprises the sarcomere. The thin filament has two strands of actin molecules upon which are superimposed two-strand (tropomyosin) and globular (troponin) proteins. During a muscle contraction, the tropomyosin and troponin impose their influence on the activity of actin. The thick filament is comprised of the protein myosin, which can be decomposed into light meromyosin (LMM) and heavy meromyosin (HMM) fragments. The myosin molecules contain two regions of greater flexibility, so that the HMM fragment can extend from the thick filament to within close proximity of the thin filament. Because of this interaction with actin, the HMM extension has been called the crossbridge.

Neuron and Sensory Receptors

Discussion of the musculoskeletal components of the simple joint system have so far described the rigid-link elements, the joint about which they rotate, and the muscle that can exert a force on the rigid links. Basic information about the way muscle is activated is discussed in detail in Chapter 3, therefore, only mention will be made here. The nervous system is comprised of neurons which have the common functions of receiving information, determining if a signal should be transmitted, and transmitting the electrical signal. In the simple joint system, the neural elements of greatest interest are the motoneurons because they innervate the skeletal muscles. The motor end plate (neuromuscular junction) is where the electrical energy of the nerve action potential is transferred to chemical energy in the form of a neurotransmitter. On the muscle side of the junction, the neurotransmitter (chemical energy) is converted back to electrical energy with the final product being a muscle action potential. The final component of the simple joint system is the sensory receptor. The function of sensory receptors is to provide feedback to the system about its state and the environment via conversion of energy from one form to another (transduction).

APPLICATIONS TO PRODUCTION AND CONTROL OF MOVEMENT

Control of Muscle Force

Excitation factors. Control of muscle force is dependent on the excitation of the force-generating units and the characteristics of these force-generating units (muscle mechanics and muscle architecture). Excitation factors important to regulation of muscle force include the number of motor units activated (motor-unit recruitment) and the rate at which each of the active motor units generates action potentials (rate coding). Movement is accomplished through the orderly recruitment of motor units so that as muscle force increases, additional motor units are activated. Once a motor unit is activated, it remains active until the force declines. The force reaches a plateau when no additional motor units are recruited, and is reduced by the sequential deactivation of motor units. This derecruitment occurs in the reverse order of recruitment. For some muscles (i.e., adductor pollicis), all motor units are probably recruited at 30% of maximum force level. According to Kukulka and Clamann, other muscles (i.e., biceps brachii) probably continue to recruit motor units up to 85% of maximum force level.[11] The increase in muscle force beyond the motor-unit recruitment level is due to rate coding.

Although several hypotheses have been advanced to account for orderly recruitment, there is no agreement on a single mechanism.[12] The size principle proposed by Henneman suggests that the orderly recruitment of motor units is due to variations in motoneuron size, so that the motor unit with the smallest motoneuron is recruited first and the motor unit with the largest motoneuron is recruited last.[13] Recruitment order may also be influenced by morphological and electrical characteristics of the motoneuron. Since re-cruitment order is predetermined, the brain does not have to specify which motor units are to be activated, and motor units cannot be selectively activated. Generally, the small mo-toneurons appear to innervate the slow-contracting, low-force, and fatigue resistant motor units (Type S), whereas the largest motoneurons innervate the fast-contracting, high-force, fatiguable motor units (Type FF). According to Stuart and Enoka, the considerable overlap which occurs between the motor unit types makes selective activation of only one type of motor-unit or muscle fiber type (slow-twitch vs fast-twitch) highly unlikely.[12]

The force exerted by a muscle results from variable combinations of the number of active motor units and the rate at which these motor units discharge action potentials (rate coding). The relationship between muscle force and action-potential rate (frequency) is nonlinear, with the greatest increase in force occurring at the lower action-potential rates (3-10 Hz). This relationship shifts depending on the length of the muscle, with the frequency affecting the greatest force changes being 3-7 Hz for long muscle lengths and 10-20 Hz for short muscle lengths. Gydikov and Kosarov proposed two types of motor units (tonic and phasic) which differ in their muscle force/action-potential relationships.[14] For tonic motor units, discharge rate increases as muscle force increases, but remains constant at high forces. Conversely, the discharge rate of phasic motor units increases over the entire range of muscle forces (linear relationship). In addition, the tonic motor units generate smaller action potentials, are recruited at lower muscle forces, and are less fatigable. The phasic motor units appear to be important for dynamic conditions and contribute more to muscle force than do the tonic units. Increases in muscle force result from increases in the concurrent processes of recruitment and rate coding. Harrison suggested that the relative contribution of recruit-ment and rate coding depends on the distribution of motor-unit mechanical properties.[15]

Another aspect of rate coding that affects force production is the relationship in time between an action potential and other action potentials generated by the same and other motor units (temporal patterning). Burke, Rudomin, and Zajac described the "catch" property of muscle as the dis-charge of two action potentials (a doublet) from one motor unit within a short time interval (i.e., 10 ms) which produces a substantial increase in the force exerted by the motor unit.[16] According to Gydikov and associates, the occurrence of these doublets represents a rate coding effect which probably varies from muscle to muscle and may depend upon the task (concentric vs eccentric).[17] Milner-Brown et al. proposed that an increase in motor-unit synchronization (where the motor units of a muscle discharge action potentials at similar instants in time) will also result in greater muscle force.[18]

Muscle Mechanics — The characteristics of the force generating units in the muscle influence the force that a muscle exerts and are referred to as muscle mechanics. External mechanical variables such as length, velocity, power, and force are interdependent with the internal contractile state (i.e., rate of action potential occurrence). According to the sliding-filament theory, the development of force de-pends on attach-detach cycles of the crossbridges extending from thick filaments to the thin filaments. The greater the number of these cycles, the greater the force generated. Since force exertion occurs only during the attachment phase, the thick and thin filaments must be close enough for the attachment to occur. In this way, the length of the muscle influences force generation since tension varies as the amount of overlap between thick and thin filaments within a sarcomere varies.

Force generation is not only dependent upon the active process of crossbridge cycling via changing muscle length. The connective tissue structures within muscle (i.e., sarcolemma, endomysium, perimysium, epimysium, tendon) exert a passive force when stretched. This passive force combines with the active contribution of crossbridge activity to produce the total muscle force. At shorter muscle lengths, all of the force generated is due to crossbridge activity, whereas at longer lengths most of the total muscle force is due to the passive elements. The greatest overlap of thick and thin filaments occurs at a muscle length that is about midway between the minimal and maximal lengths (typically the resting length of the muscle).

Human movement is caused primarily by rotary forces (torque), so that the relationship between muscle length and muscle torque is of primary importance. Three factors influence this relationship: fiber arrangements, number of joints, and moment arm. Most body movements are controlled by groups of muscles as opposed to a single muscle, and these muscles may have different arrangements of their fibers (i.e., fusiform, pinnate, bipinnate). This means that at any specific joint position, the fibers in the muscles crossing the joint may be at different positions on their force-length curves. Since a number of muscles cross more than one joint (i.e., rectus femoris, semitendinosus, gastrocnemius), their length and force generating abilities are influenced by more than one joint. Torque is the product of force and moment arm (perpendicular distance from the line of action of the muscle-force vector to the joint axis). Since this moment arm distance changes with joint position, variations in muscle torque represent the interaction of moment-arm and muscle-length effects.

The relationship between the net muscle torque and the torque due to a load will determine whether the lengths of active muscles shorten (concentric), lengthen (eccentric), or remain unchanged (isometric). Torque-angle relationships have been found to remain the same regardless of whether the measurements were isometric, concentric, or eccentric muscle actions. The general effect of these muscle action types is to shift the relationship up and down the vertical axis such that the greatest torques are exerted eccentrically and the least concentrically.

Concentric and eccentric muscle torques are generated with changing muscle lengths, therefore their torques are dependent on the magnitude and direction of the rate of change in length (velocity of muscle action). Although the rate of crossbridge attachment-detachment increases as the shortening speed increases, the average force exerted by each crossbridge decreases, and there may be fewer crossbridges formed as the muscle shortens more quickly. Since the energy used by the muscle increases (due to increased

crossbridge detachment) with shortening speed while the torque exerted decreases, the muscle becomes less efficient (work output/energy input) with increases in the discrepancy between the muscle and load torques. The maximum torque under the three muscle action conditions varies as eccentric is greater than isometric, which is greater than concentric.

Several theories have been advanced to explain why a muscle can exert greater torque eccentrically than concentrically, although none have been proven. The mechanism responsible for crossbridge detachment may differ, thus altering the duration of the attachment phase and the force exerted by the crossbridge. A second possibility proposed by Hoyle may involve an enhancement of the contractile machinery activity by either increasing the quantity of Ca^{++} released or by stretching the less completely activated sarcomeres within each myofibril.[19] Training studies have shown that the eccentric activation of muscle is closely associated with muscle soreness that occurs 42-48 hours after exercise.[20,21] Two theories commonly cited to account for the soreness are the muscle spasm and structural damage theories. The muscle spasm theory espoused by de Vries suggests that exercise induced ischemia allows the transfer of a substance (called P) across the muscle cell membrane and into the tissue extracellular fluid, activating pain nerve endings that elicit reflex activity in the form of a muscle spasm.[22] The structural damage theory suggests that damage to connective tissue and/or muscle fibers occurs which activates sensory neurons due to the accumulation of metabolites.[23-25]

Positive work by a muscle occurs when a muscle shortens and the force it exerts causes an object to move. Negative work occurs when a muscle lengthens while exerting a force on the object that is moved. As discussed previously, work is defined as the product of force and distance. Therefore, an isometric muscle action where the object is not moved involves no mechanical work. This does not address the metabolic work required for any muscle action including isometric. Since the rate of doing work is referred to as power, the rate of positive work or work done by the muscle is indicated as power production. Power absorption describes the rate of doing work on the muscle. Power production is limited by the rate at which energy is supplied for the muscle contraction (i.e., ATP production) and the rate at which the myofilaments can convert chemical energy into mechanical work.[26] Power is determined as the product of the force and velocity of the muscle contraction. Maximum power occurs when the force being exerted is about one-third of the maximum isometric force. Any effect on either force or velocity will alter power. Muscle temperature mainly affects contraction speed and influences the peak power production.

Muscle architecture (how sarcomeres are arranged within the muscle) affects the force exerted by the muscle on the rigid link. The three major architectural influences are the average number of sarcomeres per muscle fiber (in-series effect), the number of fibers in parallel (in-parallel effect), and the angle at which the fibers are oriented relative to the line of pull of the muscle (i.e., the degree of pinnation). The greater the number of sarcomeres in series, the greater will be the change of length of the myofibril and the rate of change in length to a given stimulus. Muscle fiber force is proportional to the number of myofibrils in parallel (cross sectional area of muscle). The advantage of pinnation (angles of muscle fiber from the line of pull of the muscle) is that a greater number of fibers, and thus sarcomeres, in parallel can be packed into a given volume of muscle.

Muscles can have fibers arranged with a common angle of pinnation (unipinnate), with two sets of fibers at different pinnation angles (bipinnate), or with many sets of fibers at a variety of angles (multipinnate). Muscle fibers aligned with a zero angle of pinnation are usually described as having fusiform or parallel arrangement. Since a muscle fiber consists of myofibrils arranged in parallel and a myofibril represents a series arrangement of sarcomeres, the muscle fibers actually comprise an in-series and an in-parallel collection of force generating units. A long, small diameter muscle fiber represents a dominant in-series effect and, conversely, a short, large diameter fiber mainly exhibits in-parallel characteristics. Muscles are designed to capitalize on these characteristics, as evidenced by the antigravity muscles which are generally twice as strong as their antagonists and demonstrate correspondingly larger physiological cross-sectional areas.

In addition to these whole muscle effects of sarcomere arrangement, at least two other design factors influence the torque a muscle can exert. These are the points of attachment of the muscle relative to the joint and the proportion of whole muscle length that contains contractile protein. The angle of pull and thus the proportion of muscle force that contributes to rotation depends on the distances from each end of the muscle to the joint, and the joint angle. The major effects of varying these parameters on the torque have been summarized by van Mameren and Drukker.[27] The torque-angle relationship has a sharper peak when the distances to each end of the muscle from the joint are equal. When either side of the muscle is a much greater distance than the other from the joint, the maximum torque values are attainable over a greater range of joint angles. Peak torque is reached closer to full extension when the muscle distances are equal and occurs closer to midrange position when the distances are markedly different. The maximum torque exerted by the muscle is greater when the distances are different and when the proportion of whole muscle length containing contractile protein is greater. Muscles that have different lengths do not gain much torque by increasing the whole muscle contractile length.

Patterns of Muscle Activation

Muscle Organization — Muscle activity patterns represent a combined effect of the type of movement desired and the functional and structural restraints of our bodies. Structural restraints refer to the organization of muscles around the joint, which varies throughout the body. The structure of the joint largely determines the quality of motion that can occur between two segments. The number of movements that a joint permits defines the degrees of freedom of the joint. Movable joints have a minimum of one (i.e., elbow) and a maximum of three (i.e., hip and shoulder) degrees of freedom. A minimum of one pair of muscles must cross a joint to control each degree of freedom, although usually several muscles contribute to the same action. The main difference between these groups of muscles is their points of attachment and thus their mechanical action.

The attachment points may vary in three ways: by moment arm, by action, and by postural position. In the first variation, the changes in moment arm distances are maximized for one muscle over one part of the range of motion and for another muscle over another part of the range. For example, the further a muscle attachment is from a joint, the greater the velocity of muscle shortening for a particular angular velocity of the limb, but the greater the variation in the moment arm. In the second variation, muscles can contribute to different actions, as in the biceps brachii assisting with elbow flexion and forearm supination because of its attachment on the radial tuberosity. In the third variation, suggested by Lexell and associates, one muscle in the group may be more ideally located to assist with the maintenance of posture so that muscles involved with maintaining upright posture tend to be closer to the long bone of the segment.[28] In addition, muscles may span more than one joint. Some investigators have asserted that two joint muscles simplify the control of movement for the central nervous system.[29,30]

Net Muscle Activity — The mechanical effect of muscular activity can be quantified as resultant muscle force and resultant muscle torque. Two limitations to this approach are the method used to determine resultant muscle torque and non-muscular contributions. Resultant muscle torque is calculated as the residual moment from the Newtonian equations of motion. Free-body and mass acceleration diagrams are composed for dynamic analysis and the moments of force are identified (Figure 3). Values for all of the terms are known except for the resultant muscle torque, and so the expression is rearranged to solve for the unknown. This unknown is referred to as the residual moment because it represents any difference in the kinematic effect and the moments of force. Two limitations associated with this procedure are that other structures (i.e., ligaments, joint capsule) in addition to muscle can contribute to the residual torque, and that residual torque does not represent the absolute quantity of muscle activity.

Despite these limitations, the mechanics of movement can still be used to deduce the net muscle activity. By comparing the directions of the resultant muscle torque vector and the segment rotation in dynamic analysis, the net muscle activity can be determined as concentric or eccentric. If the directions of the resultant muscle torque vector and the segment rotation are the same, then the muscle group is experiencing a concentric muscle action. Conversely, if the directions of the resultant muscle torque vector and the segment rotation are opposite, then the muscle group is experiencing an eccentric muscle action. In addition, the orientation of the body relative to the direction of gravity will affect the pattern of muscle activation (ie. upright standing vs. supine). These analyses apply only to quasistatic conditions where the accelerations of the system and its parts are very small. In fast movements, different types of contact forces (joint reaction, ground reaction, fluid resistance, elastic, inertial, and muscle forces) become large and substantially alter the

FIGURE 3. Free body diagram (FBD) and mass accelaration diagram (MAD) showing trunk of a person standing up from a squat.

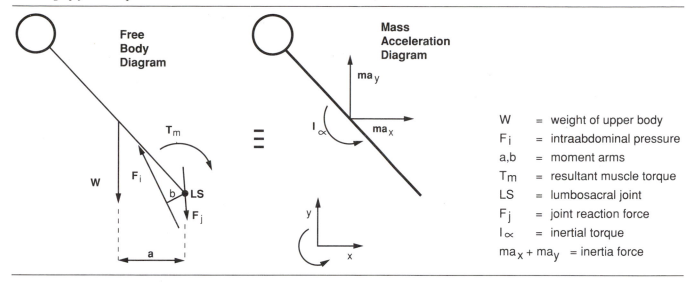

W	=	weight of upper body
F_i	=	intraabdominal pressure
a,b	=	moment arms
T_m	=	resultant muscle torque
LS	=	lumbosacral joint
F_j	=	joint reaction force
$I\alpha$	=	inertial torque
$ma_x + ma_y$	=	inertia force

pattern of muscle activity necessary to control the movement. For these fast movements, a complete dynamic analysis is required.

Measurement of electromyographic (EMG) activity provides a picture of the total neural drive to a muscle, and can provide information about force relationships that are difficult to measure using other means. Three examples (moment arm effects, three burst pattern, and cocontraction) provide an overview of the ways in which EMG can assist in the understanding of the neural signals sent by segmental centers. Although the relationship between muscle force and EMG is complex, EMG is related to force in a predictable manner under isometric conditions. Using the isometric condition, the EMG angle relationship is inversely related to the changes in moment arm. As a second example, a three burst pattern of EMG has been shown for both biphasic and unidirectional movements. The three burst pattern for unidirectional movements appears to be related to the stopping of a movement at a targeted position, but the control strategy adopted by the central nervous system has not yet been determined. The three burst pattern is drastically affected by the features of movement (i.e., instructions given to the subject) and by the mechanical conditions (i.e., orientation of the subject, inclusion of more than one muscle in a movement). Lastly, cocontraction has also been observed using EMG, and is a variable characteristic of the three burst pattern. Since cocontraction has the mechanical effect of making a joint stiffer, it would seem to be a useful feature for learning novel tasks or performing high accuracy movements. According to Husan, under certain conditions cocontraction decreases the cost of performing a movement.[31] Other investigators have found that the neural strategy involved in performing cocontraction is different from that of more normal activities (i.e., supporting a load).[32]

Posture Requirements and Responses — The execution of any movement must be accompanied by maintenance of postural stability and equilibrium. This postural stability may be static (maintenance of upright standing posture) or dynamic (maintenance of balance during movement). See Chapter 10 for a review of balance mechanisms.

Gait

Transfer Function of Muscles — The pattern of muscle activity during gait has been used as a way to observe muscle group interaction during walking. Inman et al. reported that EMG produced a waveform which reflected the muscle force waveform.[33] Winter suggested that electromechanical delays between the neural command and the muscle response are recognized by the central nervous system (CNS), as evidenced by both early activation and early deactivation of muscles.[34] These patterns are evident in the tibialis anterior (TA) and soleus (S) muscles during walking (Figure 4). TA reaches peak activity just before heel contact (HC) so dorsiflexor tension reaches its peak just after HC (so that ground reaction forces which will attempt to plantarflex the foot are resisted). Similarly, at the end of stance, TA reaches its peak activity exactly at toe-off (TO), but dorsiflexor tension does not increase to a reasonable level until about 5% after TO, when it dorsiflexes the foot for toe clearance. At the end of stance, about 200 ms before TO, the S activity reaches its peak and suddenly drops off to near-zero 100ms before TO. This sudden derecruitment of the plantarflexors reflects the need to decrease the plantarflexor force from its peak at about 100ms before TO to near-zero at TO. If this plantarflexor activation had continued until TO, there would be a large plantarflexor moment into early swing which would prevent the rapid dorsiflexion of the foot necessary for safe toe clearance.

Inertias of Limb Segments — Moments of inertia for individual segments are required for the generation of appropriate acceleration profiles. This information is especially important during the swing phase of gait when the thigh and

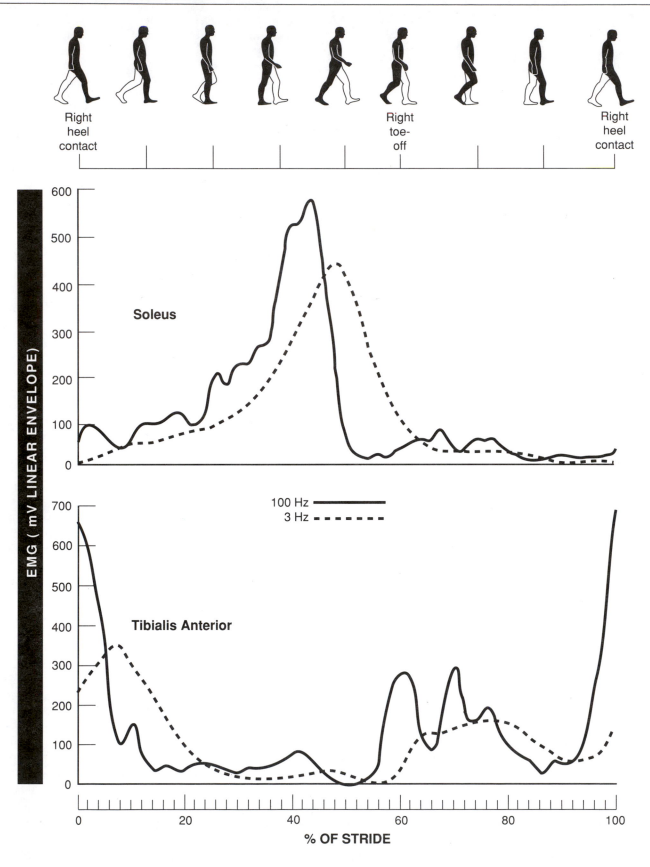

FIGURE 4. Electromyographic patterns of the soleus and tibialis anterior during walking. Adapted from Winter with permission of Gordon and Breach Science Publishers, S.A., © 1989.

leg/foot segments are initially accelerated and then decelerated prior to HC. The moments of force cannot be too high or too low if correct trajectories are to be achieved. For example, the foot segment must achieve a low but safe toe clearance and the heel must decelerate to near zero velocity prior to HC. The trajectory patterns during swing are extremely consistent as evidenced by the intra-subject repeat assessment done days apart or minutes apart by Winter.[35] This consistency suggests that the CNS accounted for the segment inertias and generated the appropriate moment of force. Ralston and Lukin added weight to the leg and reported increased kinetic energy changes of the leg and foot.[36]

Gravitation Forces — Another factor evident from the consistent swing phase trajectories is the contribution of gravitational forces to the acceleration and deceleration of the swinging leg. During the swing phase of gait, the thigh and leg/foot form a double pendulum system which is influenced by gravitational moments. During early swing, gravity assists the forward acceleration of the leg and foot, and at the end of swing it assists in its decelerating prior to HC. The knee's gravitational moment increases from TO to a maximum during early swing (at maximum knee flexion). Here, gravity assists in decelerating the backward rotating leg and then is the major contributor to its forward acceleration. During late swing the leg is decelerated until HC, with the gravitational component being somewhat less, but still important. The active contribution of the knee extensors is only about 20% to the leg's acceleration with gravity adding about 50% and the knee acceleration couple about 30%. However, during the deceleration in late swing, the knee flexors are responsible for about 80% of the joint moment of force. The CNS must recognize these non-muscular contributions since the gravitational component remains constant when walking is slow, but total inertial moment decreases.

Inter-limb Coupling — A third contributor to the leg's acceleration during walking is inter-limb coupling. During the swing phase, the angular acceleration of the thigh by the hip flexors/extensors causes a linear acceleration at the knee. This acceleration results in a reaction force at the knee, so that a couple is created to assist in the leg's acceleration and deceleration. This acceleration component is usually more important than the active muscle moment, so that the hip extensors must become active to create a reaction force at the knee that assists in the acceleration of the distal segments. This coupling strategy is used by persons with above-knee amputations to swing their prosthetic leg.

During the stance phase of gait, control of the knee joint is essential for safe and efficient weight bearing. The ankle and hip joints assist in the control of the knee joint, creating a total limb synergy referred to by Winter as the support moment.[37] This support moment is calculated to recognize inter-limb coupling such that above or below normal extensor moments at the hip and ankle have a direct control of the knee joint. For example, hyperactivity of the plantar flexors during mid stance will slow down or stop the forward rotation of the leg over the foot, and thereby reduce knee flexion (or even cause the knee to hyperextend). Similarly, hyperactivity of the hip extensors early in stance will cause a backward rotation of the thigh and knee flexion is again reduced. Such inter-limb coupling gives greater flexibility to the CNS to accomplish the same knee control in more than one way.

Eccentric-concentric Muscle Action — As previously mentioned, muscle force decreases as the velocity of shortening (concentric muscle action) increases, and increases as the velocity of lengthening (eccentric muscle action) increases. In order to generate the correct muscle force, the CNS activation must be altered depending on the lengthening or shortening velocity. The same level of activation may result in markedly different levels of force. This velocity effect is less important during slow walking than during faster gaits.

Overall Control of Gait — In addition to these control factors, a total control strategy must be incorporated which supports the body during stance (prevents collapse of the lower limb), maintains upright posture and balance of the trunk in both anterior-posterior and medial-lateral directions, and controls the foot trajectory to achieve safe ground clearance and gentle heel or toe landing. The first two tasks are regulatory, occur during the stance phase of gait, and involve high forces. The third task in cyclical, occurs primarily during the swing phase of gait, and involves low forces.

SUMMARY

The musculoskeletal system exhibits characteristics which influence the production and control of any movement. Kinematics and kinetics are basic to an understanding of the role that these musculoskeletal characteristics play in movement production and control. Three approaches can be used to solve kinetic problems with the approach of choice dependent on the information available. The role that the musculoskeletal components play is also influenced by their individual structures and by the way that the individual structures work together during different types of movement. The control of muscle force and the patterns of muscle activation create numerous strategies available to the CNS for execution of movement. Walking is an example of one activity which demonstrates the interaction of musculoskeletal components in movement production and control. ❑

REFERENCES

1. Winter DA: Biomechanics and Motor Control of Human Movement, ed 2. New York, NY, John Wiley & Sons, Inc, 1990
2. Frankel VH, Burstein AH: Orthopaedic Biomechanics - the Application of Engineering to the Musculoskeletal System. Philadelphia, PA, Lea & Febiger, 1970
3. Frankel VH: Biomechanics of the locomotor system. In CD Ray (ed): Medical Engineering, Chicago, IL, Year Book Medical Publisher, 1974, pp 505-516
4. Noyes FR, Torvik PJ, Hyde WB, et al: Biomechanics of ligament failure. J Bone Joint Surg 56A:1406-1418, 1974
5. Enoka RM: Neuromechanical Basis of Kinesiology. Champaign, IL, Human Kinetics Books, 1988
6. Cowin SC: The mechanical and stress adaptive properties of bone. Ann Biomed Eng 11:263-295, 1983
7. Alexander RM: Optimal strengths for bones liable to fatigue and accidental fracture. J Theor Biol 109:621-636, 1984
8. Lanyon LE, Rubin CT: Static vs dynamic loads as an influence on bone remodelling. J Biomech 17:897-905, 1984
9. Woo SL-Y, Ritter MA, Amiel D, et al: The biomechanical and biochemical properties of swine tendons- Long term effects of exercise on the digital extensors. Connect Tissue Res 7:177-183, 1980
10. Vailas AC, Tipton CM, Matthes RD, et al: Physical activity and its influence on the repair process of medial collateral ligaments. Connect Tissue Res 9:25-31, 1981
11. Kukulka CG, Clamann HP: Comparison of the recruitment and discharge properties of motor units in human brachial biceps and adductor pollicis during isometric contractions. Brain Res 219:45-55, 1981
12. Stuart DG, Enoka RM: Motoneurons, motor units and the size principle. In WD Willis (ed): The Clinical Neurosciences: Sec. 5 Neurobiology. New York, NY, Churchill Livingston, 1983, pp 471-517
13. Henneman E: Relation between size of neurons and their susceptibility to discharge. Science 126:1345-1347, 1957
14. Gydikov A, Kosarov D: Physiological characteristics of the tonic and phasic motor units in human muscles. In AA Gydikov, NT Tankov, DS Kosarov (eds): Motor Control New York, NY, Plenum, 1973, pp 75-94
15. Harrison PJ: The relationship between the distribution of the motor unit mechanical properties and the forces due to recruitment and to rate coding for the generation of muscle force. Brain Res 264:311-315, 1983
16. Burke RE, Rundomin P, Zajac FE: The effect of activation history on tension production by individual muscle units. Brain Res 109:515-529, 1976
17. Gydikov AA, Kossev AR, Kosarov DS, et al: Investigations of single motor units firing during movements against elastic resistance. In B. Jonsson (ed): Biomechanics X-A. Champaign, IL, Human Kinetics, 1987, pp 227-232
18. Milner-Brown HS, Stein RB, Lee RG: Synchronization of human motor units: Possible roles of exercise and supraspinal reflexes. Electroencephalogr Clin Neurophysiol 38:245-254, 1975
19. Hoyle G: Muscles and Their Neural Control. New York, NY, Wiley, 1983
20. Armstrong RB, Ogilvie RW, Schwane JA: Eccentric exercise-induced injury to rat skeletal muscle. J Appl Physiol 54:80-93, 1983
21. Komi PV, Buskirk ER: Effect of eccentric and concentric muscle conditioning on tension and electrical activity of human muscle. Ergonomics 15:417-434, 1972
22. de Vries HA: Quantitative electromyographic investigation of the spasm theory of muscle pain. Am J Phys Med Rehabil 45:119-134, 1966
23. Abraham DWM: Factors in delayed muscle soreness. Med Sci Sports Exerc 9:11-20, 1977
24. Kuipers H, Drukker J, Frederik PM, et al: Muscle degeneration after exercise in rats. Int J Sports Med 4:45-59, 1983
25. Armstrong RB: Mechanisms of exercise-induced delayed onset muscular soreness: A brief review. Med Sci Sports Exerc 16:529-538, 1984
26. Weis-Fogh T, Alexander RM: The sustained power output from striated muscle. In TJ Pedley (ed): Scale Effects in Animal Locomotion. London, England, Academic Press, 1977, pp 511-525
27. van Mameren H, Drukker J: Attachment and composition of skeletal muscle in relation to their function. J Biomech 12:859-867, 1979
28. Lexell J, Henriksson-Larsen K, Sjostrom M: Distribution of different fibre types in human skeletal muscle: 2. A study of cross-sections of whole muscles vastus lateralis. Acta Physiol Scand 117:115-122, 1983
29. Fujiwara M, Basmajian JV: Electromyographic study of two-joint muscles. Am J Phys Med Rehabil 54:234-242, 1975
30. Mussa-Ivaldi FA, Hogan N, Bizzi E: Neural, mechanical and geometric factors subserving arm posture in humans. J Neurosci 5:2732-2743, 1985
31. Husan Z: Optimized movement trajectories and joint stiffness in unperturbed, inertially loaded movements. Biol Cybern 53:373-382, 1986
32. Gydikov A, Kossev A, Radicheva N, et al: Interaction between reflexes and voluntary motor activity in man revealed by discharges of separate motor units. Exp Neurol 73:331-344, 1981
33. Inman VT, Ralston HJ, Saunders JB, et al: Relation of human electromyogram to muscular tension. Electroencephalogr Clin Neurophysiol 4:187-194, 1952
34. Winter DA: CNS strategies in human gait: Implications for FES control. Automedica 11:163-174, 1989
35. Winter DA: The Biomechanics and Motor Control of Human Gait. University of Waterloo Press, Waterloo, Canada, 1987
36. Ralston HJ, Lukin L: Energy levels of human body segments during level walking. Ergonomics 12:39-46, 1969
37. Winter DA: Overall principle of lower limb support during stance phase of gait. J Biomech 13:923-927, 1980

SUGGESTED READINGS

Beer FP, Johnston ER: Vector Mechanics for Engineers - Static and Dynamics, ed 3. Baltimore M.D., Williams & Wilkins, 1986

Cavanagh PR, Lafortune MA: Ground reaction forces in distance running. J Biomech 13:397-406, 1979

Cochran G: A Primer of Orthopaedic Biomechanics. New York, NY, Churchill Livingston, 1982

Dhanjoo NG: Osteoarthromechanics. Washington, DC, Hemisphere Pub Co, 1982

Frankel VH, Nordin M (eds): Basic Biomechanics of the Skeletal System. Philadelphia, PA, Lea & Febiger, 1980

Friederich JA, Brand RA: Muscle fiber architecture in the human lower limb. J Biomech, 23(1):91-95, 1990

Frost HM: An Introduction to Biomechanics. Springfield, IL, Charles C. Thomas, Pub, 1980

Fung YC: Biomechanics: Mechanical Properties of Living Tissues. New York, NY, Springer-Verlag, 1981

Hay JG: The Biomechanics of Sports Techniques, ed 2. Englewood Cliffs, NJ, Prentice-Hall Inc, 1966

LeVeau BF: Williams and Lissner: Biomechanics of Human Motion, ed 2. Philadelphia, PA, WB Saunders Co, 1977

Miller DI, Nelson RC: Biomechanics of Sports. Philadelphia, PA, Lea & Febiger, 1976

Radin EL, Simon SR, Rose RM, et al: Practical Biomechanics for the Orthopedic Surgeon. New York, NY, John Wiley & Sons, 1979

Rodgers MM, Cavanagh PR: Glossary of biomechanical terms, concepts, and units. Phys Ther 64:1886-1902, 1984

Schafer RC: Clinical Biomechanics: Musculoskeletal Actions and Reactions, ed 2. Baltimore, MD, Williams & Wilkins, 1987

Shames IH: Engineering Mechanics, ed 2. Englewood Cliffs, NJ, Prentice-Hall Inc, 1966

Soderberg GL: Kinesiology: Application to Pathological Motion. Baltimore, M.D., Williams & Wilkins, 1986

Wiktorin C, Nordin M: Introduction to Problem Solving in Biomechanics. Philadelphia, PA, Lea & Febiger, 1986

Chapter 5
Case Studies

Patricia C. Montgomery, Ph.D., PT
Barbara H. Connolly, Ed.D., PT

INTRODUCTION

One of the major problems experienced by the student, new graduate, or clinician inexperienced in the treatment of patients with neurologic dysfunction is integrating theory with practice. A problem solving approach can be helpful in developing skills in the practical application of assessment and treatment techniques. To facilitate a problem solving approach, we have selected four case studies that represent common problems encountered by the clinician. Contributing authors were asked to address the problems observed in each of these patients and to develop goals and objectives for an "ideal" treatment program. A composite clinical picture of each patient is presented in this chapter and should be reviewed briefly before proceeding to the subsequent chapters.

CASE STUDY #1
MRS. JANE SMITH

CURRENT STATUS

Mrs. Smith is a 74 year old woman who is six months post onset of her cardiovascular accident (CVA) and comes into a rehabilitation facility 2X/week as an outpatient to receive physical, occupational, and speech therapy.

HISTORY

Mrs. Smith has a medical history of hypertension, peripheral vascular disease, and bilateral endarterectomies. She is retired, but has remained active with her hobbies including gardening, sewing, and bowling. She is married with two grown children and four grandchildren.

Six months ago, Mrs. Smith woke up in the morning with a right hemiparesis and marked aphasia. Her husband brought her into the emergency room of the local hospital where she received medical treatment.

Four days following onset of her CVA, Mrs. Smith was evaluated by physical, occupational, and speech therapists. The initial physical therapy evaluation noted that she was oriented and cooperative, but with severe expressive aphasia. She could say "yes" and "no," but her responses were unreliable. Her right upper extremity was flaccid; she had adductor and extensor stiffness in the right lower extremity. She needed maximal assistance to roll, for all transfers and ADL's, and could not stand and bear weight on the right leg. Her sitting balance was fair and she had poor sensation on the right side of her body. Her occupational and speech therapy assessments indicated that her limb apraxia interfered with performance on language and ADL tasks. She had severe verbal apraxia with moderate to marked aphasia. Verbal production was limited to isolated episodes of automatic speech.

Three weeks following onset, Mrs. Smith was transferred to the rehabilitation unit in another facility. The physical therapy assessment at this time indicated Grade 2 strength in the right hip and knee musculature with muscles around the ankle and foot at Grade 1. Rolling to the right could be accomplished with minimal assistance and to the left with moderate assistance of one other adult. Mrs. Smith needed assistance in pivot transfers, coming from sit to stand, balancing in standing, and with maneuvering her wheelchair. She required frequent verbal cues because of severe neglect of the right side. A hinged ankle-foot orthosis (AFO) was ordered for her right lower extremity. She also was demonstrating perseveration in dressing and difficulty with sequencing tasks. Reading comprehension was good, but she was able only to use gestures and automatic speech to communicate.

Mrs. Smith was in the rehabilitation unit for 3 weeks. She then returned home and was seen daily for one week by PT, OT, and speech, then 3X week by each therapist for an additional two weeks.

COGNITIVE

Mrs. Smith continues to demonstrate severe verbal apraxia, with moderate aphasia. She is 85% accurate with "yes" and "no" to complex questions and 50% accurate to 2 step verbal commands. She can sing familiar tunes, but cannot use sentences. She communicates via facial expressions and gestures. She demonstrates some impulsivity during treatment, is often frustrated, and occasionally will throw things. She has problems identifying tactile and somatosensory input due to sensory dysfunction. Deficits in response selection (making decisions) and response programming during motor tasks are evident. Mrs. Smith has poor balance, especially during transfers and in standing. She has a decreased awareness of her balance problems and poor appreciation of safety factors.

SENSORY/PERCEPTUAL

Generally poor sensory appreciation of the right limbs is present to tactile and somatosensory input. She reports that her right side feels numb and tends to neglect the hemiplegic limbs and the right side of space. She has a right visual field deficit. Auditory perception appears intact.

RANGE OF MOTION/MOBILITY/STRENGTH

Passive range of motion is within normal limits in all joints with the exception of limited ankle dorsiflexion, associated with tightness in the gastrocnemius. Weakness is present in the right lower and upper extremities as well as in the trunk. Mrs. Smith does not always move through the range of motion available to her.

MOVEMENT PATTERNS

Mrs. Smith has difficulty combining limb synergies within and between the upper and lower extremities. She cannot vary her speed, tending to move slowly. She has poor reciprocal limb movement (i.e., flexion/extension of elbow). A flexion synergy often is used in the right upper extremity. She has voluntary hand grasp with poor release. She is independent in feeding skills using her left upper extremity.

BALANCE

Balance when attempting transfers and in standing is poor. She does not regain her balance well and would fall if unsupported by her walker or another adult. She has an asymmetrical body alignment, and is able to only partially bear weight on the right leg.

GAIT

Mrs. Smith is ambulating in the parallel bars and approximately 30 feet with a hemi-walker. She has active hip flexion, but poor right foot placement. Mrs. Smith lacks knee flexion during gait, circumducting the right leg. She tends to lead with the left side with the right side of her pelvis retracted. Step length on the right is decreased. Mrs. Smith continues to wear a hinged AFO on the right side.

CASE STUDY #2
MR. DANIEL JOHNSON

CURRENT STATUS

Mr. Johnson has been diagnosed with Parkinson's disease for the past 4 years. He has increased severity of symptoms and was referred to physical therapy for treatment and a home program. He is on sinemet and bromocriptine. He reports bouts of dyskinesia about 1/2 hour after taking his medication. This consists of involuntary writhing around the neck and shoulders and is thought to be a side effect of sinemet.

HISTORY

Mr. Johnson was referred to a neurologist by his family practice physician approximately four years ago, at age 55. Up until that time, he had been healthy with no major surgeries or disease processes noted. His initial symptoms included left upper extremity tremor and facial masking with complaints of general fatigue. He received a diagnosis of mild Parkinson's disease at that time.

One year later he was referred to physical therapy because of shoulder pain, apparently related to the rigidity associated with the Parkinson's disease. He was complaining of myoclonic jerking of his body, usually at night. He had a bilateral upper extremity tremor, exacerbated when he was stressed. He also was noting difficulty when rising from a low chair and began shuffling his feet when tired. He had a mildly stooped posture with moderate tremoring of the left hand. Grade 1 rigidity in the upper extremities was noted (slight or detectable only when activated by mirror or other movements). Performance on a finger tapping test was normal. He had decreased voice volume. At this time, Mr. Johnson was still working as a school teacher and was active in physical activities, such as swimming and walking.

Mr. Johnson was followed periodically by physical therapy and provided with a home program. Approximately three years after onset, Mr. Johnson noted severe problems with constipation due to decreased motility. His physician placed him on a regimen of enemas and suppositories which relieved this problem. He also noted increased problems with hesitancy in his speech and reported bouts of frequent depression. He had a grade 2 rigidity of the upper extremities (mild to moderate) and grade 1 rigidity of the lower extremities. Finger tapping was mildly impaired. He reported upper back and neck pain when walking. At this point in time, Mr. Johnson began a medical leave from his teaching position.

COGNITIVE

Mr. Johnson is displaying problems in short-term memory. Because he is noting mild memory impairment, he is not given anti-cholinergic drugs, as they often exaggerate a memory deficit. Mr. Johnson is showing more signs of depression, is less interested in social activities, and reports frequent insomnia.

SENSORY/PERCEPTUAL

There are no indications of sensory or perceptual problems.

RANGE OF MOTION/MOBILITY/STRENGTH

Range of motion of the extremities is within normal limits, although Mr. Johnson does not always use full range available during functional movements. He does have decreased range and flexibility of the trunk and pelvis. General strength and endurance are less than anticipated probably due to less overall activity.

MOVEMENT PATTERNS

Mr. Johnson demonstrates the classic motor symptoms of Parkinson's disease including akinesia (difficulty initiating movement), bradykinesia (slow movement), and dyskinesia (poor synergistic organization of movement). He has increased bilateral tremoring which is constant rather than intermittent. He is having more difficulty with transfers, particularly in and out of a chair and in and out of a bed. He turns "en block" and trunk rotation is particularly difficult.

BALANCE

Increasing problems with balance are noted. Mr. Johnson's body alignment is forward, increasing his tendency to fall forward. He has slow reactions to loss of balance, particularly in standing.

GAIT

Although Mr. Johnson is still ambulating independently, he has a shuffling gait and lacks a reciprocal arm swing.

CASE STUDY # 3
MS. SHIRLEY TEAL

CURRENT STATUS

Ms. Teal is a 21 year old woman who is 10 months post motor vehicle accident (MVA). She has been in an extended care facility since 2 months post MVA. She receives physical and occupational therapy at the facility but becomes very combative in therapy and strikes out or curses at the therapist(s) frequently. She is scheduled for discharge from the facility within the next 2 months.

HISTORY

At the time of admission to the hospital following the MVA, Ms. Teal was decerebrate and had intracranial bleeding into the right occipital horn. She was comatose and received a tracheostomy and a gastrostomy immediately after admission to the hospital. At 2 months post trauma, she was transferred to an extended care facility. At that time, she was able to open her eyes to verbal and tactile stimuli but was unable to visually track. She was able to move her upper and lower extremities spontaneously but not on command. The initial physical therapy evaluation noted that she had mild to moderate increase in tone in her left upper extremity, severe spasticity in her right upper extremity, and severe spasticity in her lower extremities. She was limited in passive range of motion in right elbow extension (- 30 degrees), right knee extension (- 20 degrees), and right hip extension (- 15 degrees). Other ranges of motion were passively within normal limits. She exhibited bilateral ankle clonus (right greater than left) when minimal stretch was applied. She exhibited poor head and trunk control when supported sitting was attempted.

At the time of the accident, she was a single parent with a 2 year old child. She lived alone with her child and supported herself by working in a beauty salon. She had a high school education plus some training as a beautician.

COGNITIVE

Ms. Teal continues to demonstrate problems with cognition. She has difficulty with maintenance of concentration and demonstrates an inability to switch attention between tasks or objects within the environment. She is able to follow simple instructions but occasionally forgets what is asked of her. Ms. Teal is aware of sensory input but is unable to discern common objects consistently for stereognosis discrimination.

SENSORY/PERCEPTUAL

Ms. Teal is aware of sensory input to all extremities. However, she is unable to discriminate common objects that are placed in her hands. She has an excessive dependence on vision for her balance control in sitting and in standing. Auditory perception appears intact. She has benign paroxysmal positional nystagmus (BPPN) and vertigo.

RANGE OF MOTION/MOBILITY/STRENGTH

She has decreased range of motion in the right lower extremity, including a 40 degree plantar flexion contracture and - 10 degrees of full knee and hip extension. She has full range of motion actively in the left extremities. Ms. Teal has increased muscle tonus bilaterally (right greater than left). Her strength is decreased in the right lower extremity and she has an inability to sustain knee extension during stance.

MOVEMENT PATTERNS

Ms. Teal has good head control in all positions. She is able to sit independently, although she lists to the right. She is able to come to sitting by rolling to the side and with minimal assistance from the therapist. She requires supervision and occasional minimal assistance with rolling. She is able to perform standing pivot transfers with only minimal assistance from the therapist.

She is able to move her right wrist, fingers, elbow, and shoulder free of synergist patterns but with decreased strength and coordination. Additionally, her coordination patterns in the left extremities are impaired. She is unable to reach directly to an object that is held out to her and she has foot placement problems with the left leg in sitting or in standing.

BALANCE

In sitting, Ms. Teal has difficulty in maintaining weight equally on both buttocks. She tends to list to the right side while placing weight primarily on her left buttock. She is able to stand in parallel bars but has to be reminded to place weight on her right lower extremity. She tends to lose her balance easily if she moves quickly and she demonstrates positional dizziness due to BPPN and vertigo.

GAIT

Ms. Teal is able to perform pivot transfers and stands in the parallel bars for 5 minutes with minimal assistance. She does not initiate ambulation on her own. She is independent in a wheelchair by using the left arm for pushing.

CASE STUDY # 4
SHAWNA WELLS

CURRENT STATUS

Shawna is a 4 year old child with a diagnosis of spastic quadriparesis and mild mental retardation. Her IQ is estimated to be about 70. She occasionally has temper tantrums during her physical and occupational therapy sessions, but most of the time she is cooperative. When she is agitated, she thrusts herself into extension but she can be easily calmed. She performs well if food reinforcers are offered.

She had a heelcord release on the right foot approximately one year ago. She has good head and trunk control in sitting and in standing. She is able to use her arms purposely but has increased flexor tone bilaterally. She has no difficulty with feeding but has problems with speech (breathiness) and with respiratory patterns (lacks full inspiration and expiration). She is able to ambulate with a posterior control walker.

HISTORY

Shawna was born at full term to a 27 year old mother who had experienced a normal pregnancy. Problems were noted at birth due to a breech position of the infant. She had APGARS of 3 and 5 at one and five minutes. She has a history of failure to thrive during her first year of life.

Shawna was enrolled in an early intervention program (EIP) at 4 months of age. She has been receiving physical therapy, occupational therapy, and speech therapy each on a twice weekly basis through the EIP since that time. For the past 3 months, Shawna has been mainstreamed into a full day preschool program but is continuing to receive therapies on a twice weekly basis.

COGNITIVE

Shawna demonstrates good identification ability to auditory stimuli. She is able to visually locate and point to common objects without difficulty. She has minimal difficulty in discriminating somatosensory stimuli and has avoidance reactions with some sensory inputs. She has difficulty with selective attention and has perseveration of responses. Her response programming ability appears to be within normal limits. Shawna has poor short-term and long-term memory for motor learning.

SENSORY/PERCEPTUAL

Shawna does not like being handled initially in therapy but becomes less resistant during the therapy session. She has had difficulties with tactile hypersensitivity since birth. Additionally, she demonstrates autonomic distress with movement. She is hesitant to play on moveable toys and becomes agitated when she is moved in space by the therapist.

RANGE OF MOTION/MOBILITY/STRENGTH

Resistance to passive range of motion in ankle dorsiflexion and knee extension is noted indicating tightness in the gastrocnemius/soleus and hamstrings bilaterally. She also has decreased trunk and upper extremity flexibility. She is able to reach for objects with either hand but is unable to actively flex at the shoulder beyond 115 degrees. She is able to reach out to the side but she tends to elevate her shoulder and thus has decreased range of motion in abduction.

Shawna has difficulty in reciprocating her lower extremities during creeping and during walking. Additionally, she is unable to sustain full knee extension on the stance leg during gait due to increased tone or decreased strength.

MOVEMENT PATTERNS

Shawna has good head control in all positions. She is able to sit independently, although with increased flexion in the trunk when her legs are extended. She is able to come to sitting independently either by rotating to the side or by assuming a "W" sitting position. She does not need her arms for support in sitting unless she attempts to reach with one arm for a toy. Shawna is able to roll using trunk rotation. Shawna's primary means of locomotion is through creeping. She uses an homologous pattern unless she is reminded and then uses a poorly coordinated cross diagonal pattern.

Shawna has an abnormal movement pattern for arm reaching and substitutes shoulder elevation for glenohumeral movement.

BALANCE

Shawna demonstrates adequate righting responses of her head and trunk when she is tilted in space. She has slow responses in protective extension forwards, sidewards , and backwards. Adequate responses to slow tilting are seen in prone and supine but are inadequate for maintenance of balance in sitting. She is unable to maintain her posture in any position when she is moved quickly. In standing, she is unable to maintain her balance on any surface that is not flat and firm. She uses a stepping pattern in response to external perturbation when she is standing. She appears to have a decreased cone of perceived stability and relies heavily on visual inputs.

GAIT

Shawna ambulates with a posterior control walker and with minimal assistance from the therapist. She demonstrates poor disassociation of the lower extremities during ambulation and uses a hinged AFO on the right. With the brace, she has minimal heel strike.

CONCLUSION

The preceding descriptions can be used to guide you through the information in Chapters 6 - 11. Chapter 12 will provide an integrated approach to the assessment and treatment of each of the four patients used in the case studies.

❏

Chapter 6
Motor Control Assessment

Patricia Leahy, M.S., PT

INTRODUCTION

In addressing motor control assessment, it is important to differentiate between measurement and assessment. The term "measure" is sometimes confusing because it is both a noun and a verb. As a verb, it means to ascertain the extent or quantity of something by comparing it with a fixed unit or known size. As a noun, measure is defined as a basis or standard of comparison. In physical therapy, we speak of measurement when we discuss testing or evaluating a patient. A commonly employed measurement is range of motion (ROM) where the patient's joint range is determined and compared with known norms. Assessment means to determine the importance, size, or value. In the example of ROM, the assessment involves determining if any deficits are important. In the case of a patient with paraplegia, 15 degree hip flexion contractures might be considered very significant because they may interfere with gait training with orthoses. However, in a non-ambulatory patient with longstanding contractures, 15 degree hip flexion contractures may not be considered a major problem. Generally, assessment follows measurement, but at times, physical therapists rely purely on assessment, without the benefit of measurement. This presents significant problems in reliability and therefore should be avoided if at all possible. In this chapter, we will examine methods of assessment that are now used. Wherever possible, I will include objective measurement tools. However, the state of the art and science of physical therapy is such that clinical assessment tools exist that rely on judgments of professionals without the use of a measurement tool. Many physical therapists think that these assessments are valid and reliable. Unfortunately, there is little scientific research to support this assumption. By providing informa-tion about electromechanical instrumentation along with the more commonly used clinical tools, studies examining concurrent validity and reliability should be fostered.

The most important consideration in choosing a test or measurement is the determination of what is to be measured. Then it is important to determine if the chosen test will accurately reflect the performance level of the individual with respect to the particular objective being examined. In other words, does the test measure what it is supposed to measure? This is called validity. Sometimes the justification of the use of a test is on the basis of logical or face validity. This is true when it is possible to measure levels of performance by a single, direct test of the goal. For instance, if the goal is to measure the patient's ability to distinguish right from left, then a test measuring the patient's ability to distinguish right from left is logically valid. However, there are many activities for which the performance to be measured does not lend itself to tests that can be justified by face validity. For example, it is difficult to design a test that measures a patient's ability to perform functional tasks at home without actually going to the patient's home.

Concurrent validity can be used to validate a new test. This refers to how the test compares with other tests proven to measure similar items. For example, if you are examining a test claiming to measure functional status, how does it compare with other tests of functional status? Given the number of factors that contribute to motor control, ranging from psychological to physiological states, and given the complexity of each of these factors, it is not surprising that the assessment of motor control is a challenge.

Generally, it is far easier to find an objective tool to measure one variable than to find an instrument that will provide a measure of the "big picture." Realistically, it is often impossible to measure all the individual areas that contribute to the patient's problems. This is due, in part, to the fact that some variables are extremely difficult to measure and, if measured at one point in time, may be very different than when measured at another point in time. An example of this is patient motivation. This is an extremely difficult variable to measure at any given time as it is likely to change from hour to hour. Yet, because it may affect the patient's performance on a number of other evaluations, it might be seen as a major omission if not tested. For a factor such as this, therapists generally take note of the situation, rate it subjectively, and consider it in forming any conclusions.

In the above example of motivation, we were faced with variability. Because patients with motor control deficits often display great variability in motivation and performance, it is difficult to determine the reliability of measurements. Intra-rater reliability refers to the same person using the test on different occasions and obtaining the same results. Inter-rater reliability refers to different people using the test to measure the same thing and obtaining the same results. There is marked variability present in patients with motor control deficits. Because it is sometimes change that we are trying to measure, it is often difficult to distinguish between an unreliable test and an actual change in the factor being measured. The following sections contain tests most commonly used by physical therapists to assess motor control.

RANGE OF MOTION

The amount of motion that is available at a specific joint is called the range of motion. The evaluation of ROM is very important to any motor control assessment because adequate ROM must be present to allow functional excursions of muscle and normal biomechanical alignment and to prevent the development of secondary deficits that result from immobilization. The ROM at particular joints varies considerably among individuals and may be affected by age, sex, and other factors. Average ranges of motion for the joints of the body may be found in the handbook of the American Academy of Orthopaedic Surgeons[1] and a variety of other texts.[2,3] A summary table is found in Norkin and White.[4] However, these averages should be used with caution because the populations from which the averages were derived are undefined and the specific test positions and types of instruments that were used are not always identified.

Another factor affecting ROM is whether the motion is attained by the examiner without assistance from the patient (passive ROM) or if the motion is attained by the patient without assistance from the examiner (active ROM). Normally PROM is slightly greater than AROM because each joint has a small amount of available motion (joint play) that is not under voluntary control. The additional PROM that is available at the end of the normal AROM helps to protect joint structures, because it allows the joint to absorb extrinsic forces.

Testing PROM provides information about the integrity of the articular surfaces and the extensibility of the joint capsule, associated ligaments, and muscles. The extent of PROM is determined by the unique structure of the joint being tested. Some joints are structured so the joint capsules limit the end of ROM in a particular direction; while other joints are structured so ligaments limit the end of a particular ROM. Other limitations to motion include contact of joint surfaces (i.e., metacarpophalangeal joint flexion), muscle tension (i.e., dorsiflexion with knee extension), and soft tissue approximation (i.e., hip flexion).[4] Each specific structure that serves to limit a ROM has a characteristic feel to it, which may be detected by the examiner who is performing PROM. This feeling, which is experienced by the examiner as resistance to further motion at the end of a PROM, is called the "end-feel." End-feels may be considered normal (physiologic) or abnormal (pathologic). Clinical decisions regarding treatment often are based not only on the amount of ROM present, but also on the end-feel. End-feels are usually classified as soft, firm, hard, or empty. The first three types may be either normal or abnormal, depending on where they occur. An empty end-feel is never normal. It describes the situation in which no real end-feel is reached because the patient experiences pain before the examiner experiences an end-feel.

In addition to evaluating specific joint motions, often it is useful to test flexibility of two-joint muscles. A muscle which crosses two joints becomes taut before it reaches the limits of range of both joints over which it passes. In so doing, it prevents the simultaneous completion of movement at both joints. A common example is the difference in ankle dorsiflexion that is seen with knee flexion as opposed to knee extension. The two joint gastrocnemius muscle becomes taut when the knee is extended and the ankle joint dorsiflexed, thus decreasing the amount of dorsiflexion available. This limitation to motion at the joint caused by the available length of a muscle, rather than by the joint itself has been termed "passive insufficiency."[5] Clinically, it is often useful to compare actual joint range measurements with measurements that indicate the length of two joint muscles.

Testing AROM provides additional information about muscle strength and coordination which may be useful when it is compared to PROM. Thus, the patient's ability to use available PROM for active movement is of clinical importance. This will be discussed further under the category of strength.

The most common method of measuring ROM is goniometry. This word was derived from two Greek words, gonia, meaning angle, and metron, meaning measure. A goniometer is used to measure the angles of the joints. Electrogoniometers are very similar to their manual counterparts, but instead of a scale that is read by the examiner, there is an electrical potentiometer attached to the fulcrum.[6] An output signal representing joint angle is available and can be read by the therapist or fed into a computer for data reduction.

STRENGTH

Although strength is one of the most widely used terms in physical therapy, it remains poorly understood. Strength refers to force production. Usually, force is measured in one of two ways, the ability to produce movement or the ability to resist movement. Both manual muscle testing and dynamometry have used these two approaches to document strength. Some authorities have chosen to differentiate between strength and power, with the latter referring to the ability to produce force through a range of motion in a particular time. Only isokinetic testing allows the clinician to assess power (see Chapter 4).

Kendall does not define strength or explain the need to measure it.[6] Instead, she mentions the many factors involved in weakness and return of strength.

"Weakness may be due to nerve involvement, disuse atrophy, stretch weakness, pain, or fatigue. Return of muscle strength may be due to recovery following the disease process, return of nerve impulse after trauma and repair, hypertrophy of unaffected muscle fibers, muscular development resulting from exercises to overcome disuse atrophy, or return of strength after stretch and strain have been relieved." [6 p. 3]

Kendall's approach to muscle testing uses both of the above-mentioned methods of evaluating force production. Based on the work of Lovett, the Kendall system originally used letters to designate grades including Zero (0), Trace (T), Fair (F), Good (G), and Normal (N). Later, Kendall changed to the use of percentages for grading muscle strength, but these percentages have direct correlates in the letter system. It is common to see the information presented in terms of numbers 0 through 5. Pluses and minuses are used to increase the sensitivity of the tool. It is important to note that these symbols are interchangeable and the underlying meaning is unchanged as illustrated in Table 1.

One of the most important concepts in manual muscle testing is the effect of gravity in grading. According to Kendall, it plays a role in only about 60% of the extremity muscle tests because it is not considered in some tests (fingers and toes, supination and pronation). This is because the effects of gravity are not appreciable in comparison to the strength of some muscles. However, from a clinical perspective, the effects of gravity are considered in most manual muscle testing. Typically, a patient is tested in an anti-gravity position for grades F to N, and in a gravity-lessened position for grades F- to 0. Kendall proposed that an assistive movement in an anti-gravity position can be used for poor and poor plus grades. This involves estimating the amount of assistance given weak muscles, similar to the way in which the estimation of resistance is used in grading stronger muscles. This provides a useful alternative approach for patients who cannot be positioned in all of the gravity-lessened positions.

Another important concept in muscle testing is substitution. When a muscle or muscle group attempts to compensate for the lack of function of a weak muscle, the result is a substitution movement by these muscles. For accurate muscle testing, substitutions should not be permitted.

To quantify the evaluation of muscle strength, a number of devices have been developed to measure the

Table 1 Manual Muscle Testing Grades		
Kendall's percent	Lovett's letters	Numerals
0	0	0
5	T	1
20	P	2
50	F	3
80	G	4
100	N	5

force exerted by the body on an external body. Such devices, called force transducers, give electrical signals proportional to the applied force. There are many kinds available ranging from simple to elaborate.[6]

Dynamometers are instruments used to measure mechanical force. Hand held dynamometers are incorporated into manual muscle testing procedures (Figure 1). Instead of the examiner estimating the amount of pressure required to "break" the patient's position, the instrument provides a readout of force. In more sophisticated systems, the hand held device is attached to a computer which provides a reading in Newtons (Figure 2). This type of testing is limited to cases in which the examiner can overcome the strength of the muscle group being tested. It also requires the examiner to be aware of and prevent substitutions.

FIGURE 1. Hand held dynamometer.

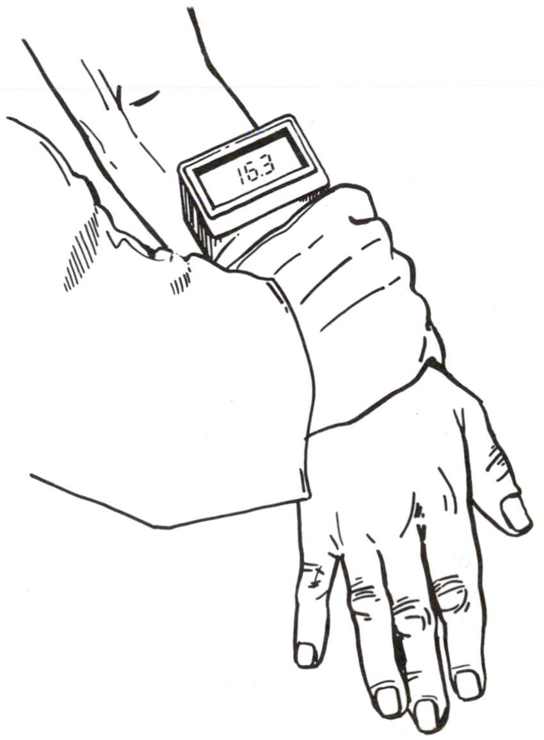

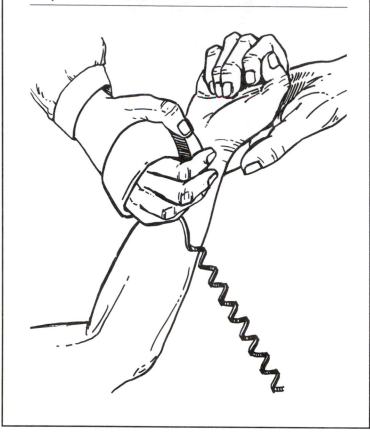

FIGURE 2. *Hand held dynamometer with computer attachment.*

twitches or the muscle force. We can measure only the resultant torque generated by the forces acting on a joint. Current methods of measuring torque (i.e., isokinetics, strain gauges) require relatively constrained movement, and cannot isolate individual muscle contributions to the torque production.

Electromyography (EMG) is a graphical representation of the electrical activity within skeletal muscle (Figure 3). The EMG signal originates after a nerve action potential has been transmitted along the axon of a motor neuron and its branches to activate the muscle fibers associated with the motor unit. The fiber action potential then propagates in both directions toward the ends of the muscle fiber. The algebraic summation of these fiber action potentials produces the motor unit action potential (MUAP), which is recorded during electromyography.[7]

Two types of electrodes are used clinically: surface electrodes and in-dwelling electrodes. Diagnostic electromyography requires the use of in-dwelling electrodes. The invasive nature of in-dwelling electrodes restricts their use primarily to diagnostic purposes, with limited clinical and research applications. Surface electrodes are easily applied and noninvasive, but they have a large pickup area and can be used only with superficial muscles. With any type of electrode, proper placement is critical to avoid "crosstalk" from other muscles and to avoid distortion of the EMG signal. Electrodes should be placed on the belly of the muscle and then placement should be checked by asking the patient to perform a functional test to isolate the muscle, if possible.

Due to the nature of the EMG signal, it contains information about the numbers of active motor units and their frequency of firing. This information represents the commands from the nervous system, so the EMG can serve as a means of monitoring the neural control of movement. The amplitude of the individual MUAP is influenced by the number of muscle fibers in the motor unit and their diameters, as well as by the degree of synchronization in the summation of single fiber action potentials.[7]

Because EMG provides a qualitative and quantitative record of muscle activation, it has the potential to enhance the evaluation of neurologically involved patients. It gives information about which muscle activity is responsible for a muscle moment and whether antagonistic activity is taking place. In attempting to assess motor control, the addition of EMG provides broader and more detailed information on which to base decisions.

Larger and more sophisticated dynamometers have been incorporated into isokinetic testing devices. As mentioned previously, these devices offer the major advantage of allowing the assessment of force production at varying speeds. In isokinetic testing, the amount of resistance changes throughout the patient's muscle contraction to match exactly the force applied by the patient. Because of this accommodation, it allows for maximal dynamic loading throughout the range of motion. As opposed to isotonic testing, where the resistance is set and the patient determines the speed, isokinetic testing sets the speed and the patient must perform at that speed to produce force. This is important because it allows evaluation of the patient's ability to produce force at high speeds, as is required for most functional activities. Although often used when evaluating patients with musculoskeletal deficits, isokinetic equipment is equally useful for the assessment of patients with neurologically based movement disorders. The inability to generate force quickly, maintain the force as desired, and terminate force are all common motor control deficits that can be evaluated on isokinetic equipment. Equipment allows for testing of the ability to produce movement (isotonic and isokinetic tests) as well as the ability to resist movement (isometric and eccentric tests).

KINESIOLOGIC ELECTROMYOGRAPHY

During a muscle contraction, the force twitches produced by the active motor units summate to produce the force output of the muscle. We cannot measure directly the force

SPASTICITY/MUSCLE TONE

Spasticity is defined as a velocity dependent increase in a muscle's resistance to passive stretch.[8] It is seen as part of the upper motor neuron syndrome, of which inability to control volitional movement is a component. Muscle tone has been used by a variety of people to mean a variety of things. In this chapter, the terms spasticity and tone will be used interchangeably, according to the definition above. There is evidence of two components of spasticity, phasic and tonic. Depending on the area and extent of the lesion producing the

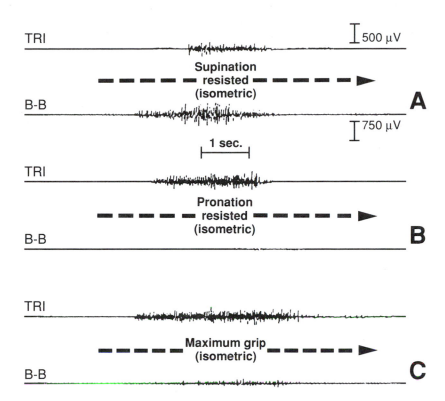

spasticity, there may be varying degrees of the phasic and tonic components. The stretch reflex also has two distinct components, phasic and tonic.

The relationship of tone to abnormal movement is not understood. Jackson categorized the dysfunction of neurologic lesions into two distinct sets of symptoms, negative and positive. Negative symptoms were defined as deficits of normal behavior such as the inability to move. Positive symptoms, such as spasticity, were viewed as a release phenomenon. Jackson concluded that the positive and negative symptoms were two entities that may be related, but do not have a cause-effect relationship.[9] Sahrmann and Norton suggested that motor deficits in patients with hemiplegia are due to limited and prolonged recruitment of the agonist and delayed cessation of the agonist contraction at the end of movement.[10] McLellan demonstrated that the response of a spastic muscle to stretch is not the same during passive motion as during active movement.[11] These and other studies indicate that clinicians should concern themselves more with the reestablishment of normal active motor control than with the reduction of the stretch reflex in response to passive movement.[12] Nevertheless, there are individuals who may find it useful to use an objective measurement of spasticity.

Examination of the deep tendon reflex (DTR) is used commonly to assess muscle tone. An increased or hyperactive DTR is indicative of the disinhibition of the stretch reflex mechanism. A decreased or hypoactive DTR indicates either interruption of the monosynaptic reflex arc or a generalized decrease in the excitability of the motoneuron pool (i.e., as seen in spinal shock). In patients with spasticity, an increased amplitude and a decreased threshold are noted. In addition to clinical assessment of DTRs using a standard reflex hammer and a subjective description of the resulting muscle contraction (using a scale of 0-4), the reflex may be measured more objectively. An electrodynamic hammer can be used to provide a standardized tap, which can be varied in terms of speed and force. The response can be objectified in a number of ways. A dynamometer can be used to evaluate the range and force if the measurement is carried out under isotonic conditions. Measurement of force developed by the muscle can be recorded in isometric and isotonic conditions by recording EMG events that accompany the tendon jerk. In this way, the threshold and amplitude of the tendon jerk response and the relative contributions of specific muscles may be determined.

A similar measure of reflex activity is the Hoffman (H) reflex. The H-reflex is essentially an electrically elicited tendon jerk, which is independent of the muscle spindle activity. An electrical pulse is used to stimulate large diameter Ia afferents instead of the tendon tap. Measurement of response is as described previously.

Clinically, the most common method of measuring spasticity is subjective evaluation of the muscle's resistance to passive stretch. It is important to vary the velocity of stretch and to observe for both phasic and tonic responses. "Clasp-knife phenomenon" represents a phasic response, without a tonic response. A more continuous resistance to passive stretch throughout the range represents the tonic component.[8] The Ashworth Scale,[13] and later a modification[14] were developed to quantify the resistance to passive stretch. In these tests, a grading scale is provided and therapists use the scale to describe the amount of resistance noted when stretch is delivered in a controlled manner. Trained investigators were able to achieve 86.7% agreement when testing elbow flexor spasticity in 30 neurologically impaired patients.[14]

Another clinical tool used to assess the muscle's response to stretch is the "pendulum test." Originally described in 1954 by Boczko et al,[15] this test is conducted by positioning the patient in a chair or on an examination table with the thigh supported in such a manner that when the leg is lifted to a horizontal position and dropped, the leg may move freely (Figure 4). In neurologically intact subjects and in patients with hypotonia, the leg oscillates freely for some time.[8] In patients with spastic muscles, different patterns of restricted movement can be observed. To quantify this test, it can be done on isokinetic equipment such as the Cybex* or KIN-COM+. The use of such equipment allows for control of the rate of stretch and the measurement of the force of reflexively induced muscle resistance. The latter system allows not only the recording of mechanical events (torque and angle) but also recording of two EMG signals.[8]

POSTURAL ALIGNMENT AND STABILITY/BALANCE

Posture refers to the maintenance of an upright position against the forces of gravity. Balance refers to the maintenance of the center of mass over the base of support (see Chapter 10). Ideal posture involves a minimal amount of stress which is conducive to maximal efficiency in the use of the body. Static posture is evaluated by comparing skeletal alignment of the patient to an ideal posture. Usually, this is done by using a plumb line to determine whether the points of reference of the individual being tested are in the same alignment as the corresponding points in the standard posture. For testing, the subject steps up to a suspended plumb line and is viewed from the front, back, and both sides. In back and front views, he stands so the feet are equidistant from the line, and in a side view, so the point just in front of the lateral malleolus is in line with the plumb line. The base point is the fixed reference point because the base is the only stationary or fixed part of the standing posture. In ideal alignment, viewed from the side, the plumb line will fall in alignment with the lobe of the ear, the shoulder joint, the midline of the trunk, the greater trochanter of the femur, slightly anterior to the midline of the knee, and slightly

FIGURE 4. Pendulum test.

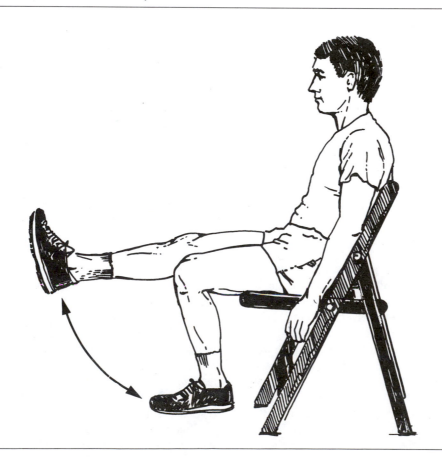

*Cybex Div. of Luxex, Inc., 2100 Smithtown Ave., Ronlonloma, NY 11779
+Chattecx Corp., P.O. Box 4278, Chattanooga, TN 37405

anterior to the lateral malleolus.[6] By comparing this ideal alignment with the actual alignment of the patient, faulty posture is identified.[5]

In individuals with motor control deficits, the assessment of postural alignment may need significant modification. Many patients are unable to maintain a standing position. Nevertheless, the principles remain the same and alignment should be evaluated in sitting. Some patients with even more significant deficits may not be able to maintain an upright position in sitting. For these individuals, the ideal alignment should be considered when designing adaptive seating systems. The ideal posture is one that requires minimal muscular activity to maintain and allows for maximal movement efficiency. Therefore, patients with significant motor control deficits should be provided with an advantageous starting point in positioning from which to relearn control of movement.

The maintenance of an upright posture requires the ability to make postural adjustments as changes occur to the center of mass, the base of support, or the support surface. For example, an individual demonstrating ideal alignment in the previously mentioned test would need to make significant adjustments if he were to hold a heavy object in front of him, stand on one foot, or stand on a changing surface, such as an air mattress. The ability to make these adjustments in order to maintain the center of mass over the base of support is known as balance.

Balance testing is performed using functional balance grades such a zero, poor, fair, good, and normal. These usually involve the evaluation of the patient's ability to remain upright with or without support, to tolerate challenges to the upright position, and to move within the upright position. Because the definition of each grade is not universally accepted, this type of scale should be accompanied by a key such as the one in Table 2.

The functional balance grades provide information about the patient's balance output, but provide no information about how the patient manages to maintain balance, or specific deficits in the patient's balance. The contribution of sensory systems to balance has been recognized for many years. The Romberg test involves maintaining standing balance with eyes open and eyes closed. If a patient can stand only with visual input, the assumption has been that the balance disorder stemmed from proprioceptive and/or vestibular deficits.[16] Analysis of sensory organization as a major component of balance has been developed further by Nashner, Shumway-Cook, Horak, and others,[17,18] and is discussed in detail in Chapter 10.

Using computerized force platforms, it is possible to measure objectively the movement of the center of pressure over the base of support. In this type of testing, the patient stands on a support surface that has force platforms built into it. The patient must stand with a prescribed base of support and the computer then integrates the information from the force plates to print out a graph of the movement of the center of pressure. This allows for evaluation of postural sway which is the very small amount of continual movement seen in so-called "static" standing. In normals, it involves about three degrees of movement in the anterior/posterior direction. In patients with motor control deficits, it may be much greater. Force platforms are useful for evaluating the cone of stability. This refers to the area around the center of mass that an individual perceives as the area of equilibrium. If sensory, perceptual, or motor abilities are impaired, the patient's perceived cone of stability may be altered so that the end limit of one or more dimensions is decreased. This increases fear, anxiety, and the risk of falling. Although physical therapists have been aware of this "shift" for many years, computerized force platforms allow quantitative assessment of this aspect of balance.

Perhaps the most sophisticated balance assessment tool available today is the EquiTest#. This computerized tool allows for standardized testing by using motorized moveable platforms and a moveable visual surround (Figure 5). The EquiTest provides measures of response latency, symmetry of weight distribution, amplitude of response in relation to the amplitude of perturbation, and pattern of muscle activation used in the balance response. The EquiTest is expensive and usually is found in research centers or clinics that specialize in the evaluation of patients with balance disorders. However, it is becoming more common in physical therapy departments that treat large numbers of patients with neurologic impairments.

The Clinical Test for Sensory Integration in Balance (CTSIB) or foam and dome testing is an affordable alternative method of using the same principles of sensory organization and motor coordination in balance assessment.[19] In this assessment, somatosensory input may be distorted by having the patient stand on thick foam, and visual input is manipulated by having the patient wear a blindfold or a "dome" that distorts visual input. Stimulation of the vestibular system is gravity dependent and thus unaffected by the testing environment. The CTSIB allows the clinician to assess the patient's ability to maintain standing balance under six different conditions involving these three sensory systems. The therapist can observe patterns of dependence on one sensory system and can assess the patient's ability to adapt to various situations. The patient's attempts to integrate multiple, simultaneous, and often conflicting sensory inputs are analyzed. Although objective data are minimal as compared to those made available by the EquiTest, the

---

Table 2
Functional Balance Grades

Normal:	Patient is able to maintain balance without support. Accepts maximal challenge and can weight shift in all directions.
Good:	Patient is able to maintain balance without support. Accepts moderate challenge and can weight shift, although limitations are evident.
Fair:	Patient is able to maintain balance without support. Cannot tolerate challenge. Cannot maintain balance while weight shifting.
Poor:	Patient requires support to maintain balance.
Zero:	Patient requires maximal assistance to maintain balance.

NeuroCom International, Inc., Clackamas, Oregon

FIGURE 5. The EquiTest® is a computerized tool used to evaluate balance under six sensory conditions.

1 Normal vision. Fixed support.

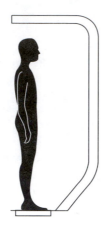

2 Absent vision. Fixed support.

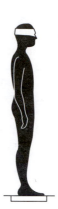

3 Sway-referenced vision. Fixed support.

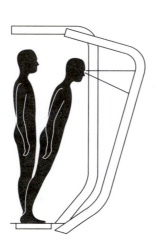

4 Normal vision. Sway-referenced support.

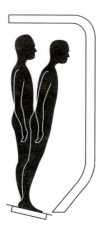

5 Absent vision. Sway-referenced support.

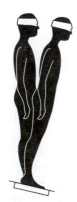

6 Sway-referenced vision and support.

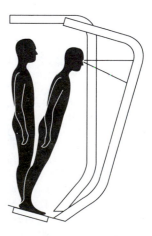

skilled clinician can obtain meaningful information about the amount of sway, the strategies used to maintain balance, and the conditions that present the most difficult problems for the patient.

COORDINATION

Coordination is defined as a harmonious working together, especially of several muscles or muscle groups, in the execution of complicated movements. Factors that the central nervous system must assess before and during coordinated movement include: starting position, amplitude of movement needed, force required, postural adjustments needed, speed required, accuracy required, and sensory and environmental conditions.

Clinical evaluation of coordination typically includes tests that require reversals of movement and accuracy in touching targets. These often include asking the patient to perform the following motions repeatedly and as quickly as possible: 1) touch his nose, then reach out and touch the examiner's finger, then alternate between these two targets as quickly as possible; 2) supinate and pronate his forearms; 3) oppose each finger to the thumb; 4) slide the heel of one foot up and down the opposite shin; and 5) tap feet together, alternately, or reciprocally.

Quantification is achieved by noting the number of repetitions that the patient can complete in a given period (i.e., six repetitions in 10 seconds). Qualitative assessment includes description of dysmetria (past pointing), dyssynergia (decomposition of movement), ataxia, dysdiodochokinesis (difficulty with reversals of movement), or tremor.

Efforts to increase reliability of coordination testing have led to the development of standardized assessments that allow for specific functions to be performed under specific conditions. A sample of these standardized tests is included below.

Jebsen Hand Function Test [20]

This test focuses on hand function. There are seven subtests of functional activities: writing, card turning, picking up small objects, simulated feeding, stacking, picking up large lightweight objects, and picking up large heavy objects. Normative data are available for age, sex, maximum time, and hand dominance.

Purdue Pegboard Test [21]

This test assesses dexterity by placement of pins in a pegboard and assembly of pins, washers, and collars. It is a test of manipulative skill incorporating right-hand, left-hand, bilateral, and assembly tasks. Norms are available.

Sensory Integration and Praxis Tests (SIPT) [22]

The SIPT is a revision of the Southern California Sensory Integration Tests, used to detect and to determine the nature of sensory integrative dysfunction in children.

Tests of eye-hand coordination, tactile functions, and various forms of praxis, such as postural, oral, and constructional praxis are included. Normative data are available

for children between 4 - 8 years of age. Reliability and validity data are available.

Test of Motor Impairment - Henderson Revision [23]

The purpose of this normed test is to differentiate children with motor impairment from normal children. It is divided into four age bands: 5 and 6 years, 7 and 8 years, 9 and 10 years, and 11 years and older. Testing consists of eight items for each age band.

Bruininks - Oseretsky Test of Motor Proficiency (BOTMP) [24]

The purpose of the BOTMP is to assess gross and fine motor skills in children between the ages of 4.5 and 14.5 years. The specific motor areas assessed by the subtests are running speed and agility, balance, bilateral coordination, strength, upper limb coordination, response speed, visual motor control, and upper limb speed and dexterity. Certain items are identified for use as a short form and can be administered for screening for purposes such as early identification of developmental problems. This test has been assessed for validity and reliability.

Computers have been used to evaluate a patient's coordination. In a typical set-up, patients begin with their hands in a set position on a touchplate. A simple switch senses whether or not the hand is on the plate. A target is projected onto the touchscreen and the patient is instructed to touch the center of the target. Spatial error is measured by comparing the patient's touch to the actual location of the target. Asymmetry calculations provide information about whether the touches were predominantly too high or too low or too far to one side. Other tasks involve moving targets. The subject is asked to touch the target when it reaches a designated destination. The touchscreen and computer timer determine the temporal error, and asymmetry calculations indicate the frequency of being too early or too late. Motor reaction time is designated as the time from the appearance of the target (or the start of target motion, depending on the test protocol) to the release of the hand from the plate, and movement time is designated as the time from the release of the hand from the plate to its contact with the touchscreen (see Chapter 7). A further variation of this type of task is accomplished by the addition of the EMG to the sensors. Cognitive reaction time is defined as the time from the presentation of the stimulus to the beginning of the nonresting-state EMG signal. The ability to separate motor reaction time as described above from cognitive reaction time is important in determining whether the problem is motoric or one of information processing. An abnormally long cognitive reaction time implies the latter state, whereas a normal cognitive reaction time coupled with an abnormally long motor reaction time implies a physical problem.[25] A wide variety of sophisticated testing is available using this type of technology. It is important to note that not only is it possible to test both upper and lower extremities, but also eye and head movement can be monitored.[26,27] This is very important because incoordination may result from deficits of the visual and vestibular systems, but without sophisticated testing, the therapist may assume the problem stems from the upper extremity.

GAIT

A specific coordinated activity that is a cornerstone of physical therapy evaluation and treatment is gait. The ability to walk requires adequate motor control and is one of the functional activities to which almost all patients aspire. Because the task is complex, its analysis is challenging.

In certain situations only a superficial gait assessment is indicated. Such an assessment would include a description of variables, such as the amount of assistance the patient requires, the use of assistive devices, the gait pattern used, the distance the patient can traverse, the speed with which he does so, and a brief description of any gait deviations. This type of assessment is used most often in settings where function is the primary objective and time does not allow a thorough quantitative analysis of the patient's gait. Efforts to quantify this type of analysis include the use of such scales as the Functional Ambulation Profile and the Locomotion Scale of the Functional Independence Measure.[28,29]

In all clinical gait analyses, the energy costs of ambulation should be considered. Efficiency is important if patients are to tolerate a return to functional activities. This has been illustrated dramatically in research on the percentage of patients with paraplegia who choose not to ambulate with crutches and long leg braces after returning to the community. The energy requirements are such that it leaves the individuals with little energy to do anything BUT walk.[30] Energy cost is most accurately assessed by measurement of oxygen consumption, carbon dioxide production, and pulmonary ventilation used during ambulation. Although accurate, these measures are not commonly available in clinical situations. The monitoring of heart rate before and after ambulation, with continued monitoring until the heart rate returns to baseline, gives an indication of energy consumption and is highly recommended. Winter has identified four major causes of inefficiency commonly seen in patients with motor control deficits.[6] These include inappropriate cocontraction, isometric contractions against gravity, jerky movements, and generation of energy at one joint with simultaneous absorption of energy at another.

There are times when gait analysis is a primary concern and more sophisticated assessment is indicated. In these instances, the type of gait analysis that is selected depends on the purpose of the analysis, the type of equipment that is available, and the knowledge and skill level of the examiner. The purpose of a gait analysis may be to determine what deviations are present in order to develop treatment to eliminate them; to compare gait with different orthoses; to compare gait following different interventions; or to describe normal values for a particular group of individuals.

The most commonly employed gait analysis is termed "observational gait analysis." This involves systematic observation of each segment of the body during each phase of gait. To assist the therapist in performing an observational gait analysis, there are a number of published protocols that outline the necessary observations and provide methods of describing what is observed.[31-33] For example, the Rancho

Los Amigos protocol instructs the examiner to observe the foot, ankle, knee, hip, pelvis, and trunk. Additionally, the therapist notes the presence or absence, as well as the timing, of deviations such as toe drag, excessive plantarflexion, and hip hiking. This type of analysis requires considerable skill on the part of the examiner. It also requires continuous walking on the patient's part, due to the number of variables under observation. The use of videotape can circumvent this requirement by allowing the therapist to view recorded samples of the patient's gait, rather than requiring the patient to walk repeatedly. However, standard videotaping for this purpose has limitations. Unless a special setup allows the camera to move as the patient does, the examiner quickly loses the direct side view as the patient moves forward and the camera position remains unchanged. Additionally, unless care is taken to delineate specific bony landmarks, visualization of particular gait deviations is difficult. Of importance, studies of intertester reliability during observational gait analysis have yielded only moderate levels of reliability, even when experienced therapists have used this tool.[34,35] Yet, because it requires little or no instrumentation, observational gait analysis remains the most commonly used type of gait analysis in clinical situations.

FUNCTIONAL ABILITIES

The usual reason a patient with motor control deficits seeks medical and rehabilitative care is because he is faced with a deficit in functional abilities. Functional activities are those identified by an individual as essential to physical and psychological well-being as well as to a personal sense of meaningful living. Four main categories of function have been delineated: physical, mental, affective, and social function.[36] Because this chapter focuses on motor control, only physical function is addressed. However, in discussing functional assessment, it is important to stress that all functional skills require the integration of cognitive, affective, and sensorimotor abilities. Physical function refers to those sensorimotor skills necessary for the performance of usual daily activities. Getting out of bed, walking, climbing stairs, and bathing are examples of physical functions. Tasks concerned with daily self care such as feeding, dressing, hygiene, and physical mobility are called basic daily living skills. Advanced skills that are considered vital to an individual's independent living in the community are termed instrumental daily living skills. These include shopping, cooking, and driving.

When evaluating individual patients for the purpose of setting goals and creating a treatment plan, physical therapists often develop functional assessments that are designed to meet the specific needs of the patient. They generally describe the patient's ability to perform specific activities and the amount of assistance needed. The assessment also would describe those tasks which the patient cannot perform. For example, the physical therapist may note that the patient is independent in all bed mobility except when moving from supine to sit, which requires minimal assistance. The patient requires minimal assistance for wheelchair to bed transfers; moderate assistance for wheelchair to commode transfers; and maximal assistance for floor transfers. When this type of descriptive assessment is performed, a key is recommended to facilitate effective communication (Table 3).

Table 3
Grades of Functional Ability
Independent: The patient can safely perform the clinical skill with no one present.
Supervision: The patient is likely to be able to perform the skill without assistance, but requires someone nearby as a precaution.
Contact Guard: The patient may require physical assistance; therefore, the assistant maintains hand contact and full attention.
Minimal Assistance: The patient requires physical assistance to perform the skill, but completes approximately 75% of the skill without assistance.
Moderate Assistance: The patient requires physical assistance to perform the skill, and the assistant provides greater than 25% of the effort.
Maximal Assistance: The patient is unable to assist or assists in less than 25% of completion of the task.

STANDARDIZED ASSESSMENTS

A large number of instruments have been developed to assess and to classify functional abilities. A sample of these instruments follows.

Standardized Assessments of Basic Daily Living Skills

The Barthel Index is a measure of a person's ability to function independently in ten self-care and mobility skills, including feeding, hygiene, dressing, transfers, and locomotion.[37] The score for each item is based on the time in performing the activity and amount of assistance needed by the patient. The index provides a score that reflects the degree of functional dependence in each skill (0-5, 10 or 15, depending on the skill) and overall (0-100). This index has been used widely to monitor functional changes in patients receiving rehabilitation. Extensive validity and reliability information are not available, but a recent study showed the Barthel to be reliable in testing functional status of patients with CVA.[38] Five therapists using the scale to rate seven patients agreed on 71.4 to 100 percent of the ratings, depending on the activity, with wheelchair transfer having the least agreement and bowel/bladder control, feeding, and stair climbing having the most agreement.

The Kenny Self-Care Evaluation is a measure of a person's ability to perform 17 basic daily living skills, divided into six major categories of bed mobility, transfers, locomotion, dressing, personal hygiene, and feeding.[39] Each area is given a grade of 0-4 ranging from completely dependent to independent. All items are equally weighted. Validity and reliability studies are not available.

The Katz Index of Activities of Daily Living is a measure of a person's ability to perform six basic daily living skills: bathing, dressing, toileting, transfers, continence, and feeding.[40] Three descriptions are provided for each category, one of which is complete independence, and the other two describe varying degrees of assistance needed. Originally developed for use with institutionalized patients, this index does not include items on ambulation or wheelchair propulsion.

Standardized Assessments of Instrumental Daily Living Skills

The Functional Status Index is a measure of the patient's perception of functional disability.[41] It is a self-report of dependence, difficulty, and pain encountered in the performance of physical and social activities. It has been used most commonly for patients with rheumatoid arthritis.

The Pediatric Evaluation of Disability Inventory (PEDI) is a standardized assessment that uses parental reporting to determine a child's comprehensive level of function.[42] Part one consists of the broad categories of self-care, mobility, and social function, with each having 13-15 items to be evaluated on a scale of 1-5. This part of the evaluation indicates the level at which the child can function without assistance. In part two, the same categories are evaluated based on the level of assistance and modifications the child typically needs to function on a daily basis. A summary profile is determined.

The Tufts Assessment of Motor Performance (TAMP) was designed specifically to examine functional motor status.[43] It is administered with standardized instructions and equipment. This is a 32-item test that involves 15 mobility, 13 activities of daily living, and four communication items. The TAMP is a criterion-referenced evaluation tool which allows each task to be analyzed and compared to a predetermined set of objective criteria. Of particular interest is the breakdown of scoring along four dimensions: assistance, approach, pattern, and proficiency. This allows the development of two separate profiles. The functional profile combines items that are functionally related. The performance profile combines tasks across different items that have similar motor characteristics and requirements. Initial attempts to determine reliability were positive.

LIMITATIONS OF MOTOR CONTROL ASSESSMENT TOOLS

A number of motor control assessment tools have been discussed in this chapter. However, the discussion has been limited to diagnosis independent tools that primarily measure the physical aspect of motor control. There are many assessment tools that have been developed for specific patient populations that have not been presented. For example, the Motor Assessment Scale,[44] the Modified Motor Assessment Scale,[45] the Modified Chart for Motor Capacity Assessment,[46] the Fugl-Meyer Assessment,[47,48] and the Evaluation of the Hemiplegic Subject Based on the Bobath Approach[49] are all scales that are used to assess motor control in stroke patients.

Many assessment tools have been developed for use with the pediatric population. In determining motor control in children, physical therapists have the additional dimension of motor development to consider. Adults with acquired motor control deficits that result from disease or injury are evaluated in terms of what they are no longer able to do. In children with motor control deficits, it is important to consider developmental aspects of motor control. For a thorough review of pediatric tests and assessments, the reader is referred to Chapter 2 in *Therapeutic Exercise in Developmental Disabilities.*[50]

The most important consideration of motor control assessment tools is the tool's usefulness in a given situation. Many of the tools discussed in this chapter were developed to provide quantitative methods to measure motor function. This is desirable when attempting to use statistical analysis to assess change. There are times, however, when qualitative information may be more useful. It is important to remember that most of the evaluations described allow assessment of performance outcome only. In evaluating patients for the purpose of planning intervention, it is often the manner in which the movement evolves that interests us. For example, in a patient with motor planning problems, it may be more useful to describe the patient's performance under varying conditions than to perform a standardized assessment. It may be that problems with planning may be better differentiated from problems with execution using qualitative rather than quantitative assessments.

Motor control is a very complex, multi-faceted skill. As movement scientists, physical therapists hope to improve our patients' abilities in this area. In order to assess our effectiveness, valid and reliable tools are needed to measure patient performance. Only with the use of such tools will we be able to determine the effects of our intervention.

ASSESSMENT CONSIDERATIONS

CASE STUDY #1
MRS. JANE SMITH

Age: 74 years
Diagnosis: Right hemiplegia,
secondary to left cerebrovascular accident
Status: Six months post onset

In preparing to evaluate this patient, there are several points to consider. Mrs. Smith is likely to have some degree of aphasia because language centers are usually found in the left (affected) hemisphere. Language dysfunction (receptive, expressive, or both) will necessitate changes in the manner in which the patient is evaluated. Secondly, it is important to monitor Mrs. Smith's vital signs. Although referred to physical therapy for a neurologic problem, it would not be surprising to find that this patient has significant cardiovascular symptomatology.

Mrs. Smith's initial evaluation would include an assessment of her passive range of motion, comparing the involved to the uninvolved side. The flexibility of the gastrocnemius muscle would be a concern, because tightness may contribute to balance and gait problems. In evaluating this patient's active range of motion, one would assess not only the patient's ability to move within the available passive range,

but also the patient's ability to vary her movements. Is the patient limited to one or two movement patterns, or is she able to selectively combine movements at each segment of her limbs?

Strength or force production should be evaluated. At six months post insult, it is likely that the patient has some degree of disuse atrophy and may benefit from strengthening exercises. However, it is important to assess each component of the muscle contraction. How quickly can the patient recruit muscle fibers? Can she maintain the contraction and does she have the ability to relax the fibers volitionally? It is unlikely that EMG would be used in the clinical situation, but it may be useful if it is unclear whether or not the patient is contracting antagonistic muscle groups in an appropriate sequence.

Some therapists would evaluate the patient's spasticity by assessing the response of muscle to passive stretch applied at different velocities. Other therapists would argue that this information is not useful and need not be addressed.

Perhaps the most crucial part of this patient's evaluation is the functional assessment. Activities such as rolling, coming to sitting, achieving standing, and ambulation are likely to be the patient's major concerns. If the patient is ambulating, the assessment would include uneven surfaces, elevations, and management of obstacles such as doors and fallen objects.

In addition to the motor control assessment, related evaluations such as sensation, perception, cognition, the home environment, and need for adaptive equipment should be included.

CASE STUDY #2
DANIEL JOHNSON

Age: 59 years
Diagnosis: Parkinson's Disease
Status: Four years post initial diagnosis

In assessing Mr. Johnson, both current and potential problems should be addressed. Because he has a progressive disease, it is crucial that he maintain his optimal condition and avoid secondary problems that would further disable him. An assessment of the patient's range of motion and flexibility is very important. Due to the paucity of movement seen in patients with Parkinson's disease, one must be concerned with potential loss of range. If loss of range occurs, the problems encountered because of the neurological deficits are compounded. Posture is an important area for this patient because many patients with Parkinson's disease develop a stooped posture that may have detrimental effects on respiration and balance. Early detection and intervention for developing postural deficits may decrease the patient's level of disability. Mr. Johnson is likely to show decreases in the speed of his movements, in his ability to initiate movement, and in his ability to reverse movements. He may have resistance to passive movement but this will not be velocity dependent and is called rigidity, not spasticity.

Again, the focus of the evaluation should be on function. Balance and gait will be important components of his assessment and identifying factors that improve his function will be stressed. Many patients with Parkinson's disease respond well to rhythmic cues such as "one, two, ready, walk" rather than elaborate descriptions of what is involved in the movement.

CASE STUDY #3
SHIRLEY TEAL

Age: 21 years

Diagnosis: Post motor vehicle accident
Closed head injury

Status: Four months post accident

To discuss the assessment of this patient, we will have to make some assumptions regarding her cognitive and behavioral status. We will assume that she has mild to moderate cognitive and behavioral deficits that allow her to interact meaningfully with her environment and follow directions. For patients with more severe cognitive and/or behavioral problems, modifications to the motor control assessment would be necessary.

Evaluation would include passive and active range of motion, posture, strength, speed, and variety of movement and functional skills. Because a patient with significant head injury is usually in a coma for a period of time, it is not unusual to develop muscle imbalances and postural deformities. Given the young age of this patient, it is important to remediate any deformities before they become fixed. Common problem areas include ankles, shoulders, and the cervical region.

When ambulatory, Ms. Teal may have difficulty with higher level balance and coordination activities. Her evaluation at that time would include ambulation on uneven surfaces, on elevations, outdoors, and in busy environments. A balance assessment (Equitest or CTSIB) would be indicated. If Ms. Teal has significant visual problems, she should receive a full evaluation by a neuro-opthomalogist. By administering the TAMP, a comprehensive functional evaluation for future comparison will be provided.

CASE STUDY #4
SHAWNA WELLS

Age: 4 years

Diagnosis: Cerebral palsy; spastic quadriparesis;
mild mental retardation

Status: Onset at birth

Evaluation would include the basic components of movement such as passive and active range of motion, force production, and functional activities. Postural abnormalities that might interfere with the development of normal motor skills would be identified. For this patient, we would be concerned with her developmental progress, noting when she reaches milestones such as sitting unsupported, standing, and walking. Current ambulation would be assessed for degree of independence and reliance on assistive devices. Administration of the PEDI would provide a comprehensive assessment of function. ❏

REFERENCES

1. American Academy of Orthopaedic Surgeons: Joint Motion: Method of Measuring and Recording. Chicago, IL, American Academy of Orthopaedic Surgeons, 1965
2. Hoppenfeld, S: Physical Examination of the Spine and Extremities. New York, NY, Appleton-Century-Crofts, 1976
3. Kapandji, IA: Physiology of the Joints, Vol. 1, ed 2. London, England, Churchill-Livingstone, 1970
4. Norkin CC, White DJ: Measurement of Joint Motion: A Guide to Goniometry. Philadelphia, PA, FA Davis, 1985
5. Winter DA: Biomechanics of Human Movement. New York, NY, Wiley & Sons, Inc, 1979
6. Kendall FP, McCreary EK: Muscles: Testing and Function, ed 3. Baltimore, MD, Williams & Wilkins, 1983
7. Brown WF: The Physiological and Technical Basis of EMG, Stoneham, MA, Butterworth, 1984
8. Dimitrijevic MM, Dimitrijevic MR, Sherwood AM, et al: Clinical neurophysiological techniques in the assessment of spasticity. In Davis R, Kondraske GV, et al(eds): Quantifying Neurologic Performance, Philadelphia, PA, Hanley & Belfus, 1989
9. Kandel ER, Schwartz JH: Principles of Neural Science, ed 2, New York, NY, Elsevier, 1985
10. Sahrmann SA, Norton BS: The relationship of voluntary movement to spasticity in the upper motoneuron syndrome. Ann Neurol 1977; 2:460-465, 1977
11. McClellan DL: Co-contraction and stretch reflex in spasticity during treatment with baclofen. Neurol Neurosurg Psychiatry 40:30-38, 1977
12. Duncan PW, Badke MB: Stroke Rehabilitation: The Recovery of Motor Control, Chicago, IL, Yearbook, 1987
13. Ashworth B: Preliminary trial of carisoprodol in multiple sclerosis. Practioner 192:540-542, 1964
14. Bohannon RW, Smith MB: Interrater reliability of a modified Ashworth scale of muscle spasticity. Phys Ther 67:206-207, 1987
15. Boczko M, Mumenthaler M: Modified pendulous test to assess tonus of thigh muscles in spasticity. Neurology 8:846-851, 1954
16. Walton J: Introduction to Clinical Neuroscience. ed 2. Philadelphia, PA, Bailliere Tindall, 1978
17. Nashner LM, Shumway-Cook A, Marin O: Stance posture control in selected groups of children with cerebral palsy: Deficits in sensory organization and muscular coordination. Exp Brain Res 197:3393-3409, 1983
18. Shumway-Cook, A, Anson D, Haller S: Postural sway biofeedback: Its effect on reestablishing stance stability in hemiplegic patients. Arch Phys Med Rehabil 69:395-400, 1988
19. Shumway-Cook A, Horak FB: Assessing the influence of sensory interaction on balance. Phys Ther 66:1548-1550, 1986
20. Jebsen RH, Taylor N, Trieschmann RB, et al: Objective and standardized test of hand function. Arch Phys Med Rehabil 50:311-319, 1969
21. Smith HD: Assessment and evaluation-specific evaluation procedures. In Hopkins HL, Smith HD (eds): Willard and Spackman's Occupational Therapy, ed 6. New York, NY, Lippincott, 1983
22. Ayres AJ: Sensory Integration and Praxis Test Manual. Los Angeles, CA, Western Psychological Services, 1988
23. Stott DH, Moyes FA, Henderson SE: Test of Motor Impairment. Henderson Revision. Guelph, Ontario, Canada, Brook Educational Publishing, Ltd., 1984
24. Bruininks RH: Bruininks Oseretsky Test of Motor Proficiency. Examiner's Manual. Circle Pines, MN, American Guidance Service, 1978
25. Maulucci RA, Eckhouse RH: A workshop for quantifying perceptuo-motor behavior. In Davis R, Kondraske GV, Tourtellotte WW, et al (eds): Quantifying Neurologic Performance, Philadelphia, PA, Hanley & Belfus, 1989
26. Eckhouse RH, Maulucci RA: Assessment of eye-head-hand coordination. In Davis R, Kondraske GV, Tourtellotte WW, et al (eds): Quantifying Neurologic Performance, Philadelphia, PA, Hanley & Belfus, 1989
27. Bizzi E: The coordination of eye-head movement. Scientific American, 231:100-106, October 1974
28. Nelson AJ: Functional ambulation profile. Phys Ther 54:1059 - 1065, 1974
29. Morton T: Uniform data system for rehab begins: First tool measures dependence level. Progress Report, APTA 15:14, October 1986
30. Cerny D, Waters R, Hislop H, et al: Walking and wheelchair energetics in persons with paraplegia. Phys Ther 60: 1131-1139, 1980
31. Lower Limb Prosthetics. New York, NY, New York University Medical Center Post-Graduate Medical School Prosthetics and Orthotics, 1981
32. Bampton S: A guide to the visual examination of pathological gait. Philadelphia, PA, Temple University Rehabilitation Research and Training Center #8, Moss Rehabilitation Hospital, 1979
33. Gronley JK, Perry J: Gait analysis techniques. Rancho Los Amigos Hospital Gait Laboratory. Phys Ther 64:1831- 1838, 1984
34. Goodkin R, Diller L: Reliability among physical therapists in diagnosis and treatment of gait deviations in hemiplegics. Percept Mot Skills 37:727-731, 1973
35. Krebs D, Edelstein J, Fishman S: Observational gait analysis reliability in disabled children. Phys Ther (Abstract) 64;741, 1984
36. Guccione AA, Cullen KE, O'Sullivan SB: Functional assessment. In Physical Rehabilitation: Assessment and Treatment, ed 2, Philadelphia, PA, FA Davis, 1988
37. Mahoney FI, Barthel DW: Functional evaluation: The Barthel index. Md State Med J 14:61-65, 1965
38. Loewen SC, Anderson BA: Reliability of the modified motor assessment scale and the Barthel index. Phys Ther 68:1077-1081, 1988
39. Schoening H, Iversen I: Numerical scoring of self-care status: A study of the Kenny self-care evaluation. Arch Phys Med Rehabil 49:221-229, 1968
40. Katz S et al: Studies of illness in the aged. The index of ADL: A standardized measure of biological and psychosocial function. JAMA 185:914-919, 1963
41. Jette A: Functional Status Index: Reliability of a chronic disease evaluation instrument. Arch Phys Med Rehabil 61:395-401, 1980
42. Haley SM, Faas RM, Coster WJ, et al: Pediatric Evaluation of Disability Inventory. Boston, MA, New England Medical Center, 1989
43. Gans BM, Haley SM, Hallenborg SC, et al: Description and interobserver reliability of the Tufts assessment of motor performance. Am J Phys Med Rehabil 0002-9491/88/6705-0202, 202-210, 1988
44. Carr HG, Shepherd RB, Nordholm L, et al: Investigation of a new motor assessment scale for stroke patients. Phys Ther 65:175-180, 1985
45. Poole JL, Whitney SL: Motor assessment scale for stroke patients: concurrent validity and interrater reliability. Arch Phys Med Rehabil 69:195-197, 1988
46. Lindmark B, Hamrin E: Evaluation of functional capacity after stroke as a basis for active intervention. Scand J Rehab Med 20:103-109, 1988
47. Fugl-Meyer AR, Jaasko L, Leyman I et al: Post-stroke hemiplegic patient: I method for evaluation of physical performance. Scand J Rehabil Med 7:13-31, 1975
48. Duncan PW, Propst M, Nelson SG: Reliability of Fugl-Meyer assessment of sensorimotor recovery following cerebrovascular accident. Phys Ther 63:1606-1610, 1983
49. Guarna F, Corriveau H, Chamberland J, et al: An evaluation of the hemiplegic subject based on the Bobath approach, parts I -III. Scand J Rehab Med 20:1-16, 1988
50. Connolly BH, Montgomery P: Therapeutic Exercise in Developmental Disabilities. Chattanooga Corp, Educational Division, Chattanooga, 1987

Chapter 7
Issues Of Cognition For Motor Control

Kathye E. Light, Ph.D., PT

INTRODUCTION

Physical therapists are involved integrally with other health care providers, such as neuropsychologists, speech pathologists, and occupational therapists who direct many interventions toward cognitive processes. As physical therapists, we recognize the role of cognitive function to speak appropriately, act appropriately, make decisions about our lives, calculate financial transactions, and become gainfully employed. We understand these cognitive functions, but our role in the rehabilitation of patients with neurologic deficits is the retraining of movement. Movement does not require much cognitive processing, or does it?

The control of movement seldom is viewed as a cognitive process. Indeed, many of our physical therapy neurophysiologic treatment techniques emphasize automatic movement ability, and discourage the use of patient attentional processes. As therapists, we often attempt to mold the movements we perceive as best by facilitation techniques, and believe that if this facilitated movement is repeated often enough, the patient will automatically begin to move in the correct way.

Although facilitation is a common therapy practice for motor retraining, are these techniques actually enhancing motor learning? By definition, motor learning is "a set of internal processes associated with practice or experience leading to relatively permanent changes in the capability for motor skill."[1 (p. 375)] Consider yourself attempting to learn a new movement. If someone facilitates and manually guides you through the whole movement, are you then capable of performing that movement without help? When are guidance and facilitation useful and when do they hinder motor control? These are important questions for physical therapists. In this chapter, the importance of cognitive or information

processing ability for motor control will be discussed. Just as we must process information to interact appropriately with our environment, so must our patients with neurologic deficits. Just as we must hold movement plans in memory and use stages of memory and learning to function within the environment, so must our patients.

Movement control involves highly integrated and interactive processing of central and peripheral neuromuscular mechanisms. Before a controlled intentional movement occurs, the brain receives, identifies, and recognizes sensory signals from the environment. Appropriate actions are chosen, and before the movement is executed, a complicated neuromuscular integration, sequencing, timing, and coordination of motor output are required. This movement control is termed information processing and is necessary for environmentally useful movements. Information processing is interactive with the stages of memory for functionally directed movement control.

The purpose of this chapter is not to encourage physical therapists to become cognitive retrainers or neuropsychologists, but to emphasize the necessity of cognitive processing in the retraining of movement control.

INFORMATION PROCESSING

The receiving, identification, and recognition of environmental stimuli followed by selection and execution of planned actions are defined by several different information processing models.[1-3] The most basic model, described by Schmidt, consists of three stages: 1) stimulus identification, 2) response selection, and 3) response programming.[1] This simple model is illustrated in Figure 1. Each of the stages of

FIGURE 1. *Stages of information processing.*

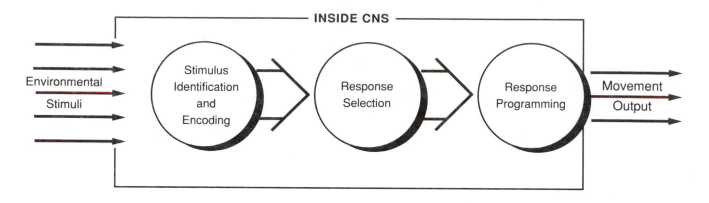

(Adapted from Schmidt, 1988)

information processing requires time, therefore the total time necessary between receiving a cued environmental stimulus and beginning a movement output is an indication of information processing ability.

Stages Defined

Stimulus identification, the first stage of the simple information processing model, entails the detection and neural encoding of sensory cues and identification and interpretation of the stimulus pattern. Basic factors known to affect processing speed within the stimulus identification stage are stimulus clarity, stimulus intensity, and pattern complexity.[1] The most easily processed sensory signal is a clear, intense cue with a simple pattern.

Response selection, the second stage of information processing, is also known as response determination.[2] In this stage, the decision is made about which response to execute. Two common factors that affect the processing time in the response selection stage are the number of stimulus-response choices available to be made and the compatibility between the stimulus and the response. Stimulus-response (S-R) compatibility can be viewed as the natural fit or match of a sensory signal to the desired motor output.[1] A simple example of S-R compatibility is the ease of matching the visual appearance of an object to the motor output of touching the object. Visual cues indicating reaching toward an object are more compatible than sound cues indicating the same action. Many of us have experienced this reality when attempting to reach for the morning alarm clock without success, until we actually opened our eyes to visually localize the target. The simplest and fastest processing will occur through response selection when there are no choices involved, i.e., a simple reaction time situation exists, and when the stimulus and response fit well together.

The last stage of information processing, response programming, is the stage in which the movement is planned, structured, and centrally activated. This occurs after the stimulus has been coded and identified, and the response selected.[1] (p. 89-90) Factors that affect response programming time are complexity of the movement, duration of the movement, and compatibility between the responses that are being performed simultaneously, in a sequence, or as choice alternatives.[4] This type of compatibility is known as response-response (R-R) compatibility.

R-R compatibility is a bit more difficult to understand than S-R compatibility. One of the most familiar examples of poor R-R compatibility is the difficulty we experience when attempting to pat our heads and rub our stomachs simultaneously. Much greater R-R compatibility exists between the two simultaneous responses of patting the head and patting the stomach or rubbing both the head and stomach.

Information processing stages are experimentally tested by chronometric techniques which involve reaction time instrumentation.[5] Because certain environmental factors affect particular stages of information processing, without affecting the processing time of other stages, experimental manipulation of those specific factors allows the central processing of particular stages to be determined.

Serial vs. Parallel Processing

How can we function efficiently within our world if all movements are dependent on information processing? How can we account for our relative ease of functional movement if all environmental stimuli are processed one at a time and in series through the stages of information processing? Certainly not all of our movements are information processing dependent. We have simple, long loop, and cortical loop reflexes; triggered reactions; and subcortical motor programs.

Various types of movement outputs differ in the amount and degree of information processing required at each stage. Some types of movements are so complicated that each stage of information processing is challenged, and only one stage can proceed at a time. Other movements may be carried out simultaneously through mechanisms of central nervous system (CNS) parallel processing. Although there are advocates who suggest that all movements are single channel processed,[6] the theoretical notion of parallel processing generally is accepted.[7,8] Parallel processing implies that environmental stimuli can be processed simultaneously or in parallel, and that at least several stages of information processing may proceed simultaneously. Parallel processing of information is hypothesized to be a higher order function than serial processing. As tasks become well learned and practiced, the possibility exists that the motor learner shifts from serial processing to parallel processing of information.

MEMORY SYSTEMS

Information processing requires memory structures. The process of memory is a neurophysiologic phenomenon involving neural activity that is not totally understood, and a review of literature on the very complicated topic of memory is beyond the scope of this chapter. The development of memory traces for newly learned information appears to be dependent on plastic circuitry which allows the passage of neural activity between the hippocampal formation and neocortical association.[9,10] If this circuitry is disrupted, the result is a loss of retrieval of recently formed memory traces and an inability to form new traces.

Working memory, however, cannot be localized to a single location with the CNS. Research suggests different neural structures are required for recall memory versus recognition.[11] In addition, memory subsystems for spatial movement tasks are not the same as those required for changing the timing and sequencing of a movement configuration.[12] Although an exact understanding of the neurophysiology of memory has not been achieved, a simplified conceptualization of how the memory processes work is depicted in Figure 2.

The cognitive processes involved in the control of movement are not just those of information processing that allow an organism to react appropriately to environmental stimuli. Memory structures also are necessary to allow signals to be recognized and movement plans developed and recalled within the CNS. Many simultaneous events occur within the environment at each moment, and, although generally we are aware of these stimuli as they enter short term sensory storage, we do not respond to all stimuli. Short term sensory storage is a memory system that allows large amounts of sensory information to be stored for periods of less than one second.[13,14]

Pertinent sensory stimuli are processed into short term memory from short term sensory storage via the mechanism of selective attention. Short term memory is a memory system with storage time up to approximately one minute and serves as a type of work area for movement plan processing.[15] Short term memory is the working space for processing the input and output that direct goal oriented movement and is considered to function similar to the buffer in a personal computer. Both the computer memory and human short term memory must be "booted up" before functioning, and require input to process the output.

Long term memory is a relatively permanent storage area for almost limitless amounts of information. Information can move into long term memory by means of rehearsal or concentrated effort. Motor programs are stored in long term memory, but must be brought into the short term memory workspace before movement output is possible.[1 (p. 96-97)]

Information processing interacts with memory storage mechanisms to control functional movement within a constantly changing environment. Alteration of any mechanism involved in information processing or memory storage will alter environmentally appropriate, functional movement. Mechanisms that affect sensory storage, selective attention,

FIGURE 2. Memory compartments for movement control.

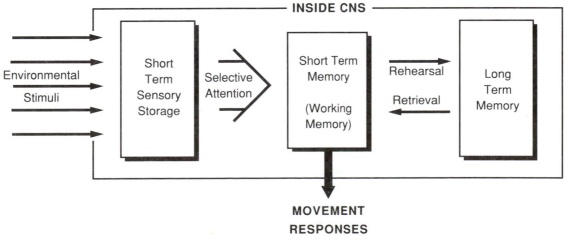

(Adapted from Schmidt, 1988)

attention switching ability to rehearse, ability to concentrate and focus, and overall states of anxiety, arousal, or activation will influence learning and controlling of movement.

BUILDING MOTOR PROGRAMS

Certainly not all of our everyday movements require attentional effort, decision making, rehearsal, intense concentration, attention switching, or other information processing and memory components mentioned previously. Most of us are capable of drinking a cup of coffee, writing our thoughts on paper, reaching quickly toward objects, and kicking a soccer ball without laboring cognitively over the movement itself. A number of motor control theorists hypothesize that the reason we can perform many movements quickly and without attentional demands is that we have developed motor programs for those tasks.

Motor programming applies particularly to fast movements considered to be movements that occur so quickly the response would not allow the time necessitated by CNS feedback control. Closed loop movements, or those movements that occur slowly and allow feedback control, are never completely controlled by a motor program. Most slow movements are controlled by some degree of feedback during the course of movement; however, with learning, many movements that are initially controlled with feedback become more automatic via motor programming.

The control of movement is an extremely complicated task. Consider the interaction among all the neural structures for inputting, processing, and outputting the appropriate neural signals. Consider as well the complicated process of moving the body's linked system, with its numerous range of motion possibilities built on an unstable base of support, i.e, two rather small feet. Now, in addition to the actual control of the organism's central and peripheral mechanisms, consider how the environment changes from moment to moment. Not only must the organism process internal control signals and move the unstable linked system about, but the organism must also be able to interpret the external signals of the environment and keep the internal control mechanisms updated with all pertinent external information. This classic motor control problem, known as the degrees of freedom problem, is discussed in Chapter 2 and was first described by a Soviet scientist, Nicolai Aleksandrovitch Bernstein in 1947. However, his work was not translated into English until 1967.[16]

The way in which degrees of freedom of the organism's central and peripheral structure are controlled, while interacting within the environment, is one of the most interesting questions facing today's motor control scientists. Schmidt promoted the schema theory of generalized motor programs to explain the way we develop efficiency of movement control.[17,18] According to Schmidt, a motor program is an abstract memory structure that is prepared in advance of a movement and, when initiated, results in the execution of efficient coordinated movement that does not require feedback or attentional demands.[1 (p. 227-266)] Schmidt hypothesized that we gain movement efficiency by developing generalized motor programs that can be applied to whole classes of movements, regardless of the body part performing the movement. A generalized motor program is thought to consist of certain variant and invariant components. The variant components are those parameters of control that apply to a specific movement at a specific moment, and which are not fixed in the motor program. Rather, the variant components are provided at the time of the required movement, and consist of parameters such as the exact muscles required to perform the movement, the overall duration of the movement, and the overall force required to produce the movement. The components considered to be fixed or invariant in the motor program are order or sequence of events, phasing or temporal structure, and relative forces required to execute the actions of the program.[1]

Another group of motor control scientists disagree that the CNS must store programs for classes of movements. These researchers promote a dynamic systems approach to the control of movement.[19] Kelso and coworkers, advocates of Bernstein's theory, emphasized that the body periphery, i.e., the biomechanical linkages of muscles and joints, plays a significant role in movement, and that the CNS learns to take advantage of the laws of physics to control movement.[20] According to dynamic systems theorists, skill in a motor task occurs through the development of a coordinative structure which writes equations of constraint between the CNS and the biomechanical linkages of the body periphery to control the degrees of freedom. More recently, Kelso and colleagues have moved away from a purely biomechanical emphasis but continue to explain movement pattern coordination according to dynamic theory.[19,21]

Regardless of how movement efficiency is developed between the CNS and periphery, motor skill in both closed and open loop tasks is established by the process of motor learning. Motor learning, or the relatively permanent change in the capacity to perform a motor task, is accomplished through basic stages often labeled as the cognitive stage, associative stage, and autonomous stage.

The cognitive stage learner struggles with understanding the motor task. At this stage the learner needs to hear and repeat verbalized instructions, decide the goal of the task, establish what makes a good performance, and understand the sequencing of the parts. In the early stages of cognitive motor learning, the preparation to begin the task and initiation of the first few movement attempts require total attention of the learner. Concern for timing and accuracy is not possible in the cognitive stage, and the teaching therapist must be aware of potential overload. During the cognitive learning stage, motor skill develops primarily as a result of verbal-cognitive changes; therefore, the role of information processing at this stage of learning is extremely important.

While the patient is in the cognitive stage of learning, the most important component of therapy is to assist the development of a reference of correctness. The learner must be clear on the goal of the movement which not only implies the outcome of the movement, but also involves the critical features of the movement performance. If, as the therapist, your goal includes symmetrical weight shift, a smooth movement trajectory, and a forward scapula, the patient must understand all of these components before a proper reference of correctness can be developed. Once the reference of correctness is achieved, the learner will be able to detect errors in the movement and make alterations by an internal locus of control.

A patient will be in the cognitive stage of learning during the first few weeks of rehabilitation following a neurologic insult; therefore, the issues of memory, information processing, and goal development are critical to early rehabilitation. During this time, the therapist's appreciation of cognitive components is important because movement ability and motor skill development progresses the most while the patient is in the cognitive learning stage.

Once the movement task is well understood, the goals and subgoals are well established, and the learner has a reference of correctness for the motor skill, a natural progression toward the associative stage of learning occurs. During the associative stage of learning, the patient refines the motor skill. Much less verbalization about the task by the therapist or patient is needed. The learner must be allowed to experiment with movement control during the associative stage in order to determine the subtleties of an efficient movement plan. The amount and speed of motor skill improvement during the associative stage are less than during the cognitive stage of motor learning. Rather, the associative stage will be marked by gradual refinements in the motor patterns, timing, coordination and movement efficiency.

The last stage of motor learning, the autonomous stage, comes about slowly after a great deal of practice and experience with the motor task. When the learner reaches the autonomous stage, performance of the motor task will appear to be automatic. Little attention will be paid to the primary motor task, but rather a type of periodic "checking in" on the performance seems to be the method of control. When the learner reaches the autonomous stage, the motor skill can be accomplished under all types of environmental settings. The learner will not be affected by distractions and will be able to attend to and perform secondary tasks simultaneously with the primary motor skill.

NEUROLOGIC DEFICITS

The clinical literature demonstrates that brain damage to different parts of the CNS results in a variety of movement control problems related to information processing. The obvious problems of stimulus identification occur when primary or association areas of sensory processing are damaged. Deficits in visual attention and loss of appropriate visual scanning result from lesions of the parieto-occipital cortex.[22] Left hemisphere cerebrovascular accidents (CVAs) have been demonstrated to cause greater response programming deficits than right CVAs.[23] Controversy exists over the role of the basal ganglia in information processing, but it appears that basal ganglia structures have little to do with memory scanning, orientation, or attention to a stimulus.[24] The basal ganglia appear to be involved in movement initiation and execution,[25] but these deficits appear to be unrelated to perceptual impairment.[26] There is disagreement about the role of the basal ganglia in movement preparation.[24,25]

Because various types of movements may involve different memory subsystems,[12] specific types of lesions result in different control problems. Working memory structures for timing and force control appear to be damaged by lesions to the cerebellum or basal ganglia.[27,28] Working memory for spatial processing and targeting is affected by posterior cortical damage.[29] Memory for mimicking or copying sequences of movements or gestures results from cortical damage, particularly of the frontal lobes.[30] Research is clear that memory for movement control is not limited to the three boxes illustrated in Figure 2. Every type of self initiated or environmentally directed movement made by an individual must, however, use the memory systems conceptualized in Figure 2. Evaluating the patient with neurologic deficits for the stages of memory, processes of selective attention and attention switching ability, and ability to rehearse or concentrate for adequate time periods will offer valuable direction to the physical therapist.

COMPENSATION vs. TRAINING

Not all neurologic deficits are resolvable. The practical problem faced each day by the rehabilitation therapist is how to spend valuable treatment time in the most efficient manner. The physical therapist has control over three different aspects of neurologic rehabilitation. We control the teaching of movement, including physical guidance, encouragement, and verbal instruction. We also control the practice schedule, deciding how much and how hard a patient should work at a task. Finally, we have control over the physical or exercise training of strength, endurance, flexibility, and coordination.

Our overall physical therapy goal is to assist functional independence at the highest level of each patient's potential. Because the environmental demands of total independence in our ever changing world are endless, we all must set limits and develop a degree of structure to the environmental challenges we undertake. As physical therapists, we help to establish those limits for our patients. We assist the patient in improving movement and functional abilities in order to take on the world, and then we help the patient and caregivers to structure that world within the capabilities of the patient.

After evaluating the patient's overall functional ability we establish rehabilitation training programs to achieve specific functional goals. Most of these goals will necessitate that the patient be able to perform certain movement patterns with appropriate timing, sequencing, and control. Many of the goals will necessitate improved strength, flexibility, and endurance. As therapists, we must not forget that the principles of exercise physiology apply to the training of strength, flexibility, and endurance of all patients, not just cardiac and orthopedic patients. In addition to exercise training, the retraining of functional movement patterns will be accomplished best by applying the principles of motor learning. The types of training appropriate depend on the patient's information processing ability and the stage of motor learning for the particular functional task being taught.

Generally, movement retraining proceeds from simple to complex. We find what the patient can do, and then we add complexity. For example, by requiring more steps, a different context, or greater accuracy of the movement, we increase the difficulty of the task requirements. The concept of simple to complex is useful in training movements controlled by information processing. Following analysis of the patient's information processing ability, the stimulus identification requirements can be made more complex after starting with clear, intense, and simple patterned stimuli. Two examples of simple stimulus identification requirements are the use of one word instructional commands given in a quiet setting or the placement of one object on a table for the patient to reach. Gradually, the stimuli should be made less intense and require greater pattern complexity, such as commands given in sentences in the middle of a busy rehabilitation gymnasium. Response selection complexity can also be increased. The simplest situation is no choice being required and the motor response being easily matched to a stimulus, such as a verbal command to reach toward a visualized object. A more complex situation is one where the patient must make decisions about which activities to do and must respond to stimuli that do not fit so easily with the motor output. Response programming is the most common stage of information processing manipulated by the physical therapist as the patient progresses in rehabilitation. Movement complexity can be kept simple initially with one-step unilateral limb responses. Progression to movements requiring multilimb compatibility coordination with movements sequenced in fast progression can then occur. Movement duration of task demands can be gradually increased. R-R compatibility can be progressed from doing only one movement at a time to movements performed synchronously with two or more limbs. Further progression involves movements performed simultaneously or in rapid succession

that do not have R-R compatibility, such as slow reaching with one limb while the opposite limb performs a ballistic hitting response (Figure 3).

The progression of the rehabilitation program should be dependent on the patient's level of motor learning for the specific task. Training protocols and methods should vary appropriately as the motor learning progresses. The principles of practice and feedback presented by Schmidt[1 (p. 377-422)] and Winstein[31] are helpful in determining what types of practice and feedback are most appropriate during the three stages of learning (see Chapters 2 and 8).

CASE STUDIES

Evaluation

Information processing and memory systems testing were performed with the four patients. The case studies present the findings of the evaluation and general treatment approaches to address identified problems.

Clinical evaluation of patients' information processing abilities would be detected best with chronometric testing equipment. Because this type of equipment is not readily available in the clinic, a simple reaction time evaluation system was developed, consisting of a telegraph key connected to a millisecond timer. Stimulus identification ability was tested by requesting a pointing response of the most easily controlled upper extremity toward a visual light stimulus, an auditory bell stimulus, and a somatosensory vibration stimulus placed within appropriate sensory fields. This test was increased in complexity by presenting combinations of two or more stimuli sequentially or simultaneously and testing ability to detect all of the stimuli presented. This testing also allowed examination of short term sensory store.

Once basic stimulus detection was tested, stimulus identification ability of the least impaired sensory fields was examined. The ability to differentiate stimuli was tested by presenting multiple stimuli and asking the patient to point toward the named stimulus. Visual discrimination was tested with five common objects: pencil, glass, key, piece of paper, and small box. Auditory discrimination was tested by presenting five sounds: music, ringing bell, buzzer, whistle, and clapping (Figure 4). Somatosensory discrimination was tested with a stereognosis test using objects from the visual discrimination test. Somatosensory discrimination was tested by simultaneous stimulus presentation of vibration, pin prick, and light touch and requesting the patient to point toward the named stimulus.

Response selection was tested first by observing simple reaction times for releasing a start switch. Using the more controlled hand, the patient was required to reach quickly to turn off a switch at the sound of a bell. Reaction time was measured as the time in milliseconds required to release the start key. The test was performed by the therapist first giving the command "Get ready" and then allowing variable warning periods between 1 and 3 seconds before saying "Go." This simple reaction speed was compared to the reaction times for releasing

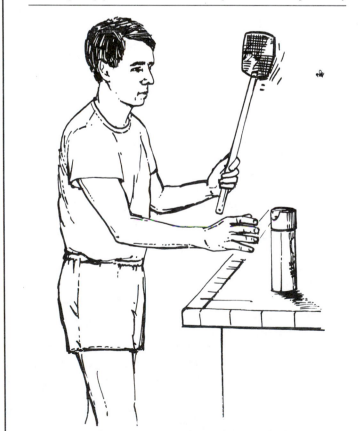

FIGURE 3. Simultaneous reaching for the fly spray while swatting the fly are movements with poor R–R compatibility.

FIGURE 4. Auditory and visual discrimination testing.

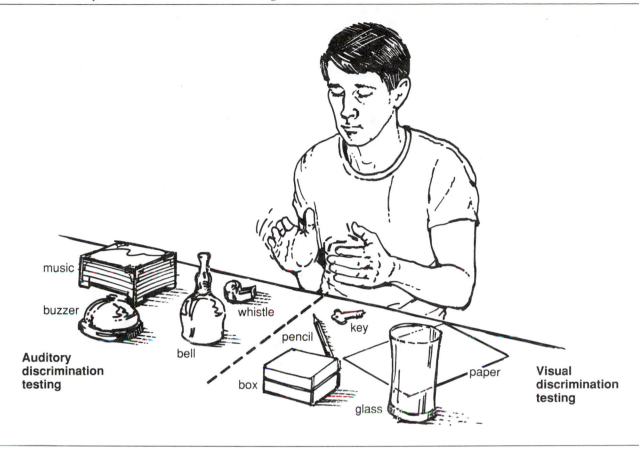

Auditory discrimination testing
music
buzzer
bell
whistle
pencil
box
key
glass
paper
Visual discrimination testing

the start switch when a choice was required. The choice was between reaching for the bell switch when it would ring versus reaching for a buzzer switch when sounded. Additional sounds were added to increase the number of choices required. Response selection ability was judged by the change in reaction time for releasing the start position key for the bell stimulus under simple and progressively more difficult choice situations. This test also helped determine the patient's short term memory for movement because the patient had to remember the appropriate reaching movement to accomplish the goal. Selective attention was evaluated with the response selection paradigm by having the patient first perform the task without distractions. Selective attention requirements were increased by adding environmental distractors of a visual, auditory, and somatosensory nature. The patient's performance was compared under the nondistracting and visual, auditory, and somatosensory distracting conditions.

Response programming ability was determined by the simple reaction time for releasing a switch under three progressively difficult tasks for movement execution. The tasks were releasing the start key; releasing the start key and reaching twelve inches; and releasing the start key and reaching first sideways to the right twelve inches, then sideways to the left twelve inches and returning to the start position.

CASE STUDY #1
JANE SMITH

Age: 74 years
Diagnosis: Right hemiplegia, secondary to left cerebrovascular accident
Status: Six months post onset

ASSESSMENT

Evaluation reveals extreme deficits in stimulus identification ability for the right visual field and somatosensory fields of the right upper extremity (RUE) and right lower leg and foot. Auditory fields appear to have no deficits. Once basic stimulus detection was tested, stimulus identification ability of the least impaired sensory fields was examined. The ability to differentiate visual stimuli appeared intact when visual objects were placed in the left visual field. Auditory discrimination appears intact overall. Somatosensory discrimination for the stereognosis test was intact with the left hand, but Mrs. Smith could not differentiate between the key and the pencil or between the small box and glass with the right hand. Somatosensory discrimination, tested by simultaneous stimulus presentation of vibration, pin prick, and light touch, revealed marked deficits on the right side.

Mrs. Smith has extreme deficits in response selection as indicated by her 500% faster performance under the simple reaction time condition versus two choice conditions. The deficit became much more apparent as more choices were added.

Mrs. Smith has difficulty with response programming for movements performed both with the right and left arms. Response programming deficits are greater for graded complexity with the RUE. The response programming problem does not appear to be as great as the problem with response selection. During response programming, testing comparisons were made between performance of the left and right arms. Mrs. Smith did not perform the movements crisply and smoothly with either arm until numerous practice trials with verbal feedback corrections were given. She then could perform the left arm movements with good coordination. However, this indicates that Mrs. Smith may not have an appropriate internal reference of correctness for the required movements with the left arm that she can hold as a standard for the right arm.

Four distinct problems were observed including stimulus identification difficulty, response selection difficulty, response programming difficulty, and poor reference of correctness. The goals, objectives, and treatment plan for Mrs. Smith's information processing problems are as follows:

GOALS

Treatment goals are for the patient to:
1. improve stimulus identification ability
2. improve response selection
3. increase accuracy in response programming
4. demonstrate improved reference of correctness.

FUNCTIONAL OBJECTIVES

Following 3 months of treatment, Mrs. Smith will:

1. identify a key, pencil, or small box placed in the right hand (without vision) with 50% accuracy; and visually follow from left to right, an object suspended from the ceiling, 4 of 5 trials.

2. demonstrate improved response selection by turning to right or left on verbal command, in sitting, with 90% accuracy; and looking to ceiling or floor on verbal command with 50% accuracy while standing in the walker.

3. in sitting, tap the right hand and right foot simultaneously for 10 seconds; and tap the right hand and left foot simultaneously for 10 seconds.

4. lift a glass to her mouth with the left hand three times and with the right hand three times without spillage.

TREATMENT RECOMMENDATIONS

Examples of treatment for goal #1 include practicing visual tracking of objects from left to right and right to left, covering all visual fields. Visual scanning practice of the environment in all visual fields also will be included. Somatosensory difficulties will be addressed by practicing identification of common objects with the right hand after first identifying them with the left hand, and receiving touch and proprioceptive input to the left and then to the right side.

An example of treatment for goal #2 would be a slow progression in the process of decision making. Initially, Mrs. Smith does not have to make choices, but carries out simple one stage commands. Then simple two choice responses are required, such as therapist names the object in the therapist's right hand, and Mrs. Smith looks toward the right hand. However, if the therapist names the object in her left hand, Mrs. Smith looks to the left. Another example of two choice responding would be if, while practicing sitting balance, the therapist tells Mrs. Smith to move as quickly as possible toward a forward lean when the therapist says "forward" and back as quickly as possible after hearing the "back" command. This task could be progressed in decision making by adding "left" and "right" commands. This type of response selection should be included throughout the therapy sessions.

The treatment plan for goal #3 includes having the therapist progress the task complexity and movement duration of the tasks used for functional training. This progression includes unilateral single step movements with the nonparetic left hand and progressing the left hand activities by adding movement steps in the activity sequence. The left hand and foot could then be worked together in a coordinated activity. After practicing with the nonparetic left limbs, the same tasks are practiced with the right extremities. Then all four limbs are coordinated in a multilimb task with progressive steps.

For goal #4, Mrs. Smith practices functional tasks with the nonparetic left extremities to improve the sense of movement requirements before practicing the identical movements with the right extremities. Movements that require bilateral activity or balance control are aided by visual feedback with a mirror, verbal feedback from the therapist, or appropriate feedback.

CASE STUDY #2
DANIEL JOHNSON

Age: 59 years
Diagnosis: Parkinson's Disease
Status: Four years post initial diagnosis

ASSESSMENT

The primary problems observed during the evaluation of Mr. Johnson were related to task execution. He appears to perceive stimuli adequately and has no notable problems with attention or response selection. As tasks were graduated in movement complexity by increasing the number of steps in the movement, increasing the length of time the movement was required, or asking him to perform two types of movement simultaneously, Mr. Johnson essentially stopped all execution attempts.

Careful examination of Mr. Johnson's responses revealed the following three major problems related to information processing: response programming deficits, short term memory difficulty, and difficulty with open loop tasks.

GOALS

Treatment goals are for the patient to:
1. demonstrate improve response programming
2. increase short term memory
3. improve performance of open loop tasks.

FUNCTIONAL OBJECTIVES

Following 3 months of therapy, Mr. Johnson will:

1. walk 30 feet in 15 seconds; and will hold a piece of paper with the left hand while cutting out a pattern with scissors with the right hand

2. accurately recall and verbally explain initial treatment activity at the end of treatment, 4 of 5 sessions; and will remember the correct sequence of a 3 part task from one session to another

3. sequentially place 15 household objects into 3 drawers placed in front of him within 20 seconds; and displace 10 spoons from a tray in 10 seconds.

TREATMENT RECOMMENDATIONS

The length of time requested for Mr. Johnson to perform repetitive tasks such as restorator cycling, ambulation, folding papers, and pulling nonresistive reciprocal pulleys will be gradually progressed (goal #1). Task requirements will be graduated first by increasing the repetition time of the same task and then increasing the number of steps in a requirement movement sequence. Task complexity will be increased further by requiring him to shift between types of movement, i.e., ballistic reaching, tying a shoestring, wrapping, carrying, bending, and kicking. Finally, the task difficulty will be enhanced by decreasing R-R compatibility. R-R compatibility will be high initially, such as requesting Mr. Johnson to clap both hands simultaneously. Then, similar types of movements of one hand and one foot will be requested, followed by requests for simultaneous dissimilar movements of the hands, such as tapping with one hand while the other hand reaches for an object or opens a drawer. R-R compatibility challenges will be progressed by providing multilimb coordination tasks with functional relevance.

For goal #2, Mr. Johnson will perform a requested movement activity during the first few minutes of therapy, go to another task requirement, and will then be asked to recall and demonstrate the first activity. After the demonstration, other activities will proceed. At the end of the therapy session, he will be asked to again demonstrate the first activity. Each session a new memory activity will be requested.

For goal #3, Mr. Johnson will perform short, quick responses such as pressing a lever to ring a bell, knocking with his fist on a door, or pulling a light switch cord to a lamp. Tasks will be progressed in open loop complexity by requiring fast two step and then 3-4 step movements. All fast movements will be performed as quickly and briskly as possible, without feedback until the task is completed.

CASE STUDY #3
SHIRLEY TEAL

Age: 21 years
Diagnosis: Post motor vehicle accident
Closed head injury
Status: Four months post accident

ASSESSMENT

During the evaluation, Ms. Teal lost interest and focus on each task presented. She failed to notice new items and tasks as attention switching requirements were challenged. Although aware of pinprick, vibration, and light touch overall, she could not discriminate common objects consistently in the stereognosis test of either hand.

Ms. Teal followed simple instructions well and did not appear to be dramatically affected when movement requests were altered in duration, complexity, or R-R compatibility. This finding suggested the need for additional evaluation of response programming. When simple and choice reaction times were compared, she had notable slowing in reaction times as the number of choices increased. At times, when choices were presented, Ms. Teal failed to react and would appear to lose attention for the task. She appeared to forget what she was doing and would begin another task.

The overall testing of information processing ability for Ms. Teal suggested the following three major problems: stimulus identification problems for stereognosis discrimination bilaterally; response selection and motor planning difficulties; and difficulty with maintenance of concentration and inability to switch attention between tasks or objects within the environment.

GOALS

Treatment goals are for the patient to:

1. improve stimulus identification ability in both hands
2. improve response selectivity and motor planning
3. increase concentration and improve attention switching ability.

FUNCTIONAL OBJECTIVES

Following three months of treatment, Ms. Teal will:

1. match 3 dimensional circle and square forms using tactile and proprioceptive cues (without vision), with 75% accuracy

2. place a hat on her head with left or right or both hands on verbal command with 50% accuracy; and imitate a wave with the left or right hand with 100% accuracy

3. draw a line with the left hand through a simple maze with 5 or fewer errors; mimic 10 upper extremity activities without being distracted from the task; and notice and attend to new objects presented, 50% of the time.

TREATMENT RECOMMENDATIONS

All treatment will be done initially in sitting. Activities will be progressed gradually to other positions, such as standing.

For goal #1, Ms. Teal will practice observing three dimensional shapes and objects, close her eyes, palpate an object with eyes closed, and locate a matching object. Common objects, such as a wash cloth, hair brush, glass, pencil, and door knob will be used for discrimination. With eyes closed, Ms. Teal will be asked to palpate a common object and then demonstrate its usage.

For goal #2, choices for response selection will be increased gradually. Initially, Ms. Teal will receive a simple one-step command for execution of a simple movement. An example is the placement of a soccer ball on the floor and asking her to "kick the ball". This will be progressed to a two choice command by using the terminology "left" or "right" to indicate which foot to use to kick the ball. Gradually, this simple activity will be progressed to a four choice situation by using the commands: "left foot," "right foot," "left hand," and "right hand".

Motor planning difficulty will be addressed by requiring a different movement output with each command. For example, to the command "right hand," Ms. Teal will strike the ball with her right hand. With the "left hand" command, she will be requested to pick up the ball and throw it with her left hand. The "left foot" command will indicate a simple kick, and the "right foot" command will require a continuous nudging of the ball with her right foot while propelling the wheelchair forward.

The treatment recommendations for goals #1 and #2 will also address goal #3. Therapy directed toward the problems of concentration maintenance and inability to appropriately switch attention will be progressed slowly to ensure patient success. For example, Ms. Teal will be asked initially to focus on the therapist. She will then be asked to mimic the therapist's left hand movements immediately after the therapist performs each movement. The therapist will begin by simply raising her left hand, then returning the hand to her left knee. This task will be repeated for 5-6 trials with variable time intervals between each movement. Then attention switching will be progressed slowly by asking Ms. Teal to focus on both the therapist's left hand and left foot. She will be required to mimic the therapist's movements of the left hand or left foot for simple lifting movements. Concentration requirements will be progressed by slowly increasing the length of time spent in the activity and by increasing the attention switching requirements. Attention switching will be progressed by having Ms. Teal mimic more and more types of movements, such that the task finally requires her to mimic quickly and immediately any activity that the therapist performs. In order to progress Ms. Teal's ability to concentrate appropriately for functional environmental demands, the length of time spent on tasks should vary intermittently.

CASE STUDY #4
SHAWNA WELLS

Age: 4 years
Diagnosis: Cerebral palsy; spastic quadriparesis; mild mental retardation
Status: Onset at birth

ASSESSMENT

As with most young children, evaluation of Shawna's information processing ability was a challenge. Shawna demonstrated good identification ability for all auditory stimuli. She could visually locate and point to all objects named during testing. The tested objects were presented in all visual fields. Shawna did not cooperate well with the evaluation of somatosensory location testing of vibration, pinprick, and light touch, but appeared to feel each sensation overall. She could discriminate the pencil, paper, and key, but could not differentiate between the glass and box during stereognosis testing. When holding objects, Shawna complained of palm itchiness, became inattentive, and wanted to get up from the test position.

When testing response selection, Shawna could perform relatively well under the simple reaction time condition. However, she often produced errors by reacting to the warning signal rather than to the stimulus signal. When two choices were presented, Shawna could not switch between the stimuli. She often persisted with the same response to both stimuli. Her responses were variable, with long delays before reacting. Under the choice condition, Shawna appeared to forget what she was supposed to do, and would frequently perform a movement unrelated to the task requirements. After a short time under the choice testing condition, Shawna became fussy and would not continue the task.

Shawna did not appear to be unduly slow in her reaction times when movement requirements became more complex. Response programming ability was, therefore, determined to be within normal limits.

Two information processing problems to be addressed in physical therapy were determined to be somatosensory stimulus detection difficulty and avoidance, and selective attention deficits.

GOALS

The goals of treatment are for the patient to:

1. improve discrimination of somatosensory stimuli and decrease avoidance responses
2. improve selective attention.

FUNCTIONAL OBJECTIVES

Following 3 months of treatment, Shawna will:

1. tolerate being swaddled in a blanket for 5 minutes without fretting; and manipulate and use appropriately a hairbrush and a toothbrush
2. attend to a table activity for 5 minutes without being distracted by two other children working at the same table.

TREATMENT RECOMMENDATIONS

To improve Shawna's willingness to experience somatosensory stimuli (goal #1), sensory experience will progress from general whole body contact to specific hand manipulation tasks. For example, therapy will begin by wrapping a cotton blanket around Shawna and then requesting Shawna to remove the blanket. Then she will wrap her own arms with a towel and unwrap the towel with guidance and assistance. This treatment will be followed by requesting Shawna to hold large solid objects, progressing to holding large soft objects, then to smaller hard objects, and finally to small soft objects. Shawna will be progressed to manipulating objects and demonstrating their usage.

To improve selective attention, therapy will progress from providing experiences in which the therapist initially controls all aspects of the environment. Specific single focus tasks will be required early in treatment within quiet, noncluttered treatment areas. Progressively, tasks will be increased in the number of attention requiring components, and the treatment environment will become less and less controlled by the therapist. ❏

REFERENCES

1. Schmidt RA: Motor Control and Learning: A Behavioral Emphasis ed 2. Champaign, IL, Human Kinetics, 1988, pp 77-97, 227-266, 375-422

2. Theios J: The components of response latency in simple human information processing tasks. In Rabbitt PMA , Dornic S (eds): Attention and Performance, Vol 5: New York, NY, Academic Press, 1975, pp 418-439

3. Salthouse TA, Somberg BL: Isolating the age deficit in speeded performance. J Geront, 37: 59-63, 1982

4. Light KE: Effects of adult aging on response programming and compatibility. Unpublished doctoral dissertation, University of Texas, Austin, TX, 1988

5. Posner MI. Chronometric Explorations of the Mind. Hillsdale, NJ, Erlbaum, 1978

6. Welford AT: The psychological refractory period and the timing of high-speed performance - A review of theory. Brit J. Psych 43: 2-19,1952

7. Keele SW: Attention and Human Performance (Chapter 4). Pacific Palisades, CA, Goodyear, 1973

8. Keele SW: Motor control. In Kaufman L, Thomas J (eds): Handbook of Perception and Performance, New York, NY, Wiley, 1986

9. Halgren E: Human hippocampal and amygdala recording and stimulation: Evidence for a neural model of recent memory. In Squire L and Butters N (eds): The Neuropsychology of Memory,New York, NY,Guilford, 1984, pp165-181

10. Squire LR, Cohen N, Nadel L: The medial temporal lobe in memory consolidation: A new hypothesis. In Weingartner H and Pardner E (eds): Memory Consolidation, Hillsdale, NJ,Erlbaum, 1984, pp 185 - 210

11. Hirst W, Johnson MK, Kim JK, et al: Recognition and recall in amnesics. J Exp Psych 12:445-451, 1986

12. Smyth MM, Pendleton LR: Working memory for movements. Quart J Exp Psych 41A (2):235 - 250, 1989

13. Sperling G: The information available in brief visual presentations. Psychological Monographs, 1960, 74 (11): whole no. 498

14. Bliss JC, Crane HD, Mansfield K, et al: Information available in brief tactile presentations. Perceptions and Psychophysics: 273 - 283, 1986

15. Atkinson RC, Shiffrin RM: The control of short term memory. Sci Amer 225: 82 - 90, 1971

16. Bernstein NA: The Coordination and Regulation of Movements,Oxford, England, Pergamon Press, 1967

17. Schmidt RA: A schema theory of discrete motor learning. Psych Rev 82: 225 - 260, 1975

18. Schmidt RA: The schema concept. In Kelso JAS (ed): Human Motor Behavior: An Introduction. Hillsdale, NJ,Erlbaum,1982, pp 219 - 235

19. Jeka JJ, Kelso JAS: The dynamic pattern approach to coordinated behavior: A tutorial review. In Wallace SA (ed): Perspectives on the Coordination of Movement. North Holland, Elsevier Science Publishers B V, 1989, pp 3-45

20. Kelso JAS: Human Motor Behavior, An Introduction. Hillsdale, NJ, Erlbaum, 1982, pp 239 - 287

21. Kelso JAS, Schoner G: Self-organization of coordinative movement patterns. Human Movement Science 7: 27 - 46, 1988

22. Lynch JL, McLaren JW: Deficits of visual attention and saccadic eye movements after lesions of parieto-occiptal cortex in monkeys. J Neurophys 61(1): 74 - 89, 1989

23. Haaland KY, Harrington DL, Yeo R: The effects of task complexity on motor performance in left and right CVA patients. Neuropsychologia 25: 783 - 794, 1987

24. Rafal RD, Posner MI, Walker JA, et al: Cognition and the basal ganglia. Brain 107: 1083 - 1094, 1984

25. Marsden CD: The mysterious motor function of the basal ganglia. The Robert Wartenberg Lecture. Neurology 32: 514 - 539, 1982

26. Stelmach GE, Phillips JG, Chau AW: Visuo-spatial processing in Parkinsonians. Neuropsychologia 27: 485 - 493, 1989

27. Keele SW, Ivry RI: Timing and force control: A modular analysis. International Research Conference on Motor Control, Moscow, March 1987

28. Margolin DI, Wing A: Agraphia and micrographia: Clinical manifestations of motor programming and performance disorders. Acta Psych 54: 263 - 283, 1983

29. DeRenzi E, Faglioni P, Previdi P: Spatial memory and hemispheric locus of lesion. Cortex 13: 424 - 433, 1977

30. Basso A, Luzzatti C, Spinnler H: Is ideomotor apraxia the outcome of damage to well defined regions of the left hemisphere? Journal of Neurology, Neurosurgery and Psychiatry 43: 118 - 126, 1980

31. Winstein CL: Motor learning considerations in stroke rehabilitation. In Duncan PW and Badke MB (eds): Stroke Rehabilitation: The Recovery of Motor Control. Chicago, IL, Year Book Medical Publishers Inc, 1987, pp 109 -134

Chapter 8
Sensory Information and Movement: Implications for Intervention

Mary Beth Badke, M.S., PT and Richard P. Di Fabio, Ph.D., PT

INTRODUCTION

The human design provides us with an adaptable neuro-motor system that uses sensory input to learn new motor functions. Sensory afference guides movement when the physical environment changes unpredictably, and sensation provides a cognitive "readiness" or set which allows us to anticipate a change in limb or body equilibrium. When pathology alters the human design, the ability to learn or relearn motor functions may be compromised. Adaptations to situations which require dynamic changes in muscle recruitment or joint motion may not occur.

In essence, pathologies affecting the use of sensory information can create serious disabilities. Deafferentation studies have revealed that a nonuse syndrome may develop quickly unless forced training follows the sensory loss.[1,2] Therefore, the use of sensory afference in the habilitation or rehabilitation process is an empirically sound approach. Physical therapists must learn to assess the functional impact of diminished, inappropriate, or untimely sensory afference so that a process of building or rebuilding sensorimotor interactions can be incorporated into appropriate therapeutic interventions.

SENSORY INFORMATION AND MOVEMENT

The interdependence of sensory afference and motor function is not fully understood. It appears that reliance on sensory afference to produce functional movement may depend on several factors, including the following:

(1) Is the movement novel or familiar to the patient? Kelso hypothesized that during early development of a motor skill, a greater reliance on sensory input is needed to effectively learn the motor task.[3] Schmidt suggested that external feedback is critical to the establishment of an internal reference of correctness.[4] For example, knowledge of performance is a practice variable that is used during treatment to facilitate a desired response.[5] Winstein suggested that an internal reference of correctness develops with practice and can take the place of extrinsic feedback. This depends on the ability to demonstrate the same change in performance when the external feedback is withdrawn.

(2) Is the movement rapid or slow? If movement, even in abnormal synergies, can be initiated by a patient, perhaps the motor pattern can be shaped through sensory feedback to produce a functional outcome.[6-8] The use of sensory information to improve functional performance takes processing time. Movements requiring inputs from visual, vestibular, auditory, and/or somatosensory systems require a latency exceeding 100 msec. This means that if someone were pushed from behind, sensory inputs would not contribute to the correction of posture until more than 100 msec had elapsed.[9,10] If movements are non-ballistic, then the chance of incorporating meaningful sensory afference to guide motion is more probable. This concept would apply to both self-initiated as well as reactive movements.[11-14]

Some motor functions can be maintained in the absence of sensory feedback.[15-17] In humans, Diener et al reported that proprioceptive input from skin, pressure, and joint receptors of the foot played a minor role in compensation of rapid surface displacements.[11] Some rapid movements may begin independently of sensory "drive," but as movement progresses, somatosensory input is thought to be used to adapt movement to the velocity and amplitude of the stimulus.[18-20]

(3) Does the patient have an expectation of the type of response that is required to achieve a functional outcome? Certain compensatory movement responses are known to be modified when the subject's expectation of the stimulus characteristics change. This phenomenon is termed "central-set" and is best conceptualized as a state of readiness with an expectation to move in a certain way. According to Schmidt,[4] central set prepares the sensory and motor systems for anticipated task conditions. Once a motion is initiated, central set can facilitate a more rapid response, but because conditions are anticipated, the response may be in error if these conditions unexpectedly change. For example, you may find yourself standing on a bus that stops every minute and then pulls forward to the next destination. After several stops you find there is no need to hold on to the safety rail because your postural adjustments are well practiced. Your expectation is that the bus will move forward after each stop. The predictable movement of the bus has helped you create a central set. If the bus unexpectedly moves backward, your incorrect anticipation of the task conditions will create an error in your balance response and the risk of falling will be increased.

ESSENTIAL ELEMENTS OF SENSORIMOTOR PROCESSING

Winstein and Schmidt described six sources of movement-related sensory information that form the basis of kinesthesis.[21] These are muscle spindles, golgi tendon organs, articular receptors, cutaneous receptors, vision, and audition. The use of sensory afference from these receptors defines limb movement and position through a complex interaction between the peripheral and central nervous systems. The importance of sensory afference is not the same for all movements (Figure 1). On one hand, spinal-mediated stretch reflexes are considered "hard-wired," meaning that a stimulus (muscle stretch) produces a response (muscle contraction) without modification from sensory afference during the course of the movement. At the opposite extreme, volitional movement is highly adaptable and can benefit from overlapping and often redundant sensory input.

In order to use sensory afference in physical therapy, it is necessary to understand the essential elements of sensorimotor processing. These elements are feedforward mechanism or open loop processing and feedback mechanism or closed loop processing (Figure 2; see Chapter 2). A feedforward mechanism creates a motor behavior which does not require sensory input during movement. For example, the reaction to a brief slip on an icy sidewalk requires rapid postural compensation which is not influenced by sensory feedback.

The advantage of a feedforward mechanism in the human design is that it provides an efficient, stereotypic response that is preprogrammed. This means that once the reaction is "triggered," the same set of muscles will be recruited with fixed latencies to adjust limb or body equilibrium. Errors in movement are corrected only after the completion of a feedforward movement. This is why preprogrammed patterns of motion are referred to as "open loop" (sensory feedback is not in the loop that generates motion).

However, sensory perception can have an influence on preprogrammed motor behavior prior to the "triggered" reaction. The patient's expectation, as well as the degree of practice, can change the stereotypic pattern of muscle discharge.[22] Nashner and Cordo demonstrated that large burst EMG activity in the lower limb during postural adjustments was attenuated dramatically when the subject placed his finger on an adjacent table.[23] The actual stabilization provided by this finger placement was insignificant, yet the underlying muscle response was modified to meet the subject's perception of greater initial stability.

In contrast, a feedback mechanism provides visual, vestibular, auditory, and/or somatosensory input to guide a movement to an appropriate outcome. For example, relearning a symmetrical gait pattern may require verbal cues or some visual monitoring of the extent of weightbearing on the

FIGURE 1. Movement continuum. Most motor patterns are characterized by some "mix" of reflex and voluntary movement.

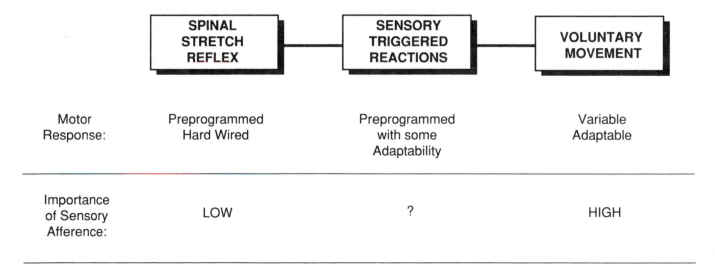

	SPINAL STRETCH REFLEX	SENSORY TRIGGERED REACTIONS	VOLUNTARY MOVEMENT
Motor Response:	Preprogrammed Hard Wired	Preprogrammed with some Adaptability	Variable Adaptable
Importance of Sensory Afference:	LOW	?	HIGH

FIGURE 2. Open and closed loop sensorimotor processing.

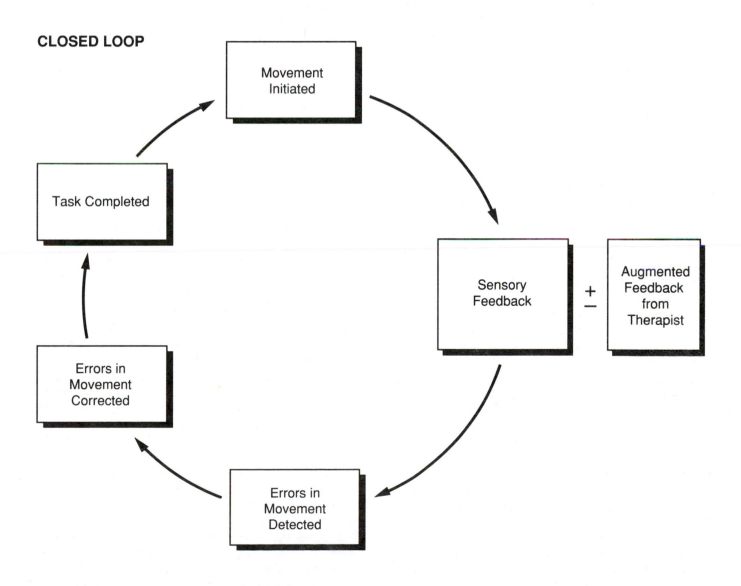

For more detailed description of the types of feedback, refer to Schmidt RA: Feedback and Knowledge of Results.
In Schmidt RA (ed): Motor Control and Learning: A Behavioral Emphasis (2nd ed.) Champaign, IL, Human Kinetics Pub Inc, 1988

paretic extremity. During ambulation, there is continuous intrinsic sensory feedback concerning performance of the gait pattern. In cases where patients have isolated sensory deficits, such as loss of position sense, other sensory modalities can be substituted to develop an appropriate motor response.

The working threshold of peripheral sensory end-organs has direct application to a discussion of sensory feedback mechanisms. Research has addressed the physiologic thresholds and working ranges of receptors, such as the muscle spindle and Golgi tendon organs, as well as visual end organs.[11,24-26] Physical therapists should consider the anatomical and physiological limitations of these receptors. For example, the patient can use visual information for continuous error-corrections (on-line feedback), whereas muscle afferents can provide the stimulus to trigger a rapid, predetermined movement (i.e., a correction in limb position following perturbation).

In the early stages of treatment, patient generated movement may be dependent predominantly on peripheral feedback. During initial phases of learning, the patient needs an external model to guide his movements. When sensory feedback is absent or distorted, other sources of information, such as electromyographic (EMG) biofeedback, can serve as an external model and inform the patient and therapist about the consequences of a movement. As learning progresses, internal control structures are developed and there is less need for peripheral feedback.

ASSESSMENT AND TREATMENT PRINCIPLES

The paresis seen in many neuromotor disorders may be caused by alterations in motor unit discharge patterns and reduced firing rate caused by damage to supraspinal descending systems. For example, patients with cerebral vascular accidents (CVA) have difficulty generating force at high velocities of movement due to their inability to recruit fast-twitch motor units.[27] Such patients should perform their neuromotor retraining initially at slow velocities. Vibration, resistance, electrical stimulation, and tactile stimulation are examples of sensory techniques which can be used to enhance motor unit recruitment. These therapeutic techniques should be used in conjunction with voluntary effort[28-30] and should be withdrawn when the patient has relearned a movement. A strengthening sequence of activities may then be used.[31-32]

A hyperactive stretch reflex causes hypertonicity or resistance to passive movement. Several inhibition techniques have been used to reduce hyperactivity. Some of these techniques are empirically based, but in others a neurophysiological basis has been determined. Techniques used to alter abnormal tone include: slow elongation of the shortened muscle group, slow stroking of the extremity, rhythmic rotation, cryotherapy, weight bearing or moving the body on the affected extremity, vibration of the antagonist muscles, and splinting or casting.[6,33-34] The reduction of spasticity by these techniques is usually temporary and does not necessarily translate into an increase in functional movement. New experimental data suggest that spasticity in patients with CNS damage is not only due to increased alpha motoneuron discharge, but also to abnormal programming and regulation of the motor neuron pool for selective and coordinated

movement.[35,36] If during active performance the patient has excessive and prolonged motor unit activity, reducing the effort of the movement and facilitating smooth, reciprocal movements should carry over to functional movements.

Hilton's law states that the same trunk of nerves furnishes a distribution to a group of muscles moving a given joint, the skin over the insertion of these muscles, and the interior of the joint being moved by the muscle group. This arrangement creates an interdependence among skin sensation, muscle action, and joint movement. The physiologic principles of Hilton's law apply most directly to movement that requires sensory feedback. The following five principles will enhance further our understanding of the interdependence between biomechanical and neurological mechanisms:[37]

1. Joints can rely on soft tissue for stability. Muscle action alone does not always account for stability.
   Example: During certain phases of pathologic gait[38] or during balance compensations[39] the knee may be hyperextended, in which case joint capsule and ligamentous structures are used to provide joint stability.

2. Kinematic parameters such as the extent, amplitude, and velocity of movement will alter proprioceptive input and change the characteristics of the motor response.
   Example: Proprioceptive input from skin, pressure, and joint receptors of the foot plays a significant role in correction of slow postural disturbances, but only a minor role in the correction of rapid balance perturbations.[11]

3. The same motor activity can be produced by action of different muscles.
   Example: During cycling activities, EMG records obtained from vastus lateralis and rectus femoris were up to 80% more variable than the foot force applied to the pedal.[40]

4. Functional joint range-of-motion (ROM) is a prerequisite for functional movement. If the neuromuscular response is learned or relearned in the absence of functional joint ROM, then the therapeutic outcome is compromised. Joint ROM should be treated from an osteokinematic and arthrokinematic perspective.[41,42]

5. Degrees of freedom influence movement complexity. As the number of joints involved in a movement increases, the complexity of demand on neurologic and biomechanic requirements increases.[43] The number of degrees of freedom associated with functional movements may not be noted by the therapist who attends only to specific isolated muscle or joint responses, and treatment, therefore, may not be planned appropriately.

From the previous examples, one may speculate that some of the motor control problems in patients with CNS damage, such as inappropriate cocontraction, difficulty initiating movement, slow velocity of movement, inability to combine limb synergies, and decreased coordination, may be attributed to disorders of sensory perception as well as to involvement of the motor system itself.[32]

The physical therapist should assess which sensory systems are functionally intact or compromised (see Chapters 7 and 10). Assessment may include classic sensory tests, such as testing appreciation of light touch, pressure, pain, and temperature. Tests of more complex perceptual functions, such as stereognosis, position in space, and perception of the vertical may also be administered. The type and amount of sensory/perceptual testing done by the physical therapist will depend on the patient's neurologic deficits as well as on information available from other team members, such as occupational therapists, neurologists, and neuropsychologists, who may have administered sensory/perceptual tests as part of their assessment of the patient. Following sensory/perceptual assessment, the therapist then selects the appropriate stimuli to provide feedback about motor performance. Most therapeutic techniques provide a combination of four types of information from vision, the vestibular system, audition, and somatosensation (skin pressure receptors, plus muscle and joint sensory receptors which signal movement of the body parts).[37] If one sensory system is impaired, other systems can substitute to provide feedback and enhance motor learning or relearning. For example, if a patient does not respond to vestibular input, or responds inappropriately, then proprioceptive or visual cues can be used in the initial intervention. Stroking, stretching, and compression are just a few examples of somatosensory feedback which may help shape a movement.

Electromyographic biofeedback is an external mode of sensory feedback that may minimize sensory deficits and augment motor performance.[44-46] However, a practical limitation is the number of muscles that can be monitored simultaneously.

Bach-y-Rita and Bailliet suggested the following general guidelines for providing sensory feedback in patients with hemiplegia:[47]

1. Establish baseline general relaxation conditions to obtain optimal use of sensory information
2. Practice slow, reciprocal motor control of the uninvolved extremity as a model to suppress unnecessary muscle activity and/or to facilitate voluntary control of the involved extremity
3. Practice voluntary, reciprocal movements of the involved side
4. Practice functional, goal-directed activities rather than isolated muscle actions. Much practice (repetition) of the sequence is needed to establish more normal control of movement.

Studies are needed to determine the therapeutic effect of sensory feedback and evaluate other relevant factors such as the influence of the amount of therapy and possible placebo effects.[33]

PRINCIPLES OF LEARNING

Variable practice sessions and schedules of withdrawing feedback when the patient has learned a movement have been proposed.[48,49] According to Schmidt, there are certain qualitative and quantitative factors that may affect any method of learning or relearning and these factors should be considered in sensory-based treatment.[4] Several principles of motor learning are listed:

1. Verbal post-response information from another person, such as a physical therapist, about task outcome (Knowledge of Results-KR) is the most important variable for motor learning.
2. Other activities should not occur in the interval between movement completion and when KR is provided. One hypothesis is that sensory "feel" of the movement needs to be retained to be associated with KR. If other movements are completed before KR is provided, it may interfere with this memory task.
3. If the interval from KR until the next response is requested is too short, learners appear to have difficulty generating a new and different movement on the next trial. For example, if the patient is asked immediately to repeat a reaching task, he may not have had sufficient time to process the KR and change the movement strategy.
4. Information-processing activities inserted in the interval from KR until the next response probably decrease performance and learning. Asking the patient to perform tasks unrelated to the movement may interfere with the process of using KR to modify and plan the next movement. An example would be talking to the patient about topics unrelated to therapy or the movement being planned.
5. Both the relative frequency of KR (the percentage of trials on which KR is given) and the absolute frequency (the number of KRs given) are important for learning. Intermittent feedback is more beneficial for learning than continuous feedback (Figure 3).
6. In adult learners, performance increases with increases in KR precision (accuracy with which the KR is given). Too much precision may be detrimental to learning in children.
7. Knowledge of performance (information about the learner's movements) can be given through videotapes, kinetic, or kinematic feedback. All appear to enhance performance and may have a positive effect on learning.
8. Prior to practice, methods such as motivation for performance, goal setting, and modeling are all beneficial to learning.
9. Variable practice sequences are slightly more effective than constant practice conditions for adults and much more effective in children. Randomly ordered practice is more effective than blocked practice.
10. Simulated activities, part-to-whole procedures, and mental practice may or may not facilitate transfer of learning to some criterion task.

CASE STUDIES

When selecting therapeutic strategies for improving functional outcomes, the elements of sensorimotor processes and the relationship of these elements to neuroanatomical and physiological concepts have formed the basis of interventions described in the case studies that follow.

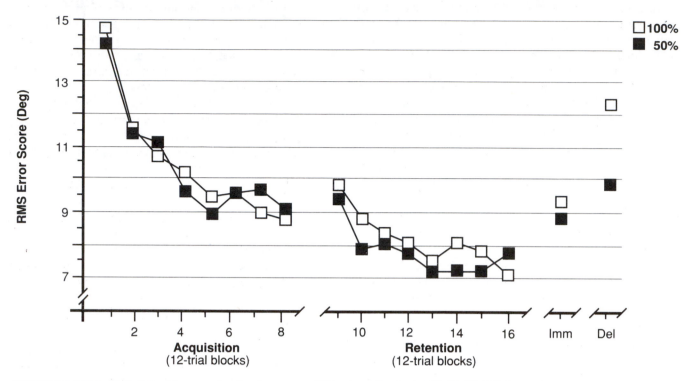

FIGURE 3. *Average root-mean squared (RMS) error for the two acquisition KR relative frequency conditions for Day 1 (Blocks 1-8), Day 2 (Blocks 9-16), immediate, and delayed no-KR retention tests. (KR = knowledge of results). Results show practive with lower relative frequencies of KR may be beneficial to longer-term retention and learning.*

(From Winstein CJ, Schmidt RA: Reduced frequency of results enhances motor skill learning. J. Exp. Psych. 16(4):677-691, 1990. Reprinted by permission of the publisher.)

CASE STUDY #1
JANE SMITH

Age: 74 years
Diagnosis: Right hemiplegia,
secondary to left cerebrovascular accident
Status: Six months post onset

ASSESSMENT

Assessment reveals the following problems related to sensory impairment: 1) right visual field deficits , 2) severe unilateral neglect of the hemiplegic side, and 3) inability to combine limb synergies in the upper extremity.

GOALS

Treatment goals are for the patient to:

1. focus attention on the neglected side

2. break down the stereotypic movement patterns into smaller components of movement, then combine and reorganize these components to increase the repertoire of movement options

3. fine tune and expand these new patterns in order to increase their flexibility.

FUNCTIONAL OBJECTIVES

Following 3 months of treatment, Mrs. Smith will be able to:

1. reach across the midline and pick up a spoon placed to the affected side of the body, 3 of 6 times

2. roll to the left independently to transfer out of bed, 100% of the time

3. reach for a glass with two hands, 3 out of 6 times

4. lift an object above the head with right elbow fully extended, 3 of 3 times.

TREATMENT RECOMMENDATIONS

Suggestions for management of Mrs. Smith's unilateral neglect include: (1) placing objects on her involved side and encouraging her to reach across the midline; (2) teaching her to roll toward her uninvolved side; (3) encouraging her to reach forward with her involved arm or leg; and (4) flashing lights or moving objects in the affected visual field to cue attention to the neglected side.[32]

The acquisition of selective control in the upper extremity requires combining the components of the flexion and extension patterns, reconstructing new movements, increasing the coordination of the movements, and incorporating the new movement patterns into functional tasks.

Examples of activities to increase the variety of movements of the involved upper extremity are:[31]

1. Sidelying — The therapist assists Mrs. Smith to flex the arm and slowly reverse into extension.

2. Supine — Mrs. Smith flexes her shoulder with elbow extension. Initially, the therapist should position the arm and ask the patient to hold the position (isometric muscle contraction) then lower the extremity against gravity (eccentric muscle contraction).

3. Supine — Mrs. Smith actively holds her shoulder in flexion as she attempts to alternately flex and extend the elbow.

4. Sitting — Mrs. Smith practices hand-to-mouth patterns.

5. Sitting — Mrs. Smith holds her arm in forward flexion with elbow extension.

6. Sitting — Mrs. Smith practices raising and lowering her arm with elbow extension (Figure 4).

7. All positions — Mrs. Smith uses the upper extremity in a variety of reaching activities, lifting activities, and in postural displacements.

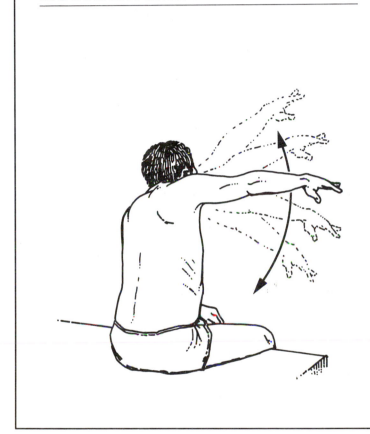

FIGURE 4. *Sitting, patient practices raising and lowering the arm with elbow extension.*

CASE STUDY #2
DANIEL JOHNSON

Age: 59 years
Diagnosis: Parkinson's Disease
Status: Four years post initial diagnosis

ASSESSMENT

Assessment reveals that use of sensory feedback and sensory feedforward systems may be helpful in addressing the following motor coordination problems: 1) poor synergistic organization of movement patterns for maintaining balance, and 2) difficulty initiating movement, particularly in rising from a chair.

GOALS

Treatment goals are for Mr. Johnson to:

1. increase his ability to respond to subtle perturbations in the standing position, particularly in the forward direction

2. increase his ability to stand up from a chair unaided.

FUNCTIONAL OBJECTIVES

Following 3 months of treatment, Mr. Johnson will be able to:

1. maintain upright stance at all times after a push on his sternum or sudden release of shoulder pressure

2. come to a standing position from a low chair, 3 of 5 times.

TREATMENT RECOMMENDATIONS

Specific training for improving balance responses should include subtle external perturbations of Mr. Johnson during stance, subtle volitional forward/backward and lateral sways in standing, and self-initiating movements that require anticipatory postural responses (i.e., standing and lifting the arm over the head). Once the responses are correct, they should be facilitated on other support surfaces and with varying visual conditions (foam and uneven surfaces; with and without vision — see Chapter 10). Velocity of the displacement and the base of support should be varied in order to increase the speed, amplitude, and adaptability of the response.

The essential components of the sit to stand task which need to be reinforced are:

1. alignment of both feet under Mr. Johnson to provide a more normal kinematic chain for shifting the weight forward and standing up

2. forward inclination of the trunk to bring the center of gravity over the feet (Figure 5)

3. hip and knee extension to allow weight-bearing through the lower extremities.

Clinically, the ability of Mr. Johnson to execute a movement may be aided greatly if appropriate anticipatory postural adjustments are made for him or if he consciously controls these normally automatic responses. Thus, he may be taught to rise from a chair by volitionally executing the normally automatic forward trunk movements in anticipation of a rise. The therapist initially may present the goal by using manual guidance, which involves passively moving the patient through the action to give him the idea of the movement.[50] Stating the goal in terms of the relationship of body parts and sequence of movements may help him organize the movement (i.e., "move your shoulders forward, then stand up"). Mr. Johnson also needs to be able to perform this task during the rest of the day when the environment changes. Adaptability of the response can be facilitated by practicing on chairs with variable heights and seating surfaces, chairs with and without arms, and on buses.

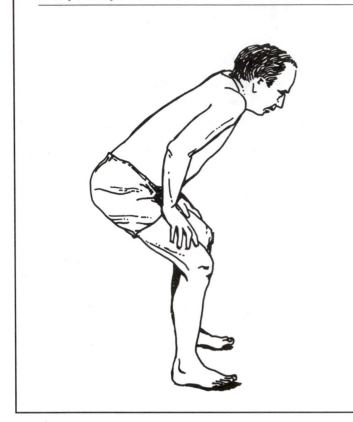

FIGURE 5. *Patient is encouraged to volitionally execute the normally automatic forward trunk movements in anticipation of a rise.*

CASE STUDY #3
SHIRLEY TEAL

Age: 21 years
Diagnosis: Post motor vehicle accident;
Closed head injury
Status: Four months post accident

ASSESSMENT

Assessment reveals the following problems which may be attributed to sensory impairment: 1) decreased weight shift over right foot and ankle during standing, and 2) excessive dependence on vision for balance control.

GOALS

Treatment goals are for Ms. Teal to:

1. improve ability to shift weight and maintain weight bearing on the right side during sitting and standing

2. improve balance and stability in the upright position without vision.

FUNCTIONAL OBJECTIVES

Following 2 months of treatment, Ms. Teal will be able to:

1. perform subtle weight shifts forward, backward, and laterally with proper alignment of hips, knees, and ankles while standing in the parallel bars, 3 of 5 times

2. maintain neutral alignment of hips and knees and with both feet flat on the floor for 30 seconds with the eyes closed while standing in the parallel bars

3. lean back on heels keeping head and trunk erect while standing in the parallel bars (Figure 6). Hold 5 seconds and return center of mass to vertical position, 3 of 5 times with eyes open and 3 of 5 times with eyes closed.

TREATMENT RECOMMENDATIONS

Standing in the parallel bars with the feet 4 inches apart, Ms. Teal will practice the following tasks:

1. look up at ceiling

2. turn head and trunk to look behind her in both directions

3. reach forward, backward, and laterally to obtain an object held by the therapist

4. stand on right foot, without leaning to side — simply shifting weight to right foot. Hold for five counts. Repeat with eyes closed

5. stand on right foot, placing left leg to the front. Hold for five counts. Repeat with eyes closed

6. throw/catch a ball

7. pick up objects from the floor.

Additional treatment strategies for visual dependence should focus on increasing proprioceptive inputs and increasing the base of support. Sensory stimulation in a weight-bearing position (i.e., stretch, joint compression, resistance, etc.) may be used to enhance feedback. Finally, the therapist should attempt to increase Ms. Teal's awareness of subtle displacements in her center of gravity while varying the base of support.

CASE STUDY #4
SHAWNA WELLS

Age: 4 years
Diagnosis: Cerebral palsy; spastic quadriparesis;
mild mental retardation
Status: Onset at birth

ASSESSMENT

Assessment suggests: 1) problems with tactile hypersensitivity, and 2) deficits in processing sensory information during movement based activities. Currently, Shawna does not like being handled initially in therapy, but becomes less resistant and more cooperative as the therapy session progresses. She is hesitant to play on moveable toys and often refuses to use her walker on surfaces other than tile floors. Her protective responses in sitting and standing are slow and often inefficient.

GOALS

Treatment goals are for Shawna to:

1. decrease possible tactile and vestibular hypersensitivity

2. improve balance and protective reactions during a variety of sensory tasks

3. participate in movement based games and activities with improved motor coordination.

FUNCTIONAL OBJECTIVES

Following 3 months of treatment, Shawna will be able to:

1. finger paint with pudding for 5 minutes without demanding that her hands be wiped

2. roll independently and quickly down a 6 foot inclined wedge

3. independently fall forward out of her walker onto a 3" thick mat, catching herself effectively with extended arms, 3 of 5 times

4. ride a tricycle independently for 100 feet within 15 minutes.

TREATMENT RECOMMENDATIONS

Shawna's physical therapy program should be coordinated with her home and school program, so similar activities are carried out at home by the parents and at school by teachers and therapists. Suggestions to decrease Shawna's tactile hypersensitivity include the following: 1) rubbing with terry cloth towels and lotion following bathing or swimming; 2) searching for toys hidden in containers of sand, rice, or beans; and 3) playing with gooey substances, such as fingerpainting with pudding, whipped cream, etc.

Shawna's poor protective reactions may be contributing to her dislike of movement-based activities. Emphasis on controlled falling from sitting and standing initially onto mats, then carpeting, and finally onto hard surfaces should be included in her program.

As Shawna is fearful of using her walker on uneven terrain, we would begin working on standing with the walker on various thickness of carpet or outside on grass. Gradually Shawna will be encouraged to walk short distances on carpeting and eventually outside on various surfaces (pavement, grass, gravel, etc.).

Problems in lower extremity dissociation and fear of movement can be addressed simultaneously by practicing independent propulsion on riding toys and/or a tricycle. Shawna will be assisted as much as necessary initially to successfully complete the task, with assistance decreased gradually. General movement activities, such as rolling up/down inclines, propelling herself prone on a scooterboard, and playing on playground equipment (swings, slides, merry-go-round) can be incorporated into her program. Shawna should be as independent as possible in each activity in controlling speed and amount of participation. The therapist should provide stability only as necessary for safety. ❏

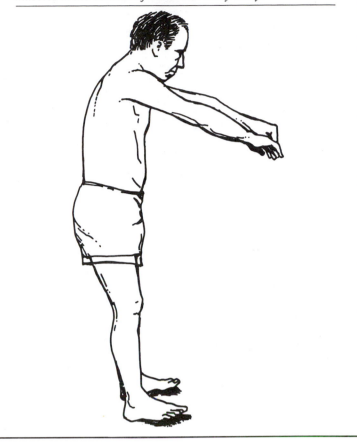

FIGURE 6. *Patient is encouraged to contract the ankle muscles in the context of volitional body sway.*

REFERENCES

1. Knapp HD, Taub E, Berman AJ: Movements in monkeys with deafferented forelimbs. Exp Neurol 7:305-315, 1963
2. Mott FW, Sherrington CS: Experiments upon the influence of sensory nerves upon movement and nutrition of the limbs. Proc R Soc Lond 57:481-488, 1985
3. Kelso JAS: The process approach to understanding human motor behavior: An introduction. In Kelso JAS (ed): Human Motor Behavior: An Introduction. Hillsdale, NJ, Lawrence Erlbaum Assoc Pub, 1982, pp 3-19
4. Schmidt RA: Motor Control and Learning. Champaign, IL, Human Kinetics Pub Inc, 1982
5. Winstein CJ: Motor learning considerations in stroke. In Duncan PW, Badke MB (eds): Stroke Rehabilitation: Recovery of Motor Control, Chicago, IL, Yearbook Med Pub, 1987, pp 109-134
6. Bobath B: Adult Hemiplegia, ed 2. London, Heinemann Medical, 1978
7. Brunnstrom S: Movement Therapy in Hemiplegia, New York, NY, Harper and Row, 1970
8. Carr JH, Sheperd RB: A Motor Relearning Program for Stroke. London, England, Aspen Systems Corp, 1983
9. Nashner LM: Adapting reflexes controlling the human posture. Exp Brain Res 26:59-72, 1976
10. Glencross D, Thornton E: Position sense following joint injury. J. Sports Med 21:23-27, 1981
11. Diener HC, Dichgans J, Guschlbauer B, et al: The significance of proprioception on postural stabilization as assessed by ischemia. Brain Res 296:103-109, 1984
12. Haas G, Diener HC, Rapp H, et al: Development of feedback and feedforward control of upright stance. Dev Med Child Neur 31:481-488, 1989
13. Cordo PJ, Nashner LM: Properties of postural adjustments associated with rapid arm movements. J Neurophysiol 47(2):287-302, 1982
14. Horak FB, Esselman P, Anderson ME, et al: The effects of movement velocity, mass displaced, and task certainty on associated postural adjustments made by normal and hemiplegic individuals. J Neurol Neurosurg Psychiatry 47:1020-1028, 1984
15. Grillner S, Rossignal S: On the initiation of the swing phase of locomotion in chronic spinal cats. Brain Res 149:503-507, 1978
16. Shik ML, Orlovsky GN: Neurophysiology of locomotor automatism. Physiol Rev 56:465-501, 1976
17. Taub E, Goldberg IA, Taub P: Deafferentation in monkeys: pointing at a target without visual feedback. Exp Neurol 46:178-186, 1975
18. Di Fabio RP, Badke MB, McEvoy A, Breunig A: Influence of local sensory afference in the calibration of human balance responses. Exp Brain Res (in press)
19. Diener HC, Horak FB, Nashner LM: Influence of stimulus parameters on human postural responses. J Neurophysiol 59:1888-1905
20. Horak FB, Diener HC, Nashner LM: Influence of central set on human postural responses. J of Neurophysiol 62(4):841-853, 1989
21. Winstein CJ, Schmidt RA: Sensorimotor feedback. In Holding D (ed): Human Skills, ed 2. Chichester, England, Wiley & Sons, 1989, pp 17-47
22. Bach-y-Rita PB, Lazarus J, Boyeson MG, et al: Neural aspects of motor function as a basis of early and post-acute rehabilitation. In DeLisa JA, Currie D, Gans B, et al (eds): Principles and Practice of Rehabilitation Medicine. Philadelphia, PA, JB Lippincott, 1988
23. Nashner LM, Cordo PJ: Relation of automatic postural responses and reaction-time voluntary movements of human leg muscles. Exp Brain Res 43:395-405, 1981
24. Poppele RE, Kennedy WR: Comparison between behaviour of human and cat muscle spindles recorded in vitro. Brain Res, 75:316-319, 1974
25. Goodwin GM, Hullinger M, Matthews WB: Studies on muscle spindle primary endings with sinusoidal stretching. In Homma S (ed): Understanding the Stretch Reflex. Progress in Brain Research, Vol. 44, Elsevier, Amsterdam, 1976, pp 89-98
26. Dichgans J, Brandt T: Visual-vestibular interaction. Effects on self-motion perception and postural control. In Held R, Leibowitz HW, Teuber HL (eds): Handbook of Sensory Physiology, Heidelberg, Springer, 1973, pp 755-804
27. Harro CC: Implications of motor unit characteristics to speed of movement in hemiplegia. Neurol Rep 9:55-60, 1985
28. Benton LA, Baker LL, Bowman BR, et al: Functional electrical stimulation - a practical clinical guide. Downey, CA, Rancho Los Amigos Rehabilitation Engineering Center, 1981
29. Bishop B: Possible application of vibration in treatment of motor dysfunction. Phys Ther 55:139-143, 1976
30. Griffin JW: Use of proprioceptive stimuli in therapeutic exercise. Phys Ther 54:1072-1079, 1974
31. Duncan PW, Badke MB: Stroke. In Payton O, Di Fabio RP, Paris SV, et al (eds): Manual of Physical Therapy - Neurology Section. New York, NY, Churchill Livingstone, 1988, pp 291-308
32. Duncan PW, Badke MB: Stroke Rehabilitation: The Recovery of Motor Control. Chicago, IL, Yearbook Medical Publishers, 1987
33. Bach-y-Rita P: Brain plasticity as a basis for the development of rehabilitation procedures for hemiplegia. Scand J Rehabil Med 13:73-83, 1981
34. Odeen I: Reduction of muscular hypertonus by long-term muscle stretch. Scand J Rehabil Med 13:93, 1981
35. Sahrmann SA, Norton BS: The relationship of voluntary movement to spasticity in the upper motoneuron syndrome. Ann Neurol 2:260-465, 1977
36. Miller S, Hammond GR: Neural control of arm movement in patients following stroke. In Van Hof MW, Mohn G, (eds): Functional Recovery from Brain Damage. Amsterdam, Elsevier/New Holland, 1981, pp 259-274
37. Badke MB, Di Fabio RP: Facilitation: a change in theoretical perspective and in clinical approach. In Basmajian J, Wolf SL (eds): Therapeutic Exercise, ed 5. Baltimore, MD, Williams and Wilkens, 1990, pp 77-92
38. Cerny K: Pathomechanics of stance, clinical concepts for analysis. Phys Ther 64:1851-1859, 1984
39. Jaeger R: Standing posture: Qualitative versus quantitative perspectives. The Behavioral and Brain Sciences 8:l, 1985
40. Brooke JD, Boyce DE, McIlroy WE, et al: Transfer of variability from electromyogram to propulsive force in human locomotion, Electromyograph Clin Neurophysiol 26: 389-400, l986
41. MacConaill MA, Basmajian JV: Muscles and Movements: a basis for human kinesiology. New York, NY, Robert E. Krieger Publishing Co, Huntington, 1977, pp 3-39l
42. Brooks S: Coma. In Payton O, Di Fabio RP, Paris SV, et al (eds): Manual of Physical Therapy, New York, NY, Churchill Livingstone, 1988, pp 215-238
43. Bernstein N: Some emergent problems of the regulation of motor acts. The Coordination and Regulation of Movements. Oxford, England, Pergamon Press, pp ll4-l42, l967
44. Brudny J, Korein J, Levidow L, et al: Sensory feedback therapy as a modality of treatment in central nervous system disorders of voluntary movement. Neurology 24:825-832, 1974
45. Brudny J, Korein J, Grynbaum BB, et al: Helping hemiparetics to help themselves: Sensory feedback therapy. JAMA 241:814-818, 1979
46. Wolf SL: Electromyographic biofeedback applications to stroke patients. Phys Ther 63:1448-1459, 1983
47. Bach-y-Rita P, Bailliet R: Recovery from stroke. In Duncan PW, Badke MB (eds): Stroke Rehabilitation: The Recovery of Motor Control. Chicago, IL, Yearbook Medical Publisher, Inc, 1987
48. Salmoni AW, Schmidt RA, Walter CB: Knowledge of results and motor learning: a review and critical reappraisal. Psychol Bull 95(3):355-386, 1984
49. Martenuik RG: Information Processing in Motor Skills. New York, NY, Holt, Rinehart and Winston, 1976
50. Carr JH, Sheperd RB: Movement Science: Foundations for Physical Therapy in Rehabilitation, Rockville, MD, Aspen Publishers, 1987

Chapter 9
Disorders in Motor Synergies, Initiation, and Termination of Movement

Carol A. Giuliani, Ph.D., PT

INTRODUCTION

We think of normal motor control as the ability to perform a well coordinated movement that involves navigating multiple limb segments in space and arriving at a target with some degree of accuracy and control. The simplest movement is often a frustrating task for patients with motor dysfunction. For therapists treating these patients, assessing the movement dysfunction and determining treatment are formidable assignments. This chapter will address the specific problems of producing movement synergies (patterns), initiating movement, and terminating movement.

Therapists commonly describe abnormal movement synergies in the summary of their neurological exam. Describing initiation and termination of movement are less commonly included. However, general descriptions, such as "past pointing" or "finger to nose test" when testing cerebellar function, and descriptions of movement difficulties in patients with Parkinson's disease or with cerebellar dysfunction may be a part of the assessment. Specific tests of motor function are used more frequently for diagnosis and identifying the area of lesion rather than for identifying motor control deficits. Describing movement dysfunction in terms of the pattern, initiation, and termination of movement may be useful for identifying movement control problems and for guiding therapists in the development of treatment plans. Measuring changes in patterns, initiation, and termination of movement are excellent methods for documenting patient response to treatment. Describing these aspects of movements may help us identify changes in the quality of movement; those things that we observe but have difficulty measuring objectively.

THEORETICAL FRAMEWORK

As described in previous chapters, motor control involves initiating and controlling voluntarily generated patterns of movements. Coordinated movement is not just a series of integrated reflexes as proposed in early theories. Functional movements are composed of a series of events involving several joints and using many muscles that are activated at the appropriate time and which produce the correct amount of force so that smooth, coordinated movement occurs. Isolated strength of an individual muscle or muscle group may have little to do with using that muscle or muscles in concert with others to perform a specific task. Sequencing and timing events are important. Not surprisingly, static tests of muscle strength do not always predict movement performance. Likewise, performance of one type of task does not predict performance of another type of task. For example, I may be skilled at walking across a balance beam, but have considerable difficulty striking a tennis ball. There are many factors that affect pattern or synergy formation, initiation, and termination of movement.

FACTORS AFFECTING THE PRODUCTION OF MOVEMENT PATTERNS OR SYNERGIES

A lack of selective joint control during attempted voluntary movement is usually described as the presence of stereotypic movement synergies or abnormal patterns.[1] Well controlled intralimb and interlimb coordination observed in normal movement may be replaced by mass limb movement patterns and difficulty coordinating movement among limbs in patients with neurologic dysfunction.[1] Although the movement patterns of each patient with a neurologic disorder are unique, physical therapists frequently use global terms to describe a characteristic pattern of body posture and limb movement for diagnostic groups. For example, movement in a patient with a CVA is described frequently as "he has a hemiplegic gait" or "he uses an upper limb synergy." Just what is meant when movement patterns are described this way, and what information does it provide for developing a treatment plan? We should be cautious when using general terms to describe movement, because patients frequently do not fit a general characterization. We must describe the patterns of movement observed in each patient at each assessment in order to recognize underlying problems.

Many factors may contribute to a patient using an abnormal movement pattern. These contributing factors may originate centrally, peripherally, or both. Central factors may include damage to the neural circuitry that generates the movement pattern, aberrant input (inhibition or facilitation) to the circuitry, or abnormal motoneuron recruitment. Peripheral factors may include muscle fiber atrophy, changes in muscle stiffness, and muscle shortening.

Producing well coordinated movement requires the interaction of both biomechanical and neuromuscular systems. Patients with hemiparesis have difficulty producing and controlling the muscle forces necessary for generating normal patterns of movement. These deficits may be related to changes in biomechanical and neuromuscular factors. For example, alterations in viscoelastic properties of muscles and tendons may increase muscle stiffness and passive restraint to movement.[2,3] Stiffness also may be a factor that inhibits speed of movement.[4] Muscle shortening may occur from immobilization due to spasticity or joint immobilization.[5] These mechanical changes may affect movement patterns. Mechanisms of neural control depend on the properties of the musculoskeletal apparatus. To appreciate the effects of small mechanical changes on movement patterns, consider the effect of increasing the length of your arm. Place a splint on one of your fingers and observe how often you make errors in movement. How long does it take you to adjust to the limb length change? Although you are aware of the apparent changes in limb length, a period of training is necessary to adjust the movement patterns appropriately.

Several researchers have reported that muscles of hemiparetic limbs have muscle fiber atrophy, predominately of the Type II fibers [6,7,8] and sometimes a hypertrophy of Type I fibers.[9] In addition to altered motor unit morphology, abnormal firing patterns were reported in subjects with hemiplegia.[10,11] Both the atrophy of fast fibers and a decreased rate of firing have been associated with reduced muscle force.[10]

Knutsson and Richards examined the EMG patterns in 23 subjects with hemiplegia.[12] They reported that each subject usually demonstrated one of three characteristic EMG patterns. The first pattern was characterized by premature activation of the triceps surae muscles during early stance, the second pattern by low levels of muscle activity with a normal temporal pattern, and the third pattern by coactivation of several muscle groups during the gait cycle. Knutsson and Richards concluded that each subject had a unique motor

control problem during locomotion that was reflected in their EMG pattern.[12]

Mechanical changes, reduced firing rates, and poor regulation of motor unit activity may help explain the difficulty in force and speed production observed in subjects with hemiparesis.[13,14] A decreased ability to regulate force at the appropriate time may result in altered or abnormal patterns of movement.

FACTORS AFFECTING THE INITIATION OF MOVEMENT

Cognitive processing will affect the initiation of movement and was discussed in Chapter 7. There may be a problem with the patient recognizing a command or signal to move, recalling and selecting the movement plan, or assembling and initiating the plan to move. All this takes place before initial movement is observed. If patients have difficulty initiating a movement, deficits in central processing must be considered.

In addition to cognitive processing, several neuromuscular factors can affect movement initiation. To move, a person must: 1) produce adequate muscle force to overcome gravity, inertial forces, or antagonist muscle restraint; 2) have an adequate rate of force production, that is the force must be produced in a certain time period; 3) have passive joint range of motion (ROM) that allows movement; 4) have an appropriate context and initial condition to perform the task; and 5) be motivated to move.

The first two factors may affect the initiation of movement as well as pattern formation and were discussed in the previous section. The third factor, sufficient ROM, is discussed in Chapter 4. How do context and initial condition, the fourth factor, affect movement initiation? These are variables affecting the expression of a behavior. That is, a person may have the capacity to initiate a movement, but may not do so. For example, if you tested reaching of a patient when he is in a standing position, he may not perform the task. It may be because he doesn't have the strength in his arm muscles, or he doesn't have adequate balance and would fall with attempted arm movement. It is also possible that he doesn't have his glasses on and cannot see the target; has bursitis and shoulder flexion is accompanied by severe pain; or is nauseated and avoids any movement.

The context involves factors such as balance ability and the interface between the patient and the environment. Therapists are familiar with the need to train patients on different walking surfaces so they learn to function in environments other than hospital clinics. The movement surface itself may affect the initiation of movement as well the pattern observed. For example, I quickly become immobilized when I step out my back door and find myself standing on a sheet of ice.

Just as important as physical factors, psychosocial factors, the final factor, can affect movement initiation. Certainly, if the patient in the previous example is not motivated to perform the movement, he may not. If he thinks it's a dumb task, or if in his culture women don't tell people what to do, he may not attempt the movement.

Many factors may affect initiation of movement. The movement may not be initiated at all or the speed and control exhibited during movement onset may be problematic for the task.

FACTORS AFFECTING THE TERMINATION OF MOVEMENT

Problems with movement termination are associated with difficulty producing alternating movements and changing directions of movement during a task. Patients may have difficulty controlling appropriate forces of the agonist at the end of a movement. This may be due to inappropriate initial scaling of agonist forces when the movement plan was generated or the inability to make modifications in force parameters. Accuracy, target acquisition, and reversing movement direction may be affected if subjects cannot control end points of movement. Sahrmann and Norton reported that patients with spastic hemiparesis had difficulty turning off agonist muscles and this was characterized by prolonged agonist activity.[15]

Difficulty terminating movement also may be due to an inability to produce adequate antagonist force at the appropriate time. Timing difficulties with muscle activation are common for patients with neurologic problems, and have been reported in patients with cerebellar, cortical, and basal ganglia disorders.[16]

Visual spatial deficits can affect movement termination. If the patient does not perceive distance or location correctly, he may create erroneous parameters that will produce inaccuracies at termination or target acquisition. For specific information about sensory deficits and movement problems refer to information presented in Chapter 8.

ASSESSMENT PRINCIPLES

The purpose of an assessment is to examine the patient and identify the problem(s), establish functional outcome goals with the patient, and determine treatment. We may want to use both voluntary and facilitated movements that are functional and goal directed. Assessment must describe accurately the movement in terms that identify the movement problem: what we see and when we see it. Why we see certain movements is less objective and requires formation of working hypotheses.

Remember that we will perform subsequent assessments to determine the effectiveness of treatment and make appropriate modifications. To ensure accurate assessment and reassessment review the information on standardized assessments in Chapter 6.

In this chapter, the assessment of movement patterns (synergies), initiation, and termination of movement will be discussed. These aspects of movement coordination are important for performing accurate functional tasks. Methods of assessment as well as treatment are suggested.

PATTERNS

When identifying movement patterns, it is important to describe the movement pattern(s), the consistency of the pattern(s), and the effect of movement speed on the pattern(s). One should describe the pattern/synergy so that another therapist reading the evaluation will have a clear picture of what the patient does. Avoid describing patterns or synergies in general terms, such as, "the patient has a lower limb extensor synergy," or "the patient has severe extensor spasticity." Use descriptive terms for identifying patient abilities. For example, when a patient gets up from a chair, does he lean forward first then push up or is he pushing into extension with his legs before he leans his trunk forward? (Figure 1)

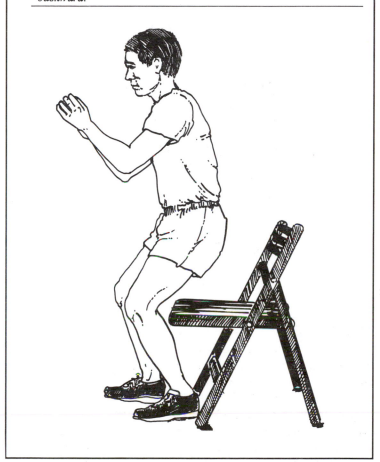

FIGURE 1. *Rising from a chair to standing. If knee extension occurs before trunk is flexed forward, the patient tends to fall backward.*

Describe the segments used to perform the movement, the order of segment movement, and associated adjustments in other segments. Have the patient perform the movement several times, if possible, without producing fatigue. Does the patient use the same movement pattern on each trial? The variability of patterns used may be just as important as the pattern itself. From a theoretical, as well as a functional standpoint, in most cases variability is better than consistency if the movement pattern is abnormal. If it is consistent and abnormal it may be more difficult to change. Observe in what other conditions/situations different patterns of movement occur.

Ask the patient to perform the task or movement at different speeds, and observe the affect of speed on the pattern and the variability of the pattern. Speed is a good probe for identifying difficulties we might not see if the patient moves at a self-selected speed. Changing movement speed will provide a better assessment of movement control.

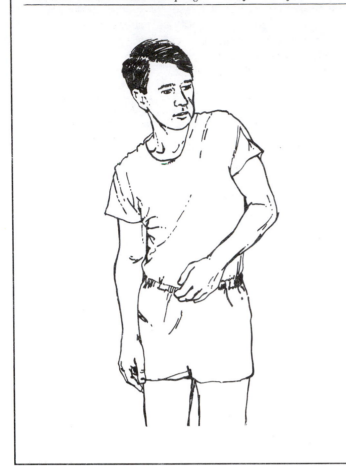

FIGURE 2. *Abnormal shoulder synergy of elbow flexion and shoulder elevation when attempting to reach for an object.*

Remember that the patterns used for movement are specific to the task and we cannot assume that the movement synergies used by the patient for one task will be used for another task. Obviously we cannot assess movement for every possible task (Figure 2). Selecting a few functional tasks that are meaningful and important to the patient will be most time efficient. Other tasks may be added to future assessments as time permits and the patient's ability improves.

Don't forget musculoskeletal assessment. Is there sufficient joint ROM? What about limb lengths and segment mass? These factors alone may all contribute to abnormal movement synergies.

INITIATION

Initiation of movement may be affected by numerous factors including environmental, biomechanical, neuromuscular, and central processing functions. It is an over simplification to attribute initiation problems only to motor deficits.

The first consideration is to ensure that we measure the performance that best reflects the patient's capacity for movement. This is especially important for movement initiation. The conditions and physical context of the assessment affect the patient's performance. The psychosocial context (environment, motivation, or social situation) are also important. Likewise, the demands and meaning of the task may affect a patient's response. One of my Taiwanese graduate students related an interesting observation: "In this country, many Chinese people are taught to use American utensils after they have had a stroke." For these people, a fork may be a novel and meaningless object. If they do not move their arm to lift when instructed to do so, we may be mistaken if we conclude that they are lacking arm control.

Commands to move may also affect the patient's response. Are the commands verbal or non-verbal? Is the terminology appropriate? Should we use lay terms? These factors may affect the initiation of movement more than the pattern or termination of movement.

How quickly does the patient respond to a command? Measuring the length of time from the command to when the patient starts to move (reaction time) may be important for identifying movement problems. If the task requires rapid movement or a quick onset of force, we must know if the patient can meet these demands. For example, patients with Parkinson's disease may initiate movement quickly, but perform movements very slowly. Reaction time (initiation time) can be measured in the clinic with a stop watch or by reviewing video tapes and counting the number of frames between the signal or command and the first movement observed.

To assess initiation ability, we must differentiate between environmental influences, central processing, and neuromuscular difficulties before determining the appropriate treatment. If the patient has a timely response to the command to move, but has difficulty producing speed and force, it is less likely to be a central processing problem. Having both processing and movement problems occurring together in a patient with a cerebral lesion or brain trauma makes assessment of motor function very difficult.

TERMINATION

For goal directed tasks, terminating a movement is important for target accuracy. Patients who have difficulty terminating movement may overshoot or undershoot the target (Figure 3). Terminating movement is just as important as initiating the movement. Problems with movement termination are best assessed by using tasks that require end-point accuracy or target acquisition. By placing a target or object at different spatial coordinates, we can determine if the difficulty is related to a spatial area, to specific muscle groups needed to move in different directions, or to visual spatial deficits. As with testing movement patterns or synergies, speed is a good probe. Patients may not have difficulty in accuracy when moving slowly, but when asked to move as quickly as possible, control may deteriorate. This is a well known phenomenon for individuals without neurologic disorders. Whenever movement speed, increases accuracy may be compromised. Patients must be able to accomplish tasks in an adequate period so that they are functional and energy is conserved.

Ask the patient to perform unidirectional and multidirectional tasks as well as those that require reversing movement direction. Observe when the endpoint control breaks down.

Most likely, it will not be the same for all tasks or all conditions. These observations will help you determine the tasks and conditions to use in treatment.

TREATMENT STRATEGIES

Once the therapist identifies the problems, and the therapist and the patient agree on goals, an appropriate treatment strategy and specific methods of treatment can be determined. Errors in problem identification may lead to prescribing and administering a treatment that is inappropriate and ineffective and thus careful observation is extremely important.

Practice must be specific to the ability we want to improve. If we want faster initiation and termination of movement, tasks must be structured to provide practice of these skills.

Vary the practice of a particular task. Practicing movements or tasks at several different speeds is especially helpful for improving movement initiation and control. Provide feedback during practice to enhance motor learning. Feedback may be verbal, visual, or tactile. However, excessive feedback or guidance may be detrimental to the positive effects of practice. Practice provides an opportunity for the patient to learn what he is doing wrong and problem solve to correct his error. If the patient learns that feedback is always available from the therapist, he may not learn to recognize his errors and apply problem solving skills. Patients perform much better during treatment than when they leave the clinic or when they return the next day. Although these patients may look better with a therapist facilitating movement, the therapist cannot be there to correct them constantly. The type of practice and the amount of feedback given to the patient will depend on the skill(s) being developed.

Changing movement patterns in patients with neurologic disorders is difficult. Movement patterns may be changed more easily by using mechanical intervention. The use of orthotics to stabilize or restrict a joint or body segment may improve or worsen a movement pattern. Likewise, adapted seating methods may improve accuracy of reach, but if applied incorrectly, functional ability may diminish.

Therapists should emphasize goal directed movement during practice. Asking the patient to use specific muscles or to control timing of muscle activity may be too confusing to the patient during most gross motor activities. Fine hand coordination or training after tendon transfer, however, requires this specific information and effort from the patient.

SUMMARY

Producing well coordinated movement involving multiple limb segments and body parts is a complex task that depends on the interaction of multiple internal and external systems. Assessing complex movement by identifying movement patterns and problems associated with initiating and terminating movement will help therapists apply effective treatments. All these skills are important for performing functional tasks. If therapists can identify motor dysfunction using concepts of motor control and direct their intervention

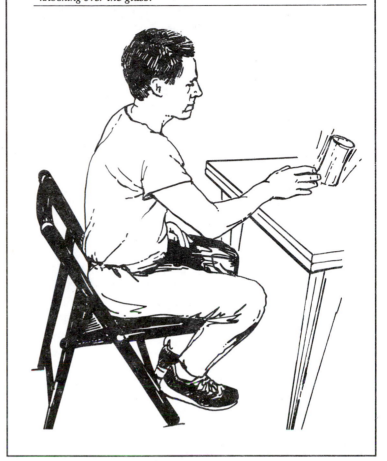

FIGURE 3. *Adult seated reaching for a glass of water. His inability to control termination of movement results in knocking over the glass.*

to the problems of control, they will be using a scientific approach to treatment. Taking this approach, I believe the time spent in treatment will be used more efficiently.

CASE STUDY #1
JANE SMITH

Age: 74 years
Diagnosis: Right hemiplegia,
secondary to left cerebrovascular accident
Status: Six months post onset

ASSESSMENT

Let's examine the information presented and try to understand what it tells us about the patient's problems, and then decide what other information we need before we can develop a treatment plan. The presence of a flexion synergy in the right arm does not tell us anything about Mrs. Smith's ability to use her arm or control arm movement. We need to know what movement pattern(s) she uses for voluntary familiar tasks. How accurate is she within her limited ability to use her arm and is the pattern the same or different for various tasks? What happens to the pattern and accuracy with a speed demand? Does she have different movement abilities in different positions, such as supine and sitting?

The description of limb control in gait also is lacking valuable information. She has active hip flexion in swing, but poor foot placement. We need to know how swing is initiated and the pattern of leg movement during the cycle. Just what is the problem with the foot placement? Is it poor because the ankle is unstable or because the ankle is in plantarflexion at footstrike? There are certainly other possibilities that could fit the "poor" description.

Mrs. Smith needs minimal assistance for transfers. What limb and trunk sequence does she use to get out of a chair? Can we determine if she has muscle strength deficits or sequencing problems? With further testing, she uses a sequence of shoulder elevation, followed by elbow flexion, and then combined shoulder flexion and elbow flexion when asked to perform hand to mouth or any movement toward her body. She moves through less than 50% of the ROM required to complete the task. When asked to reach toward an object and away from the body, she initiates elbow extension with minimal shoulder flexion in the sitting position. She cannot move at varying speeds and arm movement is slow. She can initiate finger flexion to grasp an object, but is unable to release. She has poor reciprocal joint movement at all upper limb joints, and is always stuck in the first direction of the movement. Passive ROM is within normal limits for her elbow and wrist. Passive shoulder flexion and abduction are limited to 90° by pain and there is minimal scapular movement.

Right foot heel strike during gait occurs with the ankle in inversion. During quiet standing she has her foot flat and can support her weight on the limb. She initiates swing with much effort and with the hip in flexion. Knee flexion during swing is lacking and she often circumducts her leg to advance her limb. Step length on the right is much shorter than on the left. When asked to walk as fast as possible, flexion ROM decreases in the right knee, inversion increases at the ankle, and she lengthens her step on the left leg. Passive ROM is within normal limits for all joints of the lower extremity, although she does exhibit clonus in her right ankle extensors.

Mrs. Smith is unable to get out of a chair without assistance and loses her balance during standing if she tries to move her feet. She attempts to rise from the chair in a clear movement sequence. First, she leans forward so that her shoulders are over her knees, and then needs help to lift off the seat. Her body moves up and backward so that she ends standing with her shoulders directly over her hips and feet. Movement is effortful and very slow. Several balance adjustments occur at the end of the movement as she rises to erect stance.

Mrs. Smith's problems can be described as:

1. Poor Upper Limb Control

Mrs. Smith uses sequential movement patterns through a small range of motion both for flexion and extension movements. She has weakness or lack of an ability to control muscle tension in most upper limb muscles. Although she initiates movement, she has difficulty controlling movement speed. Mrs. Smith also has difficulty reciprocating joint movement. This appears more related to difficulty shutting off the agonist than to difficulty activating the antagonist. She has shoulder pain and sensory loss which may contribute to her motor deficits.

2. Gait Abnormalities

Mrs. Smith has difficulty initiating swing and controlling movements at all three lower extremity joints. She has an inefficient gait pattern and cannot produce an increased walking speed.

3. Lack of independence in transfers.

During transfers, Mrs. Smith's movement is very segmented and slow. She lacks consistent patterns and is unable to generate sufficient momentum to lift off the chair without assistance.

GOALS

The goals are for the patient to:

1. increase strength and selective control of the right arm
2. perform independent transfers
3. improve gait pattern.

FUNCTIONAL OBJECTIVES

Following 3 months of treatment, Mrs. Smith will:

1. reach with both arms for an object overhead using shoulder flexion for 5 repetitions
2. rise from a chair to standing without using her arms to push up, 2 of 3 trials
3. ambulate with her walker for a distance of 30 feet without demonstrating hip circumduction.

TREATMENT RECOMMENDATIONS

The apparent sensory loss in Mrs. Smith's right arm and right leg may be a major factor that will impede movement accuracy and learning controlled movements. All tasks should incorporate visual feedback during exercise training to help compensate for sensory loss.

Active or active-assisted extension and flexion movement patterns of the arm, not just individual joints should be practiced, using a goal directed familiar task. Tasks and objects related to hobbies (e.g., gardening tools or flowers) should be incorporated into the program. These activities should be performed within a ROM in which the patient can initiate and control movement. Larger amplitudes of movement should be incorporated gradually and additional tasks introduced as the patient gains control. Tasks that promote strengthening and reciprocal movements should be used and movement speed varied.

Hip extension on the right limb must be increased to improve initiation of swing and increase step length. Placing Mrs. Smith on a treadmill for gait training would help stimulate hip extension during stance, but she may not have adequate balance for this approach and most clinics don't have harness suspensions to protect patients. A more conservative approach would be using proprioceptive neuromuscular facilitation (PNF) techniques of resisted gait that rotate the pelvis and force hip extension. Bicycle exercises may be useful for improving muscle strength and facilitating timing patterns of force production for reciprocal, multisegment movements.

Mrs. Smith should practice transferring from sitting to standing to sitting to improve independence. Patients have problems rising to stand from a chair because they have inadequate strength, use an inefficient pattern, or produce adequate force with the body segments in poor alignment. Mrs. Smith has problems with force production. Her strategy of leaning forward, stopping, and then attempting to stand reduces the momentum that assists in rising. Working on the movement as one continuous pattern and strengthening extensor muscles so they can produce adequate force to lift the body may be beneficial. This task provides an opportunity for practicing movement sequencing and functional strengthening. Both rising and sitting should be practiced for maximum benefit in training muscle control.

CASE STUDY #2
DANIEL JOHNSON

Age: 59 years
Diagnosis: Parkinson's disease
Status: Four years post initial diagnosis

ASSESSMENT

Mr. Johnson's major problems noted during the assessment include difficulty initiating movement, slow movement speed, and difficulty coordinating limb and trunk movements during transfers.

GOALS

The goals are for the patient to:

1. improve speed of movement initiation
2. increase speed of movement
3. improve coordination when rising from sit to stand.

FUNCTIONAL OBJECTIVES

Following 3 months of treatment, Mr. Johnson will:

1. initiate upper limb movement for reaching within 5 sec. of being requested to perform the task and initiate walking within 5 sec. of being requested to perform the task

2. walk 30 feet in less than 20 sec.

3. demonstrate coordinated trunk flexion followed by trunk and leg extension during rising from chair.

TREATMENT RECOMMENDATIONS

Mr. Johnson would benefit from a program for maintaining flexibility, strength, and reactivity. Goal directed tasks of varying speed should be used. Mr. Johnson can practice adjusting speed during the movement. It is not necessary to perfect movement at one speed before you change to another. Movement patterns are sensitive to movement speed. Working with different speeds to find one that produces the best performance is often a successful strategy. Mr. Johnson can practice movement at the most effective speed for success with occasional variance of speed for maximum learning.

Sometimes having a patient move to the beat of a metronome or music will improve timing. Changing directions of movements is another method for training timing. Adding

direction changes to the task also increases the complexity of the task and forces the patient to repeatedly initiate and terminate movement. Mr. Johnson should practice several similar functional tasks for maximum carry over to other related tasks. Working on timed tasks may improve movement initiation. Passive and active ROM exercises will maintain joint mobility and muscle length. Remember that preventing limitations of joint movement is essential for normal movement patterns to occur.

CASE STUDY #3
SHIRLEY TEAL

Age: 21 years
Diagnosis: Post motor vehicles accident
Closed head injury
Status: Four months post accident

ASSESSMENT

During assessment, Ms. Teal's major problems were found to be related to decreased strength and abnormal movement patterns in the right upper limb, trunk weakness and difficulty coordinating trunk and limb movement, and decreased strength and coordination of the lower limbs. She has problems with controlling and coordinating limb and trunk movements. This appears to be due to deficits in strength, as well as timing patterns. She appears to be progressing well and gaining in cognitive as well as physical functioning.

GOALS

The goals are for the patient to:

1. increase strength and coordination in the right upper extremity

2. increase strength in the trunk musculature

3. improve coordination between trunk and lower extremities

4. improve balance in stance.

FUNCTIONAL OBJECTIVES

Following two months of treatment, Ms. Teal will:

1. reach and grasp an object placed at shoulder height, using shoulder flexion and elbow extension for 15 trials during sitting in a chair

2. roll unassisted to either the right or left side

3. rise to standing from a chair independently

4. maintain her balance in standing for 5 seconds without holding onto the parallel bars.

TREATMENT RECOMMENDATIONS

Begin strengthening exercises for the right arm using functional goal directed tasks and resisted exercises. Use bimanual tasks to promote interlimb coordination. Emphasize simple and complex movement patterns that involve several body segments, and tasks that require speed and accuracy of

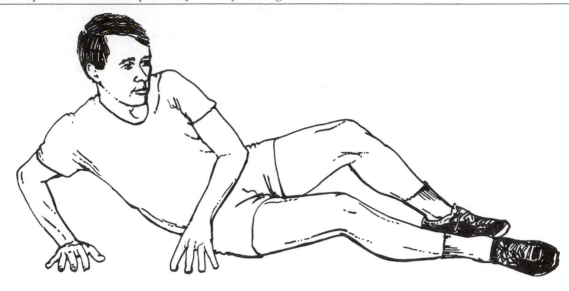

movement. Coordination requires a variety of movement speeds and directions.

Trunk flexibility and mobility tasks are appropriate for improving trunk coordination. Examples include, mat activities requiring intersegmental coordination and changes in posture such as rolling, and supine to sit (Figure 4). Sit to stand exercises emphasizing correct segmental sequencing can be done as well as bicycling, sit to stand, trampoline, walking at varying speeds with direction changes, and stair climbing. Progress with each task to increase strength, endurance, and complexity as abilities improve.

CASE STUDY #4
SHAWNA WELLS

Age: 4 years
Diagnosis: Cerebral palsy; spastic quadriparesis;
mild mental retardation
Status: Onset at birth

ASSESSMENT

Additional information is needed to assess Shawna. Information is needed on her active and passive ROM. Are there structural limitations or are her abnormal patterns due to abnormal muscle synergies? What is the strength of the limbs and trunk? Are limitations in reaching due to trunk weakness or abnormal trunk synergies that may be causing cocontraction?

Further assessment reveals that Shawna has normal passive ROM without structural limitations, therefore abnormal patterns are probably due to abnormal muscle synergies. I am concerned that she has had Achilles tendon releases, has normal passive ROM, and still has abnormal movement patterns. In this case, it appears that mechanical correction did not improve the toe walking pattern. I also found that she is able to extend her trunk using an extensor synergy pattern, but when positioned so she cannot use the synergy, she cannot extend her trunk against gravity. It is encouraging that she seems to be able to produce other patterns when she moves slowly and attends to the task. This appears to be a case of inefficient and abnormal movement patterns that may be confounded by a reduced ability to produce controlled muscle force. Her major problems are abnormal movement pattern for arm reaching, i.e., shoulder elevation rather than glenohumeral movement, difficulty producing an alternating creeping pattern, and limited poor trunk movement.

GOALS

The goals are for the patient to:
1. increase lower extremity reciprocation
2. improve active glenohumeral movement
3. increase variety of trunk movement.

FUNCTIONAL OBJECTIVES

Following 3 months of treatment, Shawna will:

1. creep 25 feet with a reciprocal pattern with verbal reminders and demonstrate longer symmetrical stride lengths during ambulation with a walker as measured by chalk prints on the floor

2. reach for an object with 90 degrees of forward flexion at the glenohumeral joint without elevating the shoulder, 2 of 3 trials

3. use a segmental trunk pattern when rolling on the floor and maintain a stable pelvis in tailor sitting on the floor while rotating to reach an object behind her.

TREATMENT RECOMMENDATIONS

Two approaches to treatment are to improve muscle strength, that is, to improve control of force production throughout joint ROM, and to improve patterns of limb movement. Initiating and terminating movement, and moving in a well coordinated pattern depend on adequate muscle strength and timing.

Tricycle exercises (adapting pedals if necessary), stair climbing, and treadmill locomotion should be encouraged for reciprocal timing and increasing muscle strength (Figure 5). Creeping and walking can be practiced with visual cueing and verbal feedback. Walking at a speed that produces the best (optimal) pattern and varying speed during the treatment session are appropriate strategies. Shawna can periodically return to the optimal walking speed for positive feedback and to decrease frustration.

Scapular mobility should be assessed during active and passive arm movement. Manual assistance of the scapula and facilitation of scapular muscles during attempted shoulder flexion can be used. Scapular and arm muscles can be strengthened through use of wheelbarrow walking, tug of war, and resisted ball activities.

Incorporation of trunk control and strengthening into activities for improving movement initiation can be done by moving the support surface (sitting on a therapeutic ball), and moving the upper body segment (reaching, throwing, and catching tasks). These activities encourage trunk control and automatic trunk responses. Another method of stimulating trunk activity is to practice rapid arm movements in a sitting position with no trunk support and in standing with minimal support so that Shawna has to stabilize her trunk to produce limb movement. ❑

FIGURE 5. *Child riding a tricycle with adapted trunk and foot support.*

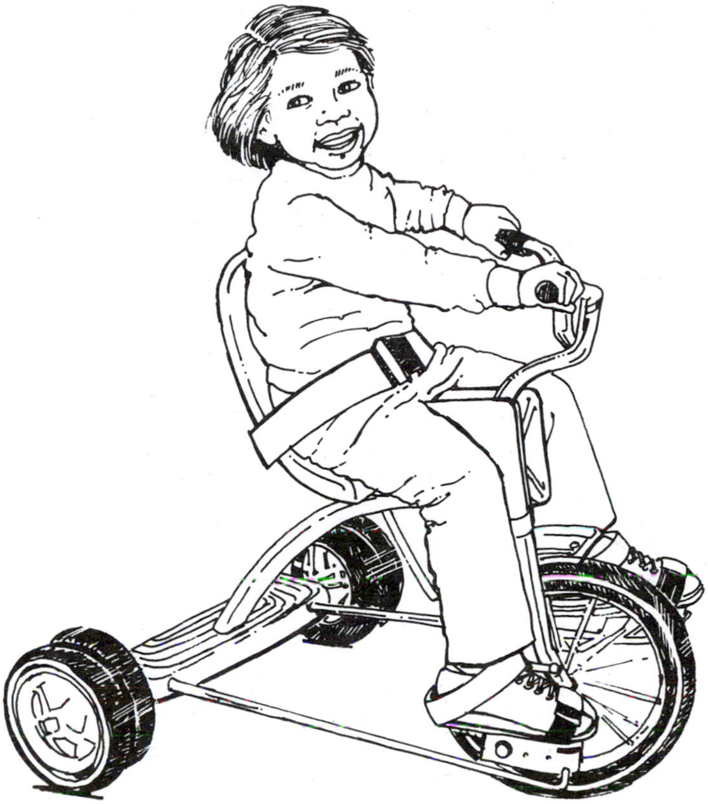

REFERENCES

1. Brunnstrom S: Recording gait patterns of adult hemiplegic patients. Phys Ther 44:11-18, 1964
2. Dietz V, Quintern J, Berger W: Electrophysiological studies of gait in spasticity and rigidity: Evidence that altered mechanical properties of muscle contribute to hypertonia. Brain 104:431-449, 1981
3. Knutsson E: Restraint of spastic muscle in different types of movement. In Feldman RG, Young RR, et al (eds): Spasticity: Disordered Motor Control. Chicago, IL, Yearbook Medical Publishers, 1980,123
4. Tang A, Rymer WZ: Abnormal force EMG relations in paretic limbs of hemiparetic human subjects. J Neurol Neurosurg Psych 44:690-698, 1981
5. Spector SA, Simard CP, Fournier M: Architectural alterations of rat hind-limb skeletal muscles immobilized at different lengths. Exp Neurol 76:94-110, 1982
6. Scelsi R, Lotta G, Lommi G: Hemiplegic atrophy: Morphological findings in the anterior tibial muscle of patients with cerebral vascular accident. Acta Neuropathol (Berl) 62:324-331,1984
7. Slager UT, Hsu JD , Jordan C: Histochemical and morphometric changes in muscles of stroke patients. Clin Ortho Rel Res 99:159-168, 1985
8. Edstrom L: Selective changes in the sizes of red and white muscle fibers in upper motor neuron lesions and parkinsonism. J Neurol Sci 11:537-550, 1970
9. McComas AJ, Sica REP, Upton ARM, et al: Functional changes in motoneurons of hemiparetic patients. J Neurol Neurosurg Psych 36:183-193., 1973
10. Rosenfalack A, Andreassen S: Impaired regulation of force and firing pattern of single motor units in patients with spasticity. J Neurol Neurosurg Psych 43: 907-916, 1980
11. Petajan JH: Motor unit control in movement disorders. Adv Neurol 39: 897-905, 1983
12. Knutsson E, Richards C: Different types of distributed motor control in gait of hemiplegic patients. Brain 102:403-430, 1979
13. Harro CC, Giuliani CA. Kinematic and EMG analysis of hemiplegic gait patterns during free and fast walking speeds. Neurol Report 11(3):57, 1987
14. Giuliani, CA: Adult hemiplegic gait. In Smidt G (ed): Normal and Abnormal Human Gait, New York, NY, Churchill Livingston, 1990, pp 253-266
15. Sahrmann SA, Norton BJ: The relationship of voluntary movement to spasticity in the upper motor neuron syndrome. Ann Neurol 2:460-465, 1977
16. Phillips JG, Muller F, Stelmach GE: Movement disorders and the neural basis of motor control. In Wallace SA (ed): Perspectives on the Coordination of Movement. North-Holland, Elsiever Science Publishers, 1989, pp 367-411.

Chapter 10
Assessment and Treatment of Balance Deficits

Anne Shumway-Cook, Ph.D., PT
Gin McCollum, Ph.D.

INTRODUCTION

While few clinicians would argue the importance of balance to independence in activities such as sitting, standing, and walking, there is no universal definition of balance, nor agreement on the neural mechanisms underlying the control of balance.[1] The purpose of this chapter is to discuss assessment and treatment of balance disorders in the neurologic patient. The term "balance" will be used interchangeably with "stability." Portions of the material presented in this chapter have been presented in previous publications.[2-5]

Over the last several decades, attention to aspects of balance disorders has shifted and broadened. The very definition of balance and stability has changed, as has our understanding of the underlying neural mechanisms responsible for the maintenance of balance. In rehabilitation science, there are at least two different conceptual models which can describe the neural control of posture and movement: the reflex/hierarchical model and the systems model (see Chapter 2).[1-3] A reflex/hierarchical model suggests that balance results from hierarchically organized reflex responses within the individual. Alternatively, the systems model suggests that balance involves an interaction between the individual and his environment. Each model has implications for assessing and treating balance disorders in the neurologic patient.

Neural models of motor control are important since they form the underpinning of clinical methods for treating movement disorders including instability. In the next sections we will discuss the more traditional reflex/hierarchical model, then the more interactive sensorimotor systems model. In final sections we outline specific assessment and treatment

strategies and apply them to case studies.

REFLEX/HIERARCHICAL CONTROL MODEL

According to the reflex/hierarchical model, balance is the ability to correctly deploy a set of interacting, hierarchically organized reflexes and reactions which support the body against gravity.[6-8] The reflex/hierarchical model of motor control is based in part on Hughlings Jackson's work describing the central nervous system (CNS) as a vertical hierarchy.[9]

During normal development, sequential maturation of ascending levels of the CNS hierarchy results in the emergence of higher levels of behavior, which in turn modify immature behaviors organized at lower levels. Therefore, during development the young child is first dominated by primitive reflexes which are controlled hierarchically at low levels within the CNS. With maturation of higher brainstem and mid-brain levels within the CNS, righting reactions emerge which modify or inhibit primitive reflexes. Finally, with maturation of the cortex, considered the "highest level of the CNS," the emergence of equilibrium reactions occurs.

Equilibrium reactions were defined by Weiss as automatic reactions by the body in response to labyrinthine inputs.[10] Equilibrium reactions, or tilting reactions, are reported to emerge first in prone, then in supine, in sitting, quadruped, and finally in standing. It is assumed that mature or partially mature equilibrium reactions must emerge at each stage of development (i.e., in sitting prior to quadruped, quadruped prior to stance) before the maturing child can achieve the next developmental milestone.[11]

Instability in the Patient With Neurologic Deficits

According to the reflex/hierarchical model, instability in this type of patient is the result of release of spinal and brainstem reflexes which are no longer modified or inhibited by higher CNS structures.[12-14] Lesions in the cerebral cortex of an adult patient result in the reappearance of primitive reflexes which dominate motor function and prevent the expression of normal equilibrium.

Therapeutic Implications

Based on the reflex/hierarchical model of motor control and development, a number of reflex profiles have been developed and integrated into clinical assessment methods.[15-18] Examination of reflexes has traditionally been considered an essential part of clinical assessment of patients with neurologic impairments, since persistence and dominance of primitive reflexes are considered to be a major deterrent to independent stability and mobility. Clinical assessment of equilibrium reactions is done most commonly by tipping or tilting a subject. Equilibrium reactions may be tested in a developmental progression of positions from supine to standing with the subject maintaining balance in response to movement of a moveable support base.[8,12,15]

Alternatively, equilibrium reactions may be tested by holding the patient about the waist and displacing the patient sideways, forwards, and backwards.[18] A number of treatment strategies have been developed for patients with primary complaints of dysequilibrium using a reflex/hierarchical model. The therapist positions and moves the patient in various ways to stimulate appropriate righting and equilibrium reactions, while inhibiting competing primitive reflexes, such as the asymmetrical tonic neck reflex.[8,12,13] Patients are often progressed through an ontogenetic sequence with righting and equilibrium reactions stimulated first in prone and supine, sitting, crawling, and finally standing. Since abnormal postural reflex activity, including abnormal tone, is thought to constrain normal righting and equilibrium reactions, time is spent in treatment inhibiting these primitive and pathologic patterns prior to stimulation of normal righting and equilibrium reactions.

SYSTEMS MODEL

An alternative to the reflex/hierarchical model is a systems model of motor control. This model is based on work by Bernstein[19] and has recently been applied to the study of postural control (see Chapter 2).[1-5] Postural stability is defined as the ability to maintain the position of the body, specifically center of body mass (COM), within specific boundaries of space, referred to as stability limits.[20] Stability limits define an area of space in which the body can maintain position without changing the base of support.[20] In a systems model, stability results from a continual interaction between the individual and the environment.

The focus of the systems approach to examining postural control in neurologically intact adults has been to determine both motor and sensory strategies used to achieve postural stability in stance[21,22] and during locomotion.[23,24] Motor strategies generate muscular forces necessary for controlling movement of the body, while sensory strategies organize sensory information for orientation and coordinate sensory information with motor aspects of postural control. The following sections briefly review movement and sensory strategies for controlling upright stance posture in a neurologically intact adult.

Movement Strategies

Balance requires the generation, scaling, and coordination of forces effective in controlling the center of mass relative to desired limits of stability. Using a moving platform to study postural motor reactions, Nashner and colleagues have identified a three-dimensional continuum of movements for controlling anterior-posterior sway: (1) an ankle movement, (2) a hip movement, and (3) a suspensory/or stepping movement.[21,22] These movements are illustrated in Figure 1. These authors also described the coordinated action of leg and trunk muscles underlying these movements.

Postural movement strategies are assumed to restore equilibrium in varied circumstances, such as in response to unexpected disturbances to equilibrium[21,22]; prior to a voluntary movement that potentially destabilizes balance[25,26]; during ambulation, specifically in response to unexpected disruptions to the gait cycle[23]; and during volitional center of mass movements in stance.[4,27]

The ankle movement strategy displaces the COM by rotating the body primarily about the ankle joints. Muscle activity and associated joint angle changes in a neurologically intact subject using an ankle movement to respond to loss of balance in the forward direction is shown in Figure 2. Motion of the platform in the backward direction causes the subject to sway forward thus producing ankle dorsiflexion and hip extension. Muscles activated in response to forward sway are shown in Figure 2A. Muscle activity begins at 90 msec in the gastrocnemius, followed by activation of the hamstring (116 msec) and paraspinal (117 msec).

Changes in joint angles at the ankle, knee, and hip associated with this pattern of muscle activity are shown in Figure 2B. Activation of the gastrocnemius produces a plantarflexion torque which slows, then reverses, the body's forward motion. Synergistic activation of the hamstrings and paraspinal muscles minimizes forward motion of the trunk, the indirect effect of the ankle torque on proximal body segments.

The ankle movement strategy is used most commonly in situations in which the perturbation to equilibrium is small and the support surface is firm. In addition, use of the ankle strategy requires intact range of motion and strength in the ankles. In contrast, the hip strategy controls motion of the COM by producing large and rapid motion at the hip joints with antiphase rotations of the ankles. The hip strategy is used in response to larger, faster perturbations or when the support surface is compliant or smaller than the feet, for example, when standing on a beam.[22] When a postural perturbation is of sufficient magnitude to displace the COM outside the base of support of the feet, a series of steps or hops

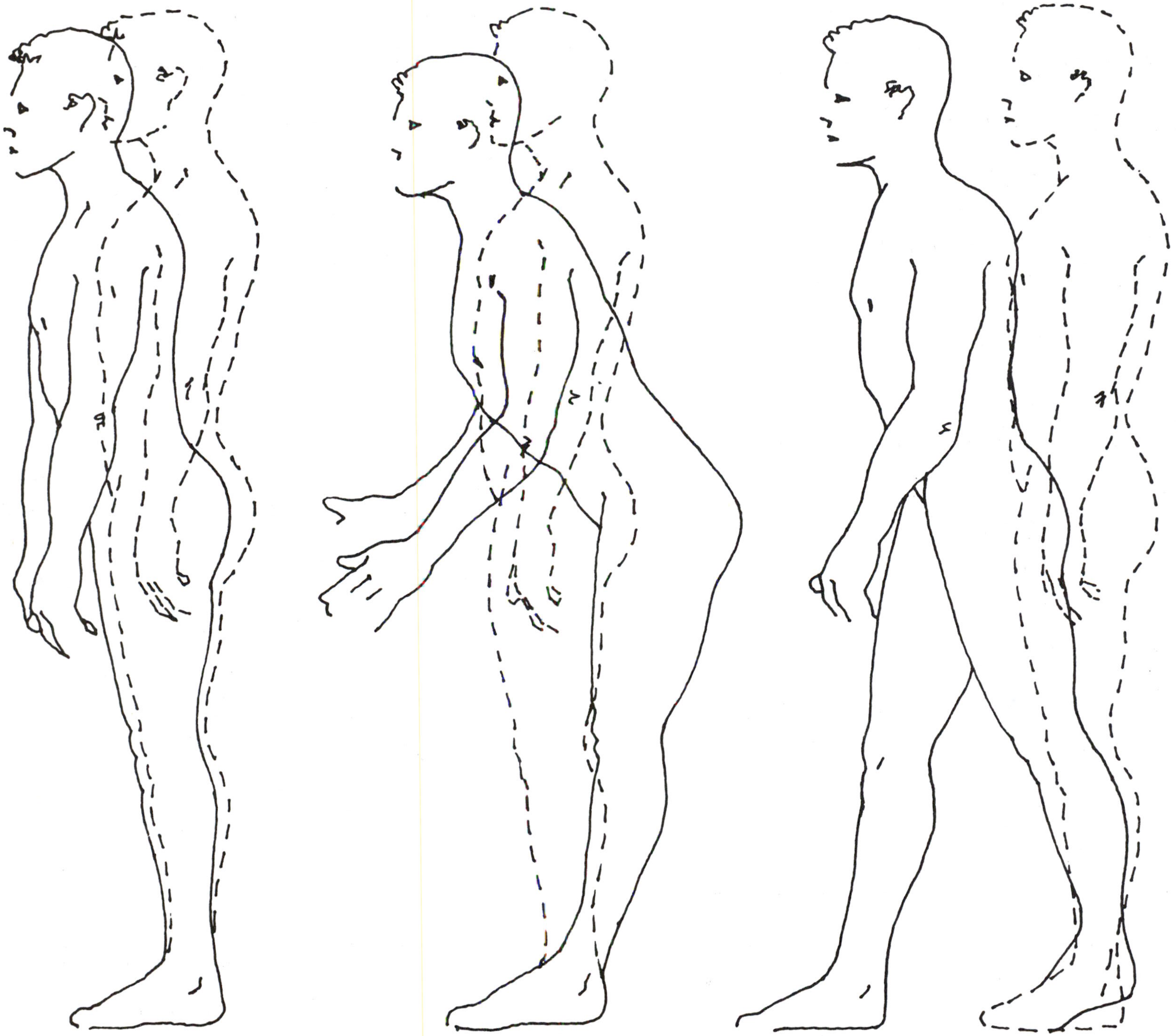

FIGURE 1. Three postural motor strategies used by normal adults for control of upright sway. Reprinted with permission from Seminars in Hearing, Vol. 10, No. 2, ©1989, Thieme Medical Publishers, Inc.

NORMAL MOTOR COORDINATION – FLAT SURFACE

A. Muscle Activity

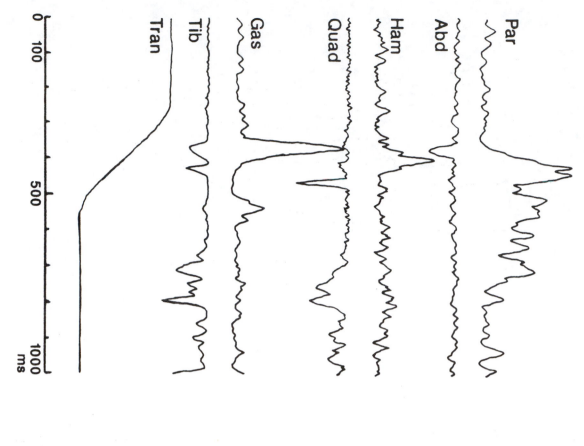

B. Joint Angles

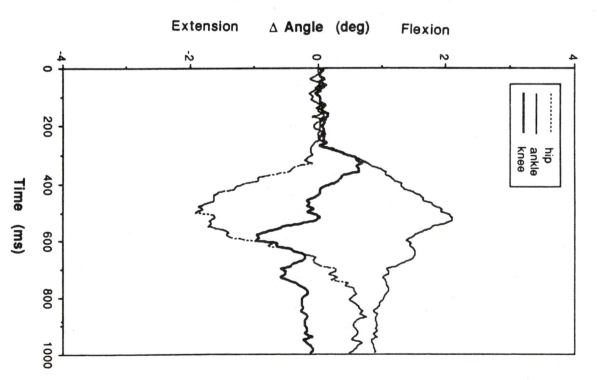

FIGURE 2. EMG and joint angle changes in a normal subject using an ankle strategy to control upright sway. Reprinted with permission from The Journal of Head Trauma Rehabilitation, Vol. 5, No. 4, © 1990, Aspen Publishers, Inc.

(the stepping strategy) is used to bring the support base back into alignment under the COM. [21]

Sensory Strategies

Examining sensory aspects of postural control involves observing the availability and accuracy of sensory information for determining the position of the body relative to gravity and the supporting surface, and developing conscious and unconscious perception of stability.

Normally, peripheral inputs from the visual, somatosensory (proprioceptive, cutaneous, and joint receptors), and vestibular systems are available to detect motion of the body with respect to gravity and the environment. Central processes integrate and determine those inputs which accurately report self-motion. In environments where a sense is not accurately reporting self motion, an alternative sense is selected for orientation. Because of the redundancy of senses available for orientation, normal individuals are able to maintain stability in a variety of environments where one or more senses are unavailable for balance.[28-30]

One approach to testing sensory components of the postural control system using a moving platform with a moving visual surround has been described in detail and will only be reviewed briefly in this chapter.[28,29] Body sway is measured while the subject stands quietly for 20 seconds under 6 different conditions which alter the availability and accuracy of visual and somatosensory inputs for postural orientation. Differences in amount of body sway in the different conditions are used to determine a subject's ability to organize and select appropriate sensory information for postural control. Many studies have been done examining the performance of normal subjects when sensory inputs for postural control are varied.[2,5,28-30] Generally, these studies have shown that adults and children over the age of 7 years easily maintain balance under all six conditions. Most individuals show gradually increasing amounts of anterior-posterior sway over the six conditions with greatest sway in conditions 5 and 6, in which primarily vestibular inputs mediate postural control.

Instability in the Patient With Neurologic Deficits

In a systems model, instability results from abnormalities within one or more of the systems controlling balance. Understanding instability in this type of patient is difficult for many reasons. The effect of a neural lesion may vary from patient to patient depending not only on the type and extent of the neural lesion, but also other interacting factors such as age, prior medical history, and current medical and rehabilitation interventions. Many of these factors will affect the capacity for compensation by the remaining intact neural systems. In addition, since instability usually results from deficits within multiple systems, it is often difficult to sort out the relative contributions of individual abnormalities to balance deficits.

Therapeutic Implications

Assessment of stability from a systems perspective focuses on evaluating the musculoskeletal and neural constraints contributing to instability. The goal of therapeutic intervention is to help the patient develop a broader range of sensory and motor strategies for implementing stability while considering musculoskeletal and neural constraints. This approach to intervention will enable a patient to maintain stability in a variety of environmental settings.

Because the development of clinical approaches to remediating instability using a systems model is just beginning, specific assessment and treatment techniques are limited. However, a number of exciting questions have been raised since there may be multiple solutions to sensory and movement problems contributing to postural instability in patients with neurologic deficits. The multiplicity of solutions potentially available depends on an understanding of the dynamic nature of stability limits and the specific nature of patients' constraints.

In the following sections we discuss in more detail stability limits and constraints underlying instability in the patient with neurologic dysfunction, and present ideas on assessment and treatment.

STABILITY LIMITS AND CONSTRAINTS

Recovery of independence in tasks such as sitting, standing, and walking demands that stability be achieved regardless of musculoskeletal and neural limitations. The definition of stability also changes depending on the task, characteristics of the individual, and the environmental conditions, such as the slipperiness of the floor.

Stability Limits

Postural stability is defined as the ability to maintain the position of the body, specifically center of body mass (COM), within specific boundaries of space, referred to as stability limits.[20] Stability limits are boundaries of an area of space in which the body can maintain its position without changing the base of support.[20] Stability limits are not fixed boundaries, but change according to the task, the individual's biomechanics, and aspects of the environment.

While stability is a requirement most tasks have in common, stability limits change with each task. For a neurologically intact adult maintaining an independent standing posture, the requirement for stability is met by maintaining the COM within stability limits defined principally by the length of the feet and the distance between them (see Figure 3). A different task, locomotion, requires that stability be preserved while the body moves forward.[24] In locomotion, stability limits extend forward of the support base determined by the stance leg, since the swing leg will be available to support the body before falling. This has led some to refer to walking as controlled falling. The task of moving from sit to stand requires moving the body from stability limits which encompass a supporting chair, to stability limits defined solely by the supporting feet. The area in which one can move safely without a change in base of support (stability limits) is dependent upon musculoskeletal and neural abilities of the individual, and the type and extent of support surface available. In an adult standing upright with no support except that from the feet, stability limits take on the form of a geometric cone as shown in Figure 3.[20] In contrast, Figure 4 shows that stability limits are asymmetric

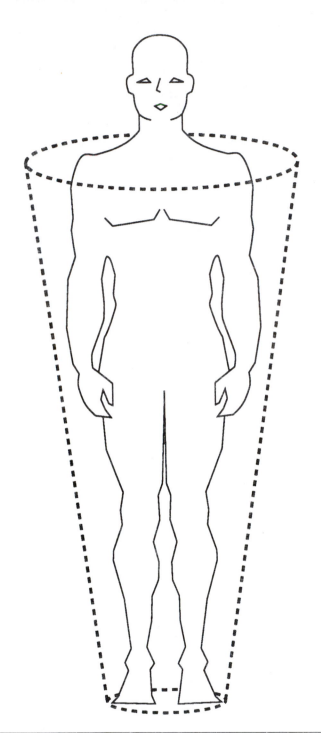

FIGURE 3. *Stability limits for the task of independent stance in a neurologically normal subject.*

It is hypothesized that the CNS has an internal representation of stability limits which contributes to a patient's conscious and unconscious perception of stability. We believe that a patient's accurate perception of stability limits is essential to the recovery of stability, since sensory and motor strategies must be developed which allow the patient to remain within his new stability limits.

Usually, an individual's "perceived" limits of stability are consistent with "actual" limits of stability, in that they lead the person to remain within the actual limits. In many patient's however, perceived stability limits may be inconsistent with actual stability limits which have changed as the result of musculoskeletal and neural limitations.

A discrepancy between perceived and actual limits of stability is a potential source of instability since patients with perceived limits of stability outside their actual limits will have a tendency to fall. We believe that discrepancies between perceived and actual stability limits are common in patients with neurologic deficits, particularly during initial stages of recovery. At this time, the patient may not be aware of the full extent of his limitations and their effects on stability limits.

During assessment, the consistency between the patient's perceived versus actual limits of stability is determined. The patient is asked to sway voluntarily as far as he can in all directions without falling, in order to determine his limits of perceived stability. In addition, the therapist uses slow displacements of the standing patient in all directions to determine the area in which the patient will allow his COM to be moved. The therapist observes the extent of COM movement in all directions and makes a subjective judgement regarding whether the patient is moving to his full stability limit in all directions.

Rehabilitation strategies involving use of postural sway biofeedback been developed to assist patients in developing consistency between perceived and actual limits of stability.[31] Alternatively, we ask seated and/or standing patients to visualize a space around them with boundaries in which they can move safely. Patients then are asked to practice moving their bodies within and to those boundaries. Boundaries may be gradually expanded with increasing sensory and motor capacities of the patient.

in an individual with hemiplegia who has unilateral weakness. As a result of his hemiparesis, the patient is unable to generate forces necessary to keep the left leg from collapsing during stance. This constraint changes how stability limits are defined for this patient. In order to maintain stance stability, the patient will be required to keep his body's COM within stability limits which are now asymmetrically centered over the intact side. In addition, stability limits now encompass an area which exceeds the supporting leg to include the cane needed by this patient for partial support when standing and walking.

Constraints On Stability

The goal of therapeutic intervention is to help the patient maintain stability in a variety of tasks and environmental settings. In order to stay within changing stability limits, the therapist must help the patient develop a broad range of sensory and motor balance strategies, and learn when to apply them. A key to achieving effective strategies for stability is understanding and modifying musculoskeletal and neural constraints. Constraints are defined as limitations within the individual which restrict sensory and movement strategies for postural control, and may be musculoskeletal, neuromuscular, sensory/perceptual, or cognitive.

Musculoskeletal Constraints — Musculoskeletal restrictions can limit movement strategies used in balance. Since use of an ankle movement strategy requires intact range of motion and strength in the ankles, constraints in ankle range or strength will limit the patient's ability to use this movement for balance. In contrast, the hip movement strategy requires large and rapid motion at the hip joints; thus musculoskeletal limitations at the hips will affect use of this strategy.

Assessment of musculoskeletal problems uses traditional physical therapy techniques to examine range of motion, strength, pain, sensation, and coordination. Treatment includes modalities such as heat, ultrasound, massage, and biofeedback. Range of motion and strengthening exercises are also used. In those patients with abnormal alignment of body segments, appropriate alignment is practiced in conjunction with forceplate and visual or auditory biofeedback to reinforce new positions.[31]

Neuromuscular Constraints — Numerous neuromuscular limitations leading to instability in the patient with a neurologic deficit have been described. Since stability requires the ability to generate forces necessary for moving the COM, upper motorneuron lesions producing limitations in strength will produce concomitant limitations in stability.[32] Abnormal muscle tonus ranging from hypotonicity to hypertonicity, is commonly reported in patients and may limit a patient's ability to recruit muscles necessary for balance.[32-34] The extent to which abnormal muscle tone is a limitation in controlling movements for balance is currently under considerable debate in the rehabilitation literature.[1,32,35]

Instability due to abnormalities of coordination within postural muscle synergies has also been reported in a wide range of patients. Examples of these limitations include: significantly delayed onset of postural responses in patients with stroke[36] or head injuries;[5] abnormal sequencing of synergistic muscles within a movement strategy in persons with hemiplegia;[36,37] abnormal timing between postural muscle synergies in patients with Parkinson's disease;[38] and delayed postural adjustments prior to potentially destabilizing voluntary arm movements.[37,39] In addition, involuntary movements and tremors can affect the ability of patients to control movements of the center of mass, thus impeding recovery of stability (Shumway-Cook & McCollum, unpublished observations).

Assessment of neuromuscular constraints includes traditional measurements of strength and abnormalities of muscle tonus.[12-14,32] In addition, assessment techniques address the presence of normally coordinated ankle, hip, and stepping strategies in stance and during dynamic gait activities. First, patients are asked to voluntarily sway in all directions while

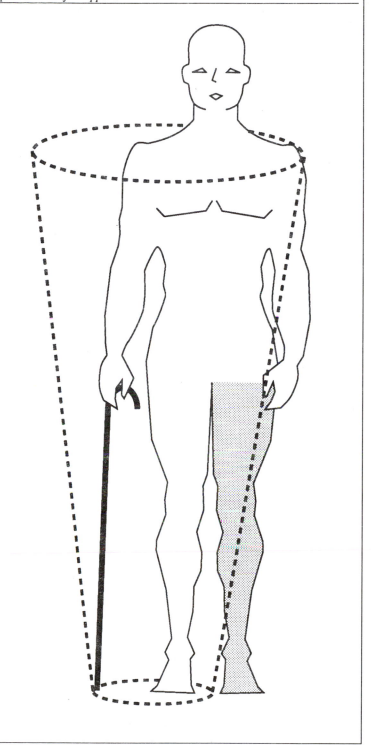

FIGURE 4. Stability limits modified in a patient with left hemiparesis who requires a cane for support.

the type of movement pattern used to maintain stability is observed. In addition, the patient is held lightly at the hips, and gently displaced in all directions while standing unsupported, and the type of movement strategy used to recover balance is observed.[18] It is important to grade carefully the extent of displacement to determine the appropriateness of movement strategy relative to the extent of displacement.

While the patient is attempting to recover balance, the therapist watches for behaviors suggestive of motor incoordination, for example, excessive flexion of the knees,

FIGURE 5. *Comparison of body motions associated with normal versus abnormal sequencing of muscle activity in response to backward sway.*

Normal Postural Correction

A

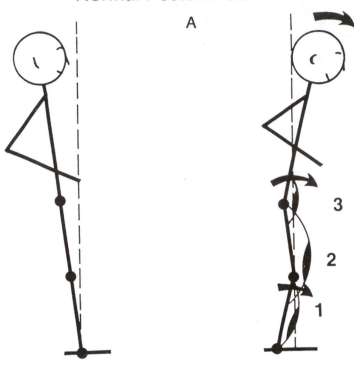

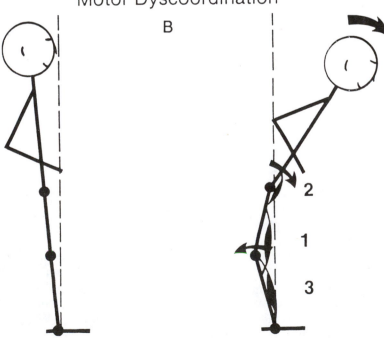

Motor Dyscoordination

B

asymmetric movements of the body, or excessive flexion or rotation of the trunk.

Figure 5 compares movement associated with normal and abnormal sequencing of muscle activity in response to backward sway. Figure 5A shows that in response to backward sway, normal muscle activation begins in the tibialis anterior (numbered 1) and moves proximally to the quadriceps muscle (numbered 2) then the abdominals (numbered 3). This pattern of muscle activity produces joint torques (shown as arrows) causing ankle centered movement propelling the COM forward.

Movement in a patient with motor incoordination resulting from abnormal sequencing of muscle activation is seen in Figure 5B. Backward sway results in activation of the quadriceps muscle first (numbered 1), followed by the abdominals (numbered 2), and finally the tibialis anterior (numbered 3). This pattern of muscle activation results in hyperextension of the knee and forward flexion of the trunk, a pattern seen commonly in patients with hemiplegia.[2,36,37]

Observing apparent incoordination through subjective analysis of movement patterns is the most common approach to evaluating muscular incoordination in the clinic. However, the underlying nature of the incoordination, that is specific timing and/or amplitude errors in synergistic muscles responding to instability, can not be determined without use of technical apparatus such as electromyography.

Treatment of neuromuscular constraints varies depending on the nature of the incoordination problem. Strengthening exercises, including the use of isokinetic equipment, has been tried successfully with the patient who has neurologic deficits.[32,40,41] A variety of treatment techniques has been proposed to remediate abnormal muscle tone in this type of patient.[12-14] The degree to which these types of treatments has affected the recovery of stability has not yet been determined.

Functional electrical stimulation and electromyographic biofeedback have been used successfully to remediate disruptions of timing among synergistic muscles within a postural synergy (Shumway-Cook, unpublished observation). Other approaches require the patient to practice various exercises including: swaying back and forth in small ranges, keeping the body straight and not bending at the hips or knees; or attempting to maintain various equilibrium positions to facilitate the appropriate use of hip and or stepping strategies.[4]

Sensory Constraints — Balance deficits in the patient who has a neurologic deficit may result from damage within individual sensory systems providing orientation inputs for postural control,[42-46] or from pathology affecting central sensory organization mechanisms which produces a sensory selection problem (see Chapter 7).[5,47,48]

Assessment of sensory constraints contributing to postural instability involves determining which sense a patient is most dependent on for sway orientation information, and how well a patient can adapt to reliance on alternative senses in situations of intersensory conflict. To provide this information, a method for clinical assessment of the influence of sensory interaction on postural stability in the standing patient with neurologic problems has been suggested.[49,50] The method requires the patient to maintain standing balance for 30 seconds under six different sensory conditions that either eliminate input or produce inaccurate visual and surface orientation inputs. Patients are tested in two positions, classic (feet together) and tandem (heel/toe position), in the sequence shown in Figure 6. Using condition 1 as a baseline reference the therapist observes the patient for changes in the amount and direction of sway over the subsequent five conditions.[49,50]

Treatment of sensory constraints uses sensory organization exercises which are designed to treat specific types of sensory disorders. In general, the exercises involve the patient maintaining balance during progressively more difficult static and dynamic movement tasks while the therapist systematically varies the availability and accuracy of one or more senses for orientation.[51] For example, patients who show increased reliance on vision for orientation are asked to maintain balance when visual cues are absent (eyes closed or blindfolded), reduced (blinders or diminished lighting), or inaccurate for orientation (petrolatum glasses, prism glasses, enhanced visual motion cues, moving rooms).

Patients who show increased reliance on the surface for orientation are asked to balance and walk over surfaces providing decreased surface cues for orientation, such as compliant foam surfaces, or various types of carpeting, or moving surfaces. Finally, in order to enhance the ability to use remaining vestibular information for postural stability, exercises are given that require the patient to balance while both visual and somatosensory inputs for orientation are simultaneously reduced, such as standing on compliant foam with eyes closed.[4,51]

An example of pathology within a single sensory system is peripheral vestibular pathology. Symptoms vary but may include nystagmus, vertigo, problems with gait stabilization, poor balance, and gait ataxia.[51] Benign paroxysmal positional nystagmus (BPPN) and vertigo are hypothesized to result from otoconia being displaced from the otolithic membrane onto the cupula of the posterior semicircular canal. Rapid repositioning of the head during exercises may dislodge the displaced otoconia back to proper position. Repetitive exercises are used as a method of habituation to help the CNS compensate for vestibular dysfunction.

Cognitive Constraints — Many patients with neurologic dysfunction exhibit deficits in attention, memory, and learning.[52-55] The extent to which these deficits affect postural stability is not known, and as a result, effective approaches for assessing and treating these types of problems have yet to be developed. Previous research with neurologically normal subjects has shown that both sensory and motor strategies for maintaining balance are adaptable. Expectation, prior experience, and practice all modify postural control through "central set."[56] Central set is defined as descending commands that modify sensory and motor systems in anticipation of a particular stimulus or task.[57]

Stability problems resulting from abnormal central set have been reported in patients with midline cerebellar lesions,[58] and in patients with diseases of the basal ganglia.[38]

FIGURE 6. Six test positions used in the Clinical Test for Sensory Interaction and Balance (CTSIT), evaluating influence of sensory interaction on balance. Reprinted from Physical Therapy, Vol. 66, No. 10, © 1986, with the permission of the American Physical Therapy Association.

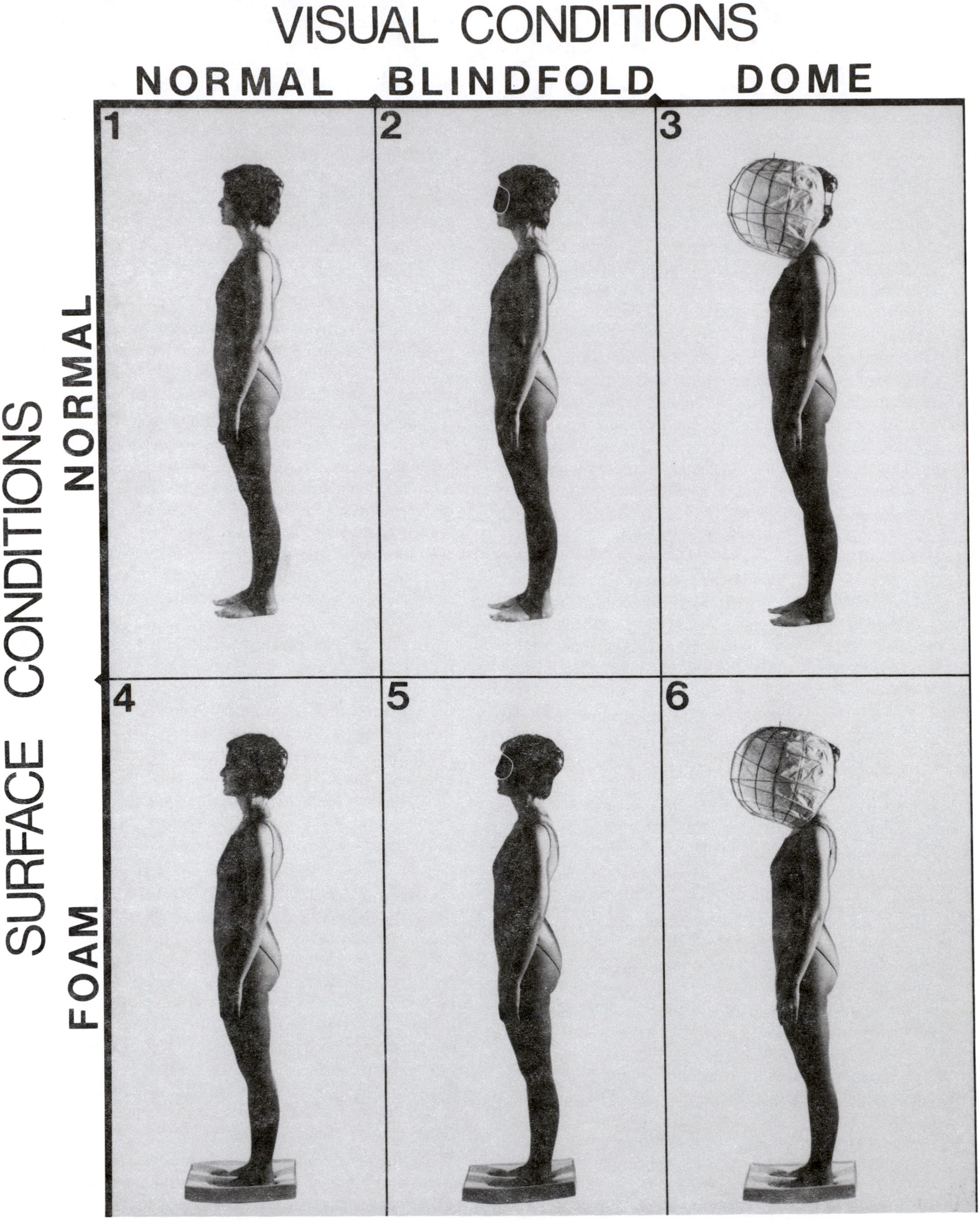

Treatment strategies to modify problems involving central set and expectation are being developed (Shumway-Cook and Horak, unpublished observation, 1990).

SUMMARY

Clinical approaches for remediating instability in the patient with neurologic deficits vary widely, reflecting, in part, fundamentally different models of neural control of posture and movement. Specific assessment methods, treatment goals, and intervention strategies reflect the therapist's underlying assumptions regarding both the neural basis for normal balance and underlying pathology contributing to instability in the patient. This chapter presented two models for the neural control of postural stability, the reflex/hierarchical model and the task/constraint model; and the clinical implications of these models. It is important to understand that a model is neither "right" nor "wrong," but rather more or less helpful in adequately describing the behaviors observed. Hence, whether one uses the reflex or systems model is less important than understanding the existence of one's model and its influence on therapeutic decisions.

CASE STUDY #1
JANE SMITH

Age: 74 years
Diagnosis: Right hemiplegia,
secondary to left cerebrovascular accident
Status: Six months post onset

ASSESSMENT

Mrs. Smith is a 74 year old woman who is 6 months post stroke, with a resultant right hemiplegia.

Functional problems include loss of independence in activities of daily living, decreased mobility skills including transfers, stance, and walking due to decreased balance. In addition, she has severe perceptual and cognitive problems reducing her awareness of her own limitations making her a safety risk with a high likelihood of falls.

The underlying constraints contributing to instability include musculoskeletal, neuromuscular, sensory perceptual, and cognitive problems. Musculoskeletal problems are limited range of motion in the right gastrocnemius and asymmetric body alignment in sit and stance, with weight shifted primarily to the left side.

Neuromuscular constraints are reduced strength in the right extremities and trunk. In stance, she is unable to sustain full weight through the right leg without collapse of the right knee. She is unable to dorsiflex her right foot during stance or gait.

She also has decreased use of an ankle strategy for controlling upright posture. Because of her reduced strength in the right ankle, Mrs. Smith relies on a hip postural movement strategy to control upright posture. In addition, she is unable to initiate a step when needed to maintain her balance and has to be caught to prevent a fall.

In the area of sensory/perceptual abilities, she has decreased somatosensation from the right extremities, severe right neglect, decreased ability to maintain balance when sensory inputs (vision or somatosensory inputs from the surface) for orientation are reduced or inaccurate, and inaccurate perception of limits of stability.

A cognitive constraint is decreased awareness of safety issues related to balance and mobility limitations. This places her at risk for a fall.

GOALS

Treatment goals are for Mrs. Smith to:

1. increase right ankle motion

2. increase strength in the right extremities, particularly right knee extensors and right ankle dorsiflexors

3. improve body alignment in sit and stance, so weight is distributed symmetrically

4. improve perception of verticality

5. improve conscious and unconscious perceptions related to limits of stability

6. improve use of movement strategies for postural control, including use of ankle strategy and stepping strategy as appropriate

7. increase ability to maintain balance when sensory inputs are reduced

8. increase awareness of safety issues related to balance.

FUNCTIONAL OBJECTIVES

Following 3 months of treatment, Mrs. Smith will:

1. demonstrate a 15 degree increase in ROM in right ankle dorsiflexion in assisted forward sway in standing

2. be able to complete 10 repetitions of resistive exercises in sitting for right knee extensors and right ankle dorsiflexors using red thera-band

3. be able to distribute weight equally in standing on two bathroom scales, 3 of 5 trials

4. align herself vertically in front of a mirror, 2 of 3 trials

5. demonstrate an increase in 5 degrees of active forward sway using an ankle strategy

6. independently take steps to regain balance when pushed outside limit of stability to right in standing, 1 of 3 trials

7. be able to maintain a symmetrical sitting posture on a foam cushion for 30 seconds

8. demonstrate a safe transfer from wheelchair to bed, 100% of the time.

TREATMENT RECOMMENDATIONS

For Goals 1 and 2, use traditional physical therapy measures to reduce range limitations and increase strength. For alignment and perception (Goals 3,4, and 5), the following activities are recommended.

In sitting, have Mrs. Smith practice maintaining a midline position. Use verbal and visual (mirror) cues to establish midline. Practice weight shifts in all directions, with Mrs. Smith returning to a midline position. Use of EMG biofeedback to establish trunk symmetry in sitting and standing might be helpful. Practice with and without vision.

In standing, have Mrs. Smith practice maintaining a midline, upright posture. Initially she could maintain stance in a corner to increase somatosensory awareness of the body in space. Provide her with objective information (biofeedback) about body position and alignment. Examples of biofeedback for alignment include: 1) use of a static forceplate retraining system to provide her with feedback about symmetrical weight bearing; 2) use of a mirror with a line down the middle, i.e., Mrs. Smith can wear a shirt with a line down the middle, and the task is to match the line on her shirt with the line on the mirror; and 3) standing on scales to achieve symmetrical weight distribution. Practice maintaining midline position with and without vision.

To improve postural movement strategies (Goals 5, 6, 7, and 8), practice an ankle strategy. From a symmetrical midline position have Mrs. Smith practice swaying forward, backward, and side to side. Begin with small amplitude sways, practice swaying from the ankles, keeping the knees and hips straight. Gradually increase the range in which she can move her body using an ankle strategy. Alternatively, hold her at the hips and move her in all directions varying the amplitude and speed of movement.

Practice a stepping strategy by holding Mrs. Smith at the hips and moving her till her center of mass is outside the base of support. Use manual assistance to help her take a step to maintain balance.

For sensory orientation (Goals 4, 5, 7, and 8), increase proprioception regarding position in space by having Mrs. Smith practice maintaining an appropriate vertical midline position in sitting and/or standing with her back against a chair or wall. She should practice without shoes and socks to increase orientation information from the bottoms of her feet. Alternate maintaining the position with and without visual cues.

CASE STUDY #2
DANIEL JOHNSON

Age: 59 years
Diagnosis: Parkinson's disease
Status: Four years post initial diagnosis

ASSESSMENT

Mr. Johnson is a 59 year old man with a diagnosis of Parkinson's disease four years post onset. Functionally, he is experiencing gradually diminishing mobility skills. These include problems in initiating transfers and maintaining a normal stance and walking pattern due to dyskinesia and impaired balance.

Musculoskeletal constraints are decreased flexibility and range of motion particularly in the trunk and pelvis. This results in decreased trunk rotation and a tendency to move "en block". Additionally, abnormal body alignment in sitting and standing is present. He stands with his head, trunk, and center of mass statically displaced forward, which increases his tendency to fall forward.

Neuromuscular problems include dyskinesia and tremor which affect his ability to make the movements necessary for balance. His bradykinesia and decreased ability to initiate movement result in slowed onset of automatic postural adjustments in response to instability.

He has no sensory/perceptual problems at this time. However, depression contributes to his decreased activity level, which in turn contributes to motor problems underlying beginning instability.

GOALS

Treatment goals are for Mr. Johnson to:

1. demonstrate fewer musculoskeletal limitations by increasing range of motion and flexibility in trunk and pelvis

2. improve trunk rotation (particularly counterrotation between upper and lower trunk) during functional movements such as rolling, moving from sit to stand, and during gait

3. improve transfer skills, including initiation and speed of transfers, i.e., sit to stand, bed to chair, etc.

4. improve postural stability in standing and walking by improving body alignment and speed of postural movement strategies

5. increase overall activity level.

FUNCTIONAL OBJECTIVES

Following 3 months of therapy, Mr. Johnson will be able to:

1. rotate his upper trunk in a sitting position to reach for an object placed out to the side and slightly behind him

2. roll up a small incline two times successively with segmentation of the trunk (does not log roll)

3. initiate sit to stand maneuver from a chair within 5 seconds of a verbal signal

4. be able to walk an obstacle course of 25 feet with 6 objects to circumvent, within 5 minutes

5. participate in a Parkinson support group exercise program two times per week.

TREATMENT RECOMMENDATIONS

Traditional physical therapy measures to improve flexibility of the trunk and to increase Mr. Johnson's ability to counterrotate between upper and lower trunk can be used to address Goals 1 and 2. Practice in maintaining a vertical posture with the head and trunk held upright and in alignment with the trunk and hips addresses Goals 3 and 4. Mr. Johnson can practice this by leaning against a wall, then moving away from the wall trying to maintain the appropriate posture. Use of a mirror and visual feedback also may help.

He should practice standing with his center of mass in a neutral position between the balls of his feet and heels, rather than forward onto the balls of his feet. Initially, he may use a small wedge to displace himself backwards. Gradually, the size of the wedge should be decreased until he is able to maintain a neutral position of the COM without cues. A static forceplate retraining system may also assist him in learning a new position.

In the treatment program, activities should be included to address increased speed of movement of the center of mass and decreased time for initiation of movement, particularly postural adjustments prior to voluntary movements. Mr. Johnson should practice timed shifts of the center of mass using a static forceplate system or practice with a metronome. He may try use of a visual and/or auditory cue prior to a voluntary timed movement of the center of mass to assist with increasing speed of performance.

CASE STUDY #3
SHIRLEY TEAL

Age: 21 years
Diagnosis: Post motor vehicle accident,
closed head injury
Status: Four months post onset

ASSESSMENT

Ms. Teal is a 21 year old woman who is 10 months post CHI. Functional problems include decreased independence in ADLs and decreased stability and mobility skills (specifically loss of independent stance and gait, secondary to impaired postural control), and positional dizziness. Ms. Teal is independent in a wheelchair.

Musculoskeletal constraints which underlie her instability include decreased range of motion in the right lower extremity, including limitation in ankle dorsiflexion and knee and hip extension. She also has asymmetric body alignment in sitting and stance, with her weight shifted primarily to the left side.

Neuromuscular constraints are increased muscle tonus bilaterally R > L, decreased coordination bilaterally R > L, and decreased strength in the right lower extremity resulting in her inability to sustain terminal knee extension during stance and gait.

Sensory/perceptual problems include inability to maintain stance balance when visual inputs are reduced or inaccurate for orientation and positional dizziness due to post-traumatic benign paroxysmal positional nystagmus (BPPN) and vertigo.

GOALS

Treatment goals are for Ms. Teal to:

1. demonstrate fewer musculoskeletal limitations
2. increase strength in the right extremities
3. improve alignment, becoming more symmetrical, with equal weight through both sides of her body in sitting and stance
4. improve symmetry of postural movement strategies in response to loss of balance
5. increase ability to maintain balance in the presence of reduced visual cues for orientation
6. decrease positional vertigo.

FUNCTIONAL OBJECTIVES

Following 2 months of therapy, Ms. Teal will:

1. demonstrate an improvement of 5 degrees of active ankle dorsiflexion and active knee extension in sitting
2. do 5 stand to semi-squat to stand exercises while holding onto a support
3. match a vertical taped line in midline of her shirt with a taped vertical line in mirror while standing in the parallel bars, 4 of 5 trials
4. demonstrate ability to regain upright/midline position when displaced 5 degrees to the left, then 5 degrees to the right while standing in a walker, 3 of 5 trials
5. maintain standing balance in the parallel bars for 5 seconds with vision occluded
6. chart amount of dizziness for same two 30 minute periods for 30 days and demonstrate a decrease in symptoms.

TREATMENT RECOMMENDATIONS

Similar activities as outlined in case studies 1 and 2 for Goals 1-5 for Ms. Teal should be used. She should be instructed in habituation exercises for BPPN. These consist of 5 repetitions, twice a day, to the left side in a modified Hallpike position (Figure 7).[59] She begins in a sitting position on the side of the bed and then tilts rapidly to her left side to recline on pillows placed on that side, allowing her head to tip slightly upward. After waiting for the dizziness to subside, or 30 seconds, she sits back up. After waiting for the dizziness to subside in an upright position, or 30 seconds, she repeats the exercise. This is an exercise designed to reduce positional dizziness through habituation.

CASE STUDY # 4
SHAWNA WELLS

Age: 4 years
Diagnosis: Cerebral palsy,
spastic quadriparesis mild mental retardation
Status: Onset at birth

ASSESSMENT

Shawna is a 4 year old child with cerebral palsy. Functional problems include: delayed postural and protective reactions during active movement and passive displacement, and reliance on a stepping pattern to regain balance in upright. She has poor tolerance for, or inadequate processing

FIGURE 7. *Modified Hallpike position.*

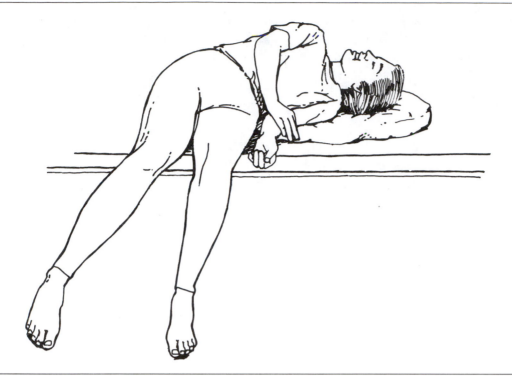

of, movement related activities. Mild mental retardation contributes to problems in cooperation during therapy sessions, as well as to learning and remembering new motor tasks.

Musculoskeletal constraints include decreased active ROM in ankle dorsiflexors and knee extensors with mild tightness in gastrocnemius/soleus and hamstrings bilaterally. She also has decreased trunk and upper extremity flexibility.

Neuromuscular problems are decreased coordination and reciprocation of lower extremities during creeping and gait, inability to sustain full knee extension on stance leg during gait; and reliance on a stepping pattern with lack of ankle or hip strategies in active movement or in response to external perturbation.

Sensory/perceptual constraints include her inability to maintain balance in standing on any surface that is not flat and firm. Additionally, she is unable to maintain balance when visual inputs are reduced or inaccurate for orientation. Her cone of perceived stability appears to be decreased.

Cognitive impairments are mild mental retardation, decreased motivation for independent movement, and poor short term and long term memory for motor learning.

GOALS

Treatment goals are for Shawna to:

1. demonstrate increased active ROM in ankle dorsiflexion and hamstrings

2. increase trunk flexibility

3. improve reciprocation of lower extremities

4. use an ankle or hip strategy in response to passive displacement

5. increase knee extension during stance

6. use an ankle strategy and demonstrate increased cone of perceived stability to forward/backward sway in active standing and weight shifting

7. improve balance in sitting and standing when visual inputs are diminished.

FUNCTIONAL OBJECTIVES

Following 3 months of treatment, Shawna will:

1. put on her socks with minimal assistance in a long sitting position on the floor (with knees held in extension)

2. perform 5 "wind mill" exercises, i.e., right hand to left toe, left hand to right toe in standing, with assistance at pelvis to maintain balance

3. march in time to slow music for 30 seconds while holding her walker

4. while holding onto walker, regain her balance in standing following slight displacements left or right without using a stepping strategy, 3 of 5 trials

5. while holding onto walker, maintain knee extension on either leg while lifting the opposite leg up and down on a step 5 times in succession

6. sway independently forward and backward in her walker using an ankle strategy, 3 of 5 trials

7. walk down a hallway with her walker at school when lights are turned off (semi-darkness) 100% of the time.

TREATMENT RECOMMENDATIONS

Active-assistive exercises to increase active ROM in gastrocnemius/soleus and hamstring muscle groups should be stressed. Daily functional activities should be devised to maintain ROM so that daily stretching does not have to be done. An example would be having Shawna sit in long sitting with sandbags over her knees in the classroom or at home for 10 minutes each day to maintain hamstring elongation.

Activities in sitting and standing to increase Shawna's cone of stability should be included in her program. These activities would include passive displacements as well as active displacements.

A variety of sensory inputs should be incorporated to increase awareness of her body parts and position in space as well as to challenge her balance. Examples would be walking barefoot, walking on different textures, and walking in rooms with variable lighting available.

Activities that are of high interest and motivating to Shawna should be used. One example is the use of music which she enjoys. Practicing active weight shifts to music (dancing) and reciprocation (marching) will be more successful if is she motivated and attending to the task. ❏

REFERENCES

1. Duncan P (ed): Balance, Proceedings of the APTA Forum. Alexandria, VA, American Physical Therapy Association, 1990
2. Shumway-Cook A: Equilibrium Deficits in Children. In Woollacott M, Shumway-Cook A: Development of Posture and Gait Across the Lifespan. Columbia, SC, University of South Carolina Press, 1989
3. Horak F, Shumway-Cook A: Clinical Implications of Posture Control Research. In Duncan P (ed): Balance, Proceedings of the APTA Forum. Alexandria, VA, APTA, 1990
4. Shumway-Cook A, Horak F: Rehabilitation Strategies for Patients with Peripheral Vestibular Disorders. Neurologic Clinics, Philadelphia, PA, Saunders Co., 1990
5. Shumway-Cook,A, Olmscheid R: A systems analysis of postural dyscontrol in traumatically brain-injured patients. J of Head Trauma Rehabilitation, in press
6. Martin JP: The basal ganglia and posture, London, England, Pitman Med Publ., 1967
7. Wyke B: The neurological basis of movement - a developmental review. In Holt K (ed): Movement and Child Development. Philadelphia, PA, Lippincott, 1975
8. Bobath B: Abnormal Postural Reflex Activity Caused by Brain Lesions. London, England, Heinemann Publishers, 1975
9. Jackson, JH: Selected writing of John Hughlings Jackson, In Taylor J (ed): John Hughlings Jackson. Vol 1, London, England, Hodder & Stoughter, 1932
10. Weiss S: Studies in equilibrium reaction. J of Nervous and Mental Disorders 88: 153-62, 1938
11. Milani Comparetti A, Gidoni E: Routine developmental examination in normal and retarded children. Dev Med & Child Neuro 9:631-38, 1967
12. Bobath, B. Adult Hemiplegia: Evaluation and Treatment. William Heinemann Medical Books, London, England, 1974
13. Davies P: Steps to Follow. New York, NY, Springer-Verlag, 1985
14. Smith S: Traumatic head injures. In D. Umphred (ed): Neurological Rehabilitation. St. Louis, MO, C V Mosby Co., 1985
15. Fiorentino MR: Reflex testing methods for evaluating CNS development, Springfield, IL, Charles C Thomas, 1973
16. Effgen SL: Integration of the plantar grasp reflex as an indicator of ambulation potential in developmentally disabled infants. Phys Ther 62:433-35, 1982
17. Haley S: Sequential analyses of postural reactions in nonhandicapped infants. Phys Ther 66:531-36, 1986
18. Carr J, Shepherd R: A motor relearning programme for stroke, Rockville, MD, Aspen Publications, 1983
19. Bernstein N: The Coordination and Regulation of Movement, London, England, Pergamon Press, 1967
20. McCollum G, Leen T: Form and Exploration of Mechanical Stability Limits in Erect Stance. J of Motor Beh 21:225-38, 1989
21. Nashner L, Mc Collum G: The organization of human postural movements: A formal basis and experimental synthesis. The Behavioral and Brain Sciences 8:135-172, 1985
22. Horak F, Nashner L: Central programming of posture control: adaptation to altered support surface configurations. J of Neuro-physiology 55:1369-81, 1986
23. Nashner L, Forssberg H: Phase dependent organization of postural adjustments associated with arm movements while walking. J of Neurophysiology. 55:1382-94, 1986
24. Das P, McCollum G: Invariant structure in locomotion. Neuroscience 25:1023-35, 1988
25. Gahery Y, Massion J: Coordination between posture and movement. In Evarts EV, Wise SP, Boousfield D (eds): The Motor System in Neurobiology. Amsterdam, Elsevier Biomedical Press, 1985
26. Cordo P, Nashner LM: Properties of postural adjustments associated with rapid arm movements. J of Neurophysiology 47: 287-298, 1982
27. Horak F, Shupert C, Mirka A: Components of postural dyscontrol in the elderly: A review. Neurobiology of Aging 10:727-745, 1989
28. Nashner L: Adaptation of human movement to altered environments. Trends in Neuroscience 5:358-61, 1982
29. Nashner L, Black FO, Wall C: Adaptation to altered support and visual conditions during stance: patients with vestibular deficits. J of Neuroscience 2:536-44, 1982
30. Shumway-Cook A, Woollacott M: The growth stability:Postural control from a developmental perspective. J of Motor Behavior 17:131-47, 1985
31. Shumway-Cook A, Anson D, Haller S: The use of postural sway biofeedback in retraining postural stability following stroke. Arch Phys Med Rehab 69:395-400, 1988
32. Duncan P: Physical therapy assessment. In M Rosenthal, Bond M, Griffith ER, Miller JD (eds): Rehabilitation of the Adult and Child with Traumatic Brain Injury, ed 2, Philadelphia, PA, FA Davis, 1990
33. Weintraub AH, Opat C: Motor and sensory dysfunction in the brain-injured adult. In Horn LJ, Cope DN (eds): Physical Medicine and Rehabilitation: Traumatic Brain Injury, 1989
34. Mercer L, Bock M: Residual sensorimotor deficits in the adult head-injured patient. Phys Ther 63:1988-1991, 1983
35. Sahrman SA, Norton BJ: The relationship of voluntary movement to spasticity in the upper motor neuron syndrome. Ann Neurol 2:240-254, 1977
36. Badke M, DeFabio R: Balance deficits in patients with hemiplegia:considerations for assessment and treatment. In Duncan P (ed): Balance, Proceedings of the APTA Forum. Alexandria, VA,,APTA, 1990
37. Nashner L, Shumway-Cook A, Marin O: Stance posture control in select groups of children with cerebral palsy: Deficits in sensory organization and muscular coordination. Exp Brain Res 49:393-409, 1983
38. Horak F, Nashner L, Nutt JB: Postural instability in Parkinson's disease: Motor coordination and sensory organization. Neurology Report 12:54-58, 1988
39. Horak F, Esselman P, Anderson M, Lynch M: The effects of movement velocity, mass displaced and task certainty on associated postural adjustments made by normal and hemiplegic individuals. J Neurol Neurosurg Psychiatry 47:1020-1028, 1984
40. Rinehart M: Strategies for improving motor performance. In M Rosenthal, Bond M, Griffith ER, Miller JD. (eds): Rehabilitation of the Adult and Child with Traumatic Brain Injury, ed 2. Philadelphia, PA, FA Davis, 1990
41. Bohannon RW, Larkin PW: Cybex II isokinetic dynamometer for the documentation of spasticity. Phys Ther 65:46-49, 1985
42. Louis M: Visual field and perceptual deficits in the brain damaged patient. Critical Care Update 8:32-34, 1981
43. Stanworth A: Defects of ocular movement and fusion after head injury. Brit J Opthal 58:266-271, 1974
44. Horak F, Nashner L, Diener H: Postural strategies associated with somatosensory and vestibular loss. Exp Brain Res. In press.
45. Lund S: Dizziness and vertigo in the posttraumatic syndrome. A Physiologic background. Acta Neurochir Suppl 36:118-21,1986
46. Healy G: Hearing loss and vertigo secondary to head injury. New England J of Med 306:1029-31, 1982
47. Newton R: Recovery of balance abilities in individuals with raumatic brain injuries. In Duncan P (ed): Balance, Proceedings of the APTA Forum. Alexandria, VA, APTA, 1990
48. DiFabio R, Badke MB: Relationship of sensory organization to balance function in patients with hemiplegia. Phys Ther 70:543-48, 1990
49. Shumway-Cook A, Horak F: Assessing the influence of sensory interaction on balance. Phys Ther 66:1548-50, 1986
50. Horak F: Clinical measurement of postural control in adults. Phys Ther 67:1881-85, 1987
51. Shumway-Cook A, Horak F: Vestibular rehabilitation: an exercise approach to managing symptoms of vestibular dysfunction. Seminars in Hearing 10:196-209, 1989
52. Alexander MP: The role of neurobehavioral syndromes in the rehabilitation and outcome of closed head injury. In Levin HS, Grafman J, Eisenberg HM (eds): Neurobehavioral Recovery from Head Injury. Oxford, Oxford University Press, 1987
53. Genarelli TA, Speilman F, Langfitt TW: Influence of the type of intracranial lesion on outcome from severe head injury: A multicenter study using a new classification system. J of Neurosurg 56:26-32, 1982
54. Auerbach SH: Neuroanatomical correlates of attention and memory disorders in TBI: An application of neuro-behavioral subtypes. J Head Trauma Rehab 1:1-11, 1986
55. Levin HS, Benton AL, Grossman RG: Neurobehavioral Consequences of Closed Head Injury. Oxford, Oxford University Press, 1982
56. Horak F, Diener C, Nashner L: Influence of central set on human postural responses. J of Neurophysiology 62:841-46, 1989
57. Schmidt R: Motor Control and Learning. Champaign, IL, Human Kinetics Publishers, 1982
58. Horak F: Comparison of cerebellar and vestibular loss on scaling of postural responses. In Brandt T (ed): X International Symposium on Disorders of Posture and Gait. Munich, Thieme Press, 1990
59. Brandt T, Daroff A: Physical therapy for benign positional vertigo. Arch Otolaryngol 106:484-85, 1980

Chapter 11
Perspectives on the Evaluation and Treatment of Gait Disorders

Carol A. Oatis, Ph.D., PT

INTRODUCTION

Evaluation of locomotion is one of the most common components of an evaluation by a physical therapist. Certainly, the restoration or improvement of locomotion is a commonly cited goal by physical therapists. Frequently, criteria for improved gait include the visual appearance of normalcy, that is, parameters such as step length or joint excursions approach normal values. Such judgments are often made using observational gait analysis, which is a systematic procedure by which the clinician views the behavior and compares it to normal values.[1] However, the basic premise of observational analysis is that a gait pattern is "good" if it looks normal, and is "not good" if it looks abnormal. Yet, there may be circumstances in which the underlying disability precludes a normal pattern of movement and achieving a normal visual appearance would increase the difficulty of walking. The purpose of this chapter is to provide a theoretical framework to analyze gait using methods including visual observation of motion.

REVIEW OF NORMAL GAIT

A clear understanding of normal locomotion is essential when analyzing gait. Parameters of gait are generally divided into two categories, kinematics and kinetics, each of which will be reviewed.

Kinematics

Much has been written about the kinematic parameters of locomotion. While kinematic parameters include displacement, velocity, and acceleration data, the vast majority of kinematic data are displacement data, particularly joint excursions of the lower extremities.[2-9] Most data describe motion in the sagittal plane, but some studies include all three planes.[10,11] A few studies include the behavior of the trunk and upper extremities. The classic standards of normal joint excursions come from Eberhart et al[2] and Murray et al.[3,12-15] The limitations of these data have been reviewed elsewhere.[16] Most of these data are from a limited number of subjects, most of whom were young adult males. This small data base decreases its applicability. For example, age has been shown by most investigators to affect joint kinematics.[12] Specifically, walking velocity appears to decrease with age[12,17] and joint excursions are generally directly proportional to velocity.[11,15,18] In other words, as walking speed decreases, joint excursions decrease while they increase with increasing gait speed. Thus, joint motion in an elderly subject may be considered abnormal because it is compared to a younger population. The standards of normalcy used during gait evaluations must be applied judiciously to avoid overstating the abnormality.

Despite these limitations in the normal kinematic data, there are basic characteristics of movement that appear to be relatively constant. A grasp of these basic elements is essential to understanding gait disorders. First, consider the basic characteristics of the movement of the lower extremities in the sagittal plane. The complexity of movement increases distally, that is, beginning at ground contact the hip joint's movement is a simple single cycle oscillation from flexion to extension to flexion again (Figure 1). Maximum extension generally occurs at 50 percent of the gait cycle, so that hip joint motion is distributed evenly across the gait cycle.[3,10,19,20] Knee joint excursion, however, demonstrates two unequal peaks of flexion, the first appearing at about 15 percent of the

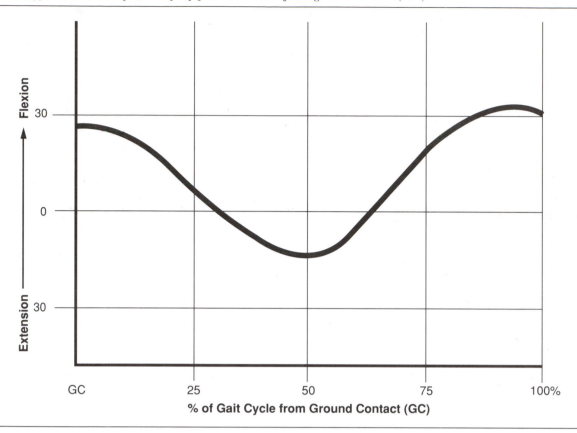

FIGURE 1. *Typical kinematic pattern of hip joint movement from ground contact (GC).*

gait cycle and the other in early swing, or at about 70-75 percent of the cycle (Figure 2).[3,20] Despite the increased complexity of the movement, there appears to be a smooth transition between flexion and extension. The ankle demonstrates two peaks of plantarflexion (Figure 3).[3] The first occurs early in the stance phase as the foot descends to the floor. The second occurs early in the swing phase as the foot is moving away from the floor. However, the transition from plantar to dorsiflexion in mid-stance is often not as smooth as in the knee, as indicated by a more variable angular velocity.[20] Thus, the pattern of joint motions increases in complexity as analysis goes from proximal to distal.

Another useful characteristic of joint kinematics is the apparent independence of joint movements in the lower extremity. Murray indicated that, for a brief instant, in early swing the ankle, knee, and hip are moving in the same direction, that is, away from the ground by flexion of the hip and knee and dorsiflexion of the ankle.[3] This kinematic independence would be interrupted by compulsory movements such as flexion or extension synergies.

Similar patterns of smooth, cyclic movement are evident in the pelvis, trunk, and upper extremities. In the sagittal plane, the pelvis moves synchronously with the two hip joints; that is, the pelvis reaches a maximum anterior tilt each time one hip reaches maximum extension.[3] Therefore, the pelvis goes through two cycles of anterior rotation, but the cycles are timed evenly through the gait cycle at zero and 50 percent.

The trunk demonstrates little isolated trunk motion in the sagittal plane. In contrast, the upper extremities exhibit almost nothing but sagittal plane motion.[3] The upper extremity moves in synchrony with the opposite lower extremity. As one lower extremity swings forward the contralateral upper extremity moves forward, while the opposite lower and upper extremities extend. The trunk rotates forward with the flexing upper extremity.[3] This movement pattern constitutes a single cycle of flexion and extension of both upper extremities and the trunk. However, the trunk is rotating forward on the side opposite from the advancing lower extremity and is opposite the transverse plane rotation of the pelvis. In other words, in the transverse plane the trunk and pelvis are 180° out of phase from one another.

By reviewing the kinematic data, certain principles seem apparent. First, there appears to be a progression of complexity from proximal to distal in the lower extremities. Second, the motions of the lower extremities require that the joints of each lower extremity be able to move independently of each other. Next, the pelvis and trunk rotate in opposite directions, so that they are 180° out of phase with each other as are the upper and lower extremities. These principles suggest that normal locomotion requires independence of the trunk and pelvis. In addition, there is a prescribed sequence of events so that the limbs and trunk move in a certain rhythm. These characteristics also are related to the kinetic parameters of locomotion. The interrelationship of kinematic and kinetic parameters may hold the key to developing a more critical approach to the analysis and treatment of gait disorders. Before the conceptual framework can be developed, our present level of understanding of the kinetic parameters must be reviewed.

Kinetics

Kinetic parameters help describe the mechanical controls of locomotion. These parameters include joint reaction forces and muscle moments at each joint as well as ground reaction forces. Kinetics also includes energy parameters such as mechanical energy and power, metabolic energy as in oxygen consumption, and muscle activity as indicated by electromyographical (EMG) data. Although the latter is not a direct measure of muscle force, it is an indicator of muscle activity and, therefore, is a relative measure of muscle load.

Ground reaction forces are the net forces exerted by the body onto the ground. They are reported generally as vertical force and forward, aft, and medio-lateral shear forces. Although Jacobs et al[21] attempted to differentiate between the gait patterns of normal subjects and those with total hip replacements using ground reaction forces, the data are frequently used to calculate joint and muscle forces and torques rather than as unique descriptors of motion.[20,21] Joint reaction forces are the net forces applied across the joint, inertial forces due to the acceleration of the limb segments,

and the ground reaction forces.[20,22] Joint reaction forces during gait have been calculated for the hips, knees, and ankles. Peak joint reaction forces at the hip have been reported to be almost seven times body weight in women and more than five times body weight in men.[23-25] Morrison,[26] Harrington,[27] and Paul[23] reported peak knee reaction forces to be as large as four times body weight. Peak ankle forces have been reported up to five and one-half times body weight.[24,28] Joint reaction forces in walking reportedly increase with increasing velocity.[11] Little is known of the impact of gait disorders on joint reaction forces, but data collected from normals remind us that walking generates large loads across joint surfaces. Techniques to minimize joint loads, such as decreasing walking speed and unloading the limbs by using an assistive device, should always be considered in the presence of joint pain or inflammation.

Joint moments are the torques applied by muscles, ligaments, and internal joint friction to control or change the angular displacement of a limb. In gait, these moments are generally attributed to muscles.[20] They are derived mathematically from inputs including ground reaction forces, kinematic data, and anthropometric characteristics of the subject including limb lengths, weights, and locations of the limb centers of mass.[20] These calculations, when compared with the corresponding joint excursions, allow us to appreciate the role of muscles in controlling the motions in gait.

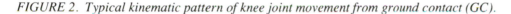

FIGURE 2. *Typical kinematic pattern of knee joint movement from ground contact (GC).*

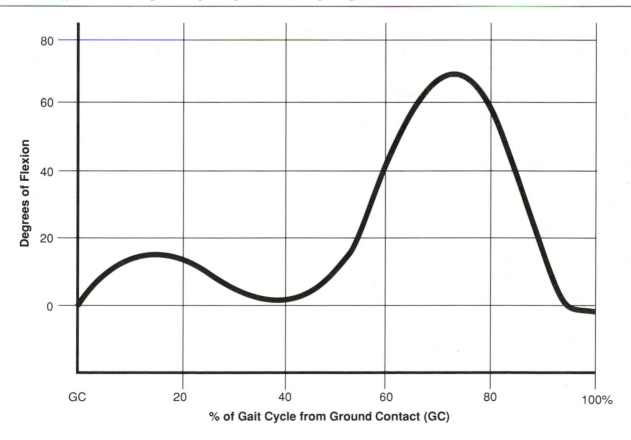

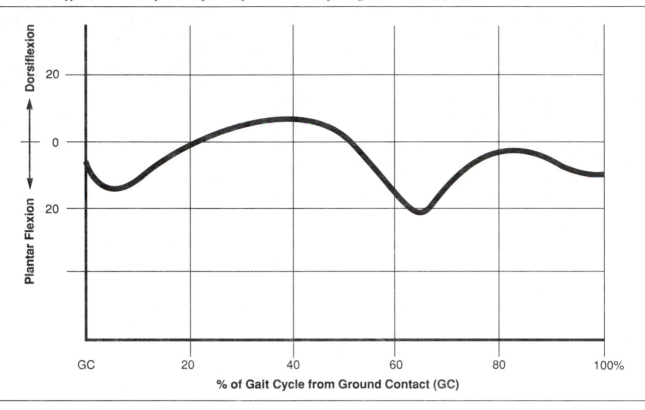

% of Gait Cycle from Ground Contact (GC)

Winter[20,29] used muscle torques to describe a "support moment" during the stance phase of gait in normal subjects. He defined the support moment as the sum of moments at the hip, knee, and ankle and operationally defined the joint moments as positive if they tended to push the body away from the ground. Thus, extensor moments at the hip and knee and plantarflexion moments at the ankle were considered positive. It was noted that the sum of these moments was consistently positive throughout most of stance, indicating the muscles' role in supporting the stance limb, and avoiding collapse of the limb. These authors also noted a synergistic relationship between the knee and hip extensors so that as one supportive component decreases the other component increases to maintain a positive support moment. Similar studies are not available for the swing phase, but the overall joint moments are smaller during swing.

Specific muscle activity in locomotion has been studied extensively, albeit in a relatively small number of subjects.[16] In general, muscles are active for very short periods of time during the gait cycle, 0.7 seconds or less.[16] Winter and Yack[30] noted that distal muscles are the most active while the proximal muscles are least active. EMG data also suggest that plantarflexors are the primary source of propulsion through mid and terminal stance.[16] The swing phase of gait is characterized by very little muscle activity. The iliacus apparently decelerates the femur in mid-stance then accelerates it in late stance and early swing.[20] The gluteus maximus helps decelerate the limb in late swing. Muscle activity at the knee is generally absent throughout swing.[31-33] At the ankle, the dorsiflexors are responsible for preventing foot drop or toe drag in swing.[34] The absence of muscle activity in swing has caused investigators to compare lower extremity motion to that of a compound or jointed pendulum[35] in which the motion of swing is dictated by gravity, given a certain initial position and velocity. Thus, muscle activity data help define three roles for muscles throughout gait. The first is that of support in the stance phase performed primarily by the hip and knee extensors (somewhat interchangeably) and by the plantarflexors. Second is propulsion performed by the plantarflexors and hip flexors, and a third is deceleration performed by the hip extensors.

Mechanical energy is probably less familiar, yet provides an insight into control of locomotion which is useful to analyze gait disorders. Mechanical energy has two forms: kinetic energy which is a function of mass and velocity, both linear and rotational, and potential energy which is a function of the distance of the body's center of mass from the ground. The principle of conservation of energy states that work must be done on an object in order to change its total energy or the sum of kinetic and potential energies (see Chapter 4). This means that if kinetic and potential energies can be changed from one form to another with no change in total energy, no work is needed in the system. In an ideal roller coaster, the car will have a maximum potential energy and minimum kinetic energy at the peak of the track. At the lowest point of the track, potential energy is at a minimum and the kinetic energy is maximized. In the ideal case, there is a complete transfer of energy so that the continued motion of the roller coaster requires no work because the total energy is unchanged. Winter, et al[36] investigated this energy transformation in the trunk, thigh, and leg. These authors reported approximately a 50% transformation in the trunk and approximately 33% exchange in the thigh, but almost no transformation in the leg. Robertson and Winter[37] investigated the energy exchange between limb segments during locomotion, which is essentially what occurs in the game of crack-the-whip in which energy is transferred from the leader along the line of children. The flow of energy between segments was significant and could account for almost all of the changes in energy in the distal limbs at the beginning and end of swing.

The use of mechanical power, which is the product of force and linear velocity, is useful to understand the role of energy storage played by muscles, particularly multi-jointed muscles. Positive power indicates a shortening or concentric contraction of a muscle by which the muscle imparts energy to the system.[37] Negative power indicates a lengthening or eccentric contraction in which energy is stored in a muscle to be released later in the gait cycle. Morrison[38] reported that two joint muscles, such as the hamstrings and quadriceps, seemed to generate considerable power at one joint when a smaller power output was required at the other joint resulting in more efficient movement. Wells[39] used this approach to quantify the efficiency of bi-articulate muscles. He reported a 7 to 29% increase in efficiency using two joint muscles which could theoretically absorb energy at one joint and release it at another.

In summary, these investigations into the kinetic characteristics of locomotion yield insights into the nature of locomotion which must be considered as we develop a framework for evaluating and treating abnormal locomotion. First, in normal locomotion the joints of the lower extremity are exposed to significant loads which may increase under abnormal conditions and contribute to joint damage or pain. Second, muscle activity, although brief, is precisely timed and muscle groups are activated in a coordinated way to provide support, propulsion, and deceleration. Third, mechanical power analysis reveals that muscle activity also is efficient in its ability to absorb and release energy to facilitate motion. Finally, analysis of mechanical energy demonstrates that the movement of some segments allows an exchange of energy forms from either kinetic or potential energy to the other and that energy actually flows from one segment to another. Since mechanical energy is dependent on velocity and position, this implies that the motion and orientation of one limb segment or joint is, at least in part, dependent on other segments. Thus, kinetic data help identify the flaws of observational gait analysis, which identifies the positions of limb segments or joints and compares these values with normal standards. The interdependence of limb segments and the controlling role of muscles can be forgotten too easily. The following section will develop a scheme to evaluate gait disorders blending this kinetic information with the more conventional kinematic data.

THEORETICAL FRAMEWORK

In the preceding section, the general principles of normal locomotion were reviewed. Identification of kinematic abnormalities has limited benefit since it ignores the interrelationships of the limb segments and the energy storage capacity of muscles. The purpose of this section is to design a scheme for using these concepts to analyze and treat locomotor disorders. Such a framework will provide a means to do more than merely identify deviations from normal. Rather, it should assist clinicians in making a judgment on the quality of gait. Winter[40] noted that evaluation consists of measurement, description, analysis, and assessment. The first three tasks comprise the data gathering phase which allows the evaluator to compare the data to normal standards. The last phase of evaluation, assessment, requires the evaluator to make a value judgment. That is, despite the abnormality of the movement, is it a "good" pattern of movement or even the "best" pattern available to the patient?

In order to determine the "goodness" of a locomotor pattern, basic tasks and requirements of locomotion must be considered. Das and McCollum[41] identified forward progression as the central task of bipedal ambulation and stated that this is implemented by the supporting legs. These investigators delineated the task of locomotion by considering swing and stance phases separately. They suggested that the stance phase has two implied tasks: to provide adequate upward support to avoid falling and to provide adequate forward and backward force for progression. These same authors offered three basic tasks for swing: safe foot clearance, placement of the swing foot onto a new and appropriate surface, and control of the transfer of angular momentum. Winter[42] also outlined three "necessary (but not sufficient)" tasks for safe ambulation. These include upward support of the body, maintenance of upright posture and balance, and control of foot movement to provide toe clearance and gentle foot contact.

Investigators recognized upward support and foot clearance as essential for safe ambulation. Physical therapists can use these basic elements as the first criteria for judging the quality of a gait. First, consider the stance phase in which support is the primary task. As detailed in the first section of this chapter, Winter[29] identified a support moment which is the sum of moments of force about the ankle, knee, and hip during the stance phase of gait. He observed that the general pattern of joint moments is a net positive or extensor moment, i.e., the sum of ankle, knee, and hip moments is a moment tending to push the subject away from the ground, providing both support and forward progression. Thus, from a clinical viewpoint, the subject must generate adequate plantarflexion force and a sufficient combination of knee and hip extensor force to prevent collapse. If this combination is present, the first basic task of the stance phase is accomplished.

We can demonstrate the advantage of regarding support as a basic criterion of the quality of gait by considering a clinical example. Using support, or the absence of falls, as a criterion for evaluating stance could lead the clinician to the conclusion that the patient with an extensor synergy has a "good" pattern of movement for the stance phase of gait. From the kinematic perspective, an extensor synergy would be a "poor" pattern of movement for the stance phase because probably it would lead to an inappropriate ground contact and inadequate ankle plantarflexion and knee flexion following contact. Yet, an attempt to normalize the kinematic behavior might interrupt the extensor synergy so that the subject could no longer provide adequate support. In this case, in the stance phase, an abnormal kinematic pattern actually is a successful mechanism to accomplish one of the basic elements of stance, that is, support.

The tasks of the swing phase are safe foot clearance,[41,42] foot advancement, and a controlled transfer of momentum.[41] Safe foot clearance essentially demands that the swinging limb is able to shorten sufficiently to allow clearance. EMG data reviewed earlier suggest that the limb shortening in swing is the result of active flexion of the thigh with a passive flexion of the knee. This passive flexion to extension of the knee is extremely rapid and requires a freely swinging knee and an adequate forward thrust of the hip to initiate the movement. The importance of a freely swinging lower extremity in swing is supported by Olgiatti, et al.[43] These investigators reported that there was a relationship between the metabolic cost of walking and the ability of subjects with multiple sclerosis to rapidly flex and extend the knee. Inability to perform rapid knee motion was considered an indicator of increased lower extremity tone, so lower extremity spasticity was significantly related to a higher energy cost of ambulation.

The increased energy expenditure with increased muscle tone reported by Olgiatti, et al[43] is consistent with Das and McCollum's second task of the swing phase of gait, transfer of momentum.[41] Joints of the lower extremity must move independently of one another, and data assessing mechanical energy transformation revealed the interdependence between limb segments and between whole limbs allowing the flow of energy between segments. Thus, some of the efficiency of the swing phase of gait depends on the apparent independence, yet coordinated movements of the adjacent limb segments.

Consider the likely effects of an extensor synergy on a patient's swing phase. First, limb shortening and foot clearance are likely to be problems since a freely swinging knee joint usually is absent in the presence of an extension synergy. Advancement of the thigh through hip flexion may be more difficult. Thus, safe foot clearance and foot placement may be impaired. In addition, if the advancement of the thigh is diminished, there will be less energy to impart to the leg and if flexion of the knee is limited by increased extensor tone, the entire synchronized motion of the lower extremity in swing is interrupted. Any significant beneficial energy flow through the lower extremity is unlikely. An extensor synergy may jeopardize seriously the patient's safety during swing and may increase the energy expenditure to clear and advance the limb. By focusing on the general tasks embedded in stance and swing phases of gait, components of the movement pattern which are beneficial and those which are deleterious can be identified and treatment can be focused appropriately.

While motor control experts and biomechanists tend to look at the quality of the movement itself, the clinician must consider the functionality of the movement. Locomotion is rarely a goal in and of itself, but rather a means to an end, that is, a means of transportation to accomplish a task such as eating, shopping, working, or sleeping. Successful locomotion must be practical. Studies have shown that patients with L1 and above paraplegia generally expend less energy transporting themselves by wheelchair than by ambulating using bilateral crutches.[44] Experience has shown that many patients who are discharged from the rehabilitation facility ambulating soon abandon ambulation for the relative ease of wheelchair transportation. While this may be regarded as failure, if the efficiency of the wheelchair allows the patient to resume an active, productive lifestyle, the wheelchair should be regarded as the "better" mode of transportation. Another study suggested that one reason for the loss of independence in the aging population is an inability to cross a street within the time allotted by a standard traffic light.[45] In other words, the overall velocity is a major contributing factor to independence. Perhaps the quality of ambulation should be judged on the person's overall ability to function as a result of walking, rather than on the pattern itself. That is, despite the appearance of the gait, can the person go grocery shopping, climb stairs, or go to school? If the gait pattern is functional, the clinician must consider carefully the value of intervening. If the intervention is directed solely toward improving the appearance of the movement, it is superfluous. However, if the intervention is designed to improve the functionality of the gait, such as increasing walking speed so the individual can cross the street safely or decreasing the energy cost of walking so the individual can walk though the school corridors and still have energy to attend class, the intervention seems worth the investment.

What is the framework with which we should evaluate gait disorders? The previous discussion suggests that task evaluation can lead to a better understanding of the quality of gait. These include tasks inherent to the movements such as support, ground clearance, and transfer of momentum, as well as to the tasks which are the goals of locomotion. Examples of such goals are transportation from point A to point B within environmental constraints, such as traffic, and with enough residual energy to perform a desired task, such as to cook dinner or shop. Traditionally, physical therapists have considered the pattern of movement as monitored by observational gait analysis rather than considering the underlying tasks embedded within the movement. Such a narrow focus makes us susceptible to the accusation that we "cannot see the forest for the trees." As in the example of the patient with an extensor synergy, it is tempting to be concerned about the absence of heelstrike or knee flexion after contact and to ignore the fact that the patient exhibits good, firm support in the stance phase. On the other hand, we should not be too hasty in discarding kinematic data which may help us understand the mechanisms underlying or controlling gait. Single elements within the movement of locomotion, such as joint excursions or joint moments, may influence the patient's ability to accomplish the tasks which, by themselves, may not be the most useful criteria to judge the quality of the movement. Instead, gait evaluation may lead to more functionally relevant goals and more successful treatments if focused on the patient's ability to perform the basic tasks inherent in locomotion. These tasks would include support, propulsion, transfer of momentum, and the ability to use locomotion for some functional outcome.

Linking standard clinical data with assessment of gait disorders can yield a judgment of the quality of the movement, possible mechanisms to explain the movement, goals of physical therapy intervention, and a treatment plan.

CLINICAL USE OF GAIT ANALYSIS

The goals of clinical gait analysis are to define a baseline pattern of behavior in order to document change, to devise a treatment plan, and ultimately to improve the behavior. To accomplish these goals the clinician must be able to disassemble the basic tasks of gait described in the previous section and to find the relationship between those elements and the other physical findings of the evaluation, such as strength, range of motion, and muscle tone. Identifying such a relationship will allow the clinician to focus on the specific components of the movement most likely to make a difference in locomotor function. No longer do physical therapists have the luxury of improving strength for its own sake, but only as it relates to function.

Strength

The relationship between muscle strength and locomotion is not well defined. Intuitively, it seems that some degree of strength is necessary to perform the motion, especially in the dorsiflexors for ground clearance and foot contact, in the quadriceps during weight acceptance, and in the gluteus medius for mid-stance. However, the level of strength required of these muscles or any others has not been determined. Only a few investigators have attempted to define a relationship between muscle strength or weakness and gait abnormalities. Krebs[46] reported moderate correlations between quadriceps muscle strength and gait function in patients with post-arthrotomy femoral neuropathies. Gait function was defined by a five point scale averaged for four activities: ambulation, stair climbing, single leg vertical jumps, and squats. Quadriceps and hamstring strength were measured by manual muscle testing and by peak isometric and isokinetic torques. An index of strength based on a summed average of the isometric and isokinetic measures revealed correlations with gait of $r = .75$ for the quadriceps and $r = .71$ for the hamstrings. Gyory et al[9] reported a correlation between quadriceps strength and knee motion during stance in patients with rheumatoid arthritis. Olgiatti, et al[43] found no significant correlation between lower extremity strength and energy cost of walking in patients with multiple sclerosis. In this latter study, strength was operationally defined as the maximum height a patient could step up. Direct comparison of these data is impossible since strength is defined differently in each study. However, the data suggest only a moderate importance of muscle strength in gait.

If muscle strength is of only moderate relevance in gait, how does the clinician use muscle strength data to formulate a treatment plan for locomotor disorders? The basic tasks imbedded in the gait cycle may provide an answer. In the stance phase, the primary task is support followed by forward progression.[41,42] According to Winter,[42] support is provided by the plantarflexors and by the hip and knee extensors. Forward progression is the role of the plantarflexors and hip extensors, although the former appear to be the primary propellant. In addition, pelvic stability is provided by the hip abductors on the stance side. Adequate strength in these muscle groups is necessary to accomplish the task of support. However, we do not know the threshold level of strength required nor do we know the relative importance of each muscle group.

The primary tasks of the swing phase are foot clearance and transfer of momentum. Foot clearance, of course, requires some strength in the dorsiflexors as well as an ability to shorten the whole limb.[11] However, EMG data suggest that limb shortening occurs from an initial thrust of the hip flexors and passive flexion of the knee.[20] Threshold energy from the thigh is then transferred to the leg and foot, facilitating knee extension. Thus, the threshold strength of importance in the swing phase appears to be in the dorsiflexor and hip flexor muscles. The astute clinician will realize that many tasks in daily life require more strength than does normal walking, such as rising from a chair or stair climbing. In terms of locomotion, perhaps muscle strength should be considered as it relates to task accomplishment in stance and swing, rather than as absolute and isolated values. Further research is required to identify the level of strength throughout the lower extremity necessary for functional ambulation.

Range of Motion

Like strength, little has been written describing the relationship between flexibility of the joints of the lower extremity and a subject's walking pattern. Gyory, et al[9] found no correlation between passive range of motion of the knee and the range of knee motion used during ambulation in subjects with arthritis. Stauffer et al[47] reported an inverse relationship between knee flexion range of motion while standing and knee motion in gait. Krebs[46] reported a moderate correlation $(r = .74)$ between percent of the patient's normal knee range of motion and ambulation index based on walking, stair climbing, jumping, and squats following knee arthrotomies. My clinical experience in patients with arthritis suggests that patients require more flexibility in the joint than is actually used during gait or conversely, patients use less joint range in walking than is present passively. Such behavior seems logical since locomotion is essentially a ballistic movement and rapid movements could damage articular structures if they occurred repeatedly at the end range. Such reasoning suggests that perhaps there is a threshold level of flexibility necessary for normal locomotion, but further research is needed to clarify the relationship of flexibility to gait and to determine those threshold values, if they exist.

Muscle Tone

Krebs[46] stated that only 25 to 50% of the variance in gait performance of patients after knee joint arthrotomies, could be accounted for by muscle strength, motor unit activity, and knee flexibility. If strength and range of motion do not completely explain locomotion performance, what other clinical factors could control locomotor behavior? As noted earlier, Olgiatti et al[43] reported that spasticity as measured by patients' ability to swing the knee rapidly was significantly related to the metabolic cost of walking. Tardieu, et al[48] also considered the effect of spasticity on locomotion patterns in children with cerebral palsy (CP). These authors examined the passive contribution of a plantar flexion contracture and the active contribution of normal activation or the excessive activation of the plantarflexor muscles during the push off period of the stance phase. By analyzing the propulsive task of stance and relating this to the passive resistance to dorsiflexion measured in a separate test at rest, these investigators identified two separate mechanisms for toe-walking in children with CP. One resulted from over activity of the triceps surae and the other was due to excessive passive shortening of the same muscle group. These data yield different intervention strategies for these two mechanisms of pathology. Thus, a careful analysis of muscle tone may lead to a better understanding of the mechanisms of gait disorders. This understanding may be enhanced further by relating information about muscle tone to the more standard measures of flexibility or strength.

Mechanical Parameters

In order to develop a clinical measure which reflected both the ballistic nature of the knee's movement in swing and the knee's energy storage role in stance, Oatis[49] presented a mechanical model of the knee as a damped spring linking two rigid segments, representing the leg-foot segment and the thigh, on which perched the mass of the head, arms, trunk, and opposite lower extremity (Figure 4). The characteristics of the damped spring, the damping and stiffness coefficients, were derived by a test in which the knee was allowed to oscillate freely after being released from an extended position. The oscillations were recorded using an electrogoniometer and the coefficients were calculated from the frequency and decay rate of the oscillations (Figure 5). The coefficients then were used to mathematically predict the kinematic behavior of the knee model using appropriate anthropometric data and the initial kinematic data of the thigh at heelstrike. The predicted behavior of the knee then was compared to the real kinematic data for subjects recorded by high-speed cinematography. Although the model was a very simple two dimensional representation of the knee and required certain adjustments to describe the varied nature of the knee's role in stance and swing, the simulated data still yielded reasonable approximations of the real motion (Figure 6). These results provided specific insight into the clinical behavior of the knee during gait, as well as another perspective on gait analysis. This study suggested that the knee's ability to oscillate, or swing, may be more relevant to its performance in locomotion then either its strength or range of motion. This study also demonstrated the usefulness of a task-oriented approach to gait analysis. The realization that

the knee movement in the swing phase required very rapid flexion and extension (344°/sec),[50] as well as recognition of its energy storage role in stance, led the author to a new measurement of knee joint function.

The studies presented in this section examined, the relationship between the functional outcome, locomotion, and some of the individual parameters of physiological activity, such as strength, range of motion, muscle tone, and the mechanical parameters of stiffness and damping. Strength and range of motion, the "gold standards" of physical assessment in physical therapy seem to have a limited influence on locomotion, while muscle tone appears to explain at least some of the mechanisms of gait pathology. The stiffness and damping coefficients can be considered composite measures of joint performance perhaps comprising resting muscle

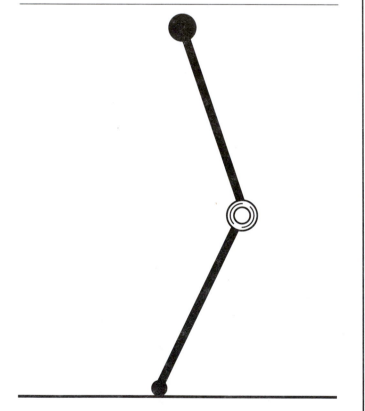

FIGURE 4. *Model of the lower extremity with the head, arms, trunk and opposite leg mounted on the thigh which articulates with the leg-foot segment via a damped torsional spring.*

tone, integrity of the articular cartilage, and joint viscosity. These factors appear to have some predictive capability for the knee joint kinematics during locomotion. It is clear, however, that none of these variables can provide the full explanation for any locomotor disorder. However, these studies should emphasize to the clinician the importance of a critical approach to the application of standard clinical variables to explain and treat gait pathologies. These reports should also encourage clinicians to be creative in their approach to gait analysis and treatment. A focus on the underlying tasks of locomotion and the patient's impaired

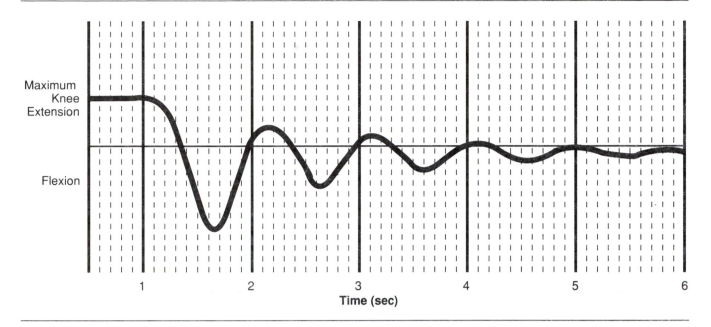

FIGURE 5. *Typical electrogoniometric data of the knee joint during free oscillations.*

Maximum
Knee
Extension

Flexion

Time (sec)

ability to accomplish those tasks may lead a clinician to define a completely new measure of performance which will be more relevant to the outcome measure, locomotion, than any variables now available.

SUMMARY

The standard approach to gait analysis in the clinic is a form of observational gait analysis which documents the subject's kinematic behavior and compares it to some standard. However, this approach ignores the mechanical factors controlling the movement. Observational gait analysis enables the clinician to discriminate between normal and abnormal, but may not provide enough information to make a judgment about the quality of the movement. An understanding of the basic tasks inherent in locomotion, that is, support and propulsion in stance, clearance of the foot, and a transfer of momentum in swing, may provide a basis by which the clinician can assess the quality of the movement. Such understanding may lead to therapeutic interventions which are related directly more to the function of gait than our standard regimen of strengthening and range of motion exercises. Clinicians must review critically their treatment procedures to analyze their relevance to the impaired task performance and researchers must help identify and explain the mechanical and physiologic requirements of the tasks embedded in the performance of gait.

CASE STUDY #1
JANE SMITH

Age: 74 years
Diagnosis: Right hemiplegia,
secondary to left cerebrovascular accident
Status: Six months post onset

ASSESSMENT

This 74 year old patient is presently undergoing out-patient physical therapy on a two times weekly basis for treatment of functional deficits secondary to a left CVA. Her complete history is presented elsewhere in this book, but certain pertinent historical data are worth noting here. An initial physical therapy evaluation was performed four days post onset of her CVA and revealed right upper extremity flaccidity, adductor and extensor stiffness in the right lower extremity, and severe expressive aphasia. She had decreased sensation throughout the right side of her body, and her sitting balance was fair. She was assisted maximally in rolling, transfers, and ADLs and was unable to stand and bear weight on the right lower extremity. The patient was transferred to a rehabilitation facility three weeks post onset, and a physical therapy re-evaluation at that time revealed significant weakness throughout the right lower extremity. She continued to need assistance in transfers, rolling, and in standing balance. She received an AFO for the right lower extremity. She remained in the rehabilitation facility for three weeks and then was followed in home care for five

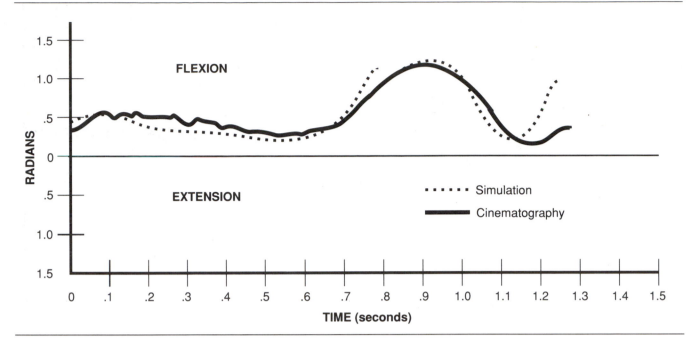

weeks. Throughout this time she received physical therapy, occupational therapy, and speech therapy.

At the present time, the patient demonstrates active hip flexion with poor right foot placement. She is able to ambulate 30 feet with a hemi-walker and requires minimal assistance in transfers. She continues to demonstrate severe verbal apraxia and moderate aphasia. She also demonstrates impulsivity during treatment, occasionally throws things, and is frequently frustrated.

The patient's problems are decreased mobility, difficulty in communication, and emotional lability including frustration and impulsivity. The goals of physical therapy are aimed at improving mobility; however, the emotional and communicative problems will influence the approach to treatment. We should create a well controlled environment and build consistency into a treatment program so the patient can discern some order in her surroundings. The exercise program which is established requires simplified tasks which can be followed easily with many repetitions. Creating such an environment may help decrease the patient's emotional outbursts as she begins to see and anticipate a well-ordered pattern in her daily routine. The physical therapist also must communicate carefully with the speech pathologist and occupational therapist in order to ensure consistency in goal setting and behavioral expectations and to avoid contradictions in approaches.

In order to establish goals for improved locomotion, the therapist must review the present pattern of movement. The patient's present status reveals a flexion synergy in the upper extremity and significant weakness in the lower extremity. There is increased tone in the trunk with scapular retraction and some trunk rotation to the right. The patient had stiffness initially in lower extremity extension and adduction and continues to demonstrate increased tone in these directions. One can visualize this patient's gait pattern in the following way. There is slow velocity with difficulty in advancing the right lower extremity. The patient advances the walker on the left and then advances the right lower extremity through hip hiking, circumduction, or posterior rotation of the pelvis. As the right limb comes forward, the right pelvis and right shoulder advance so that the pelvis and trunk are rotating in phase with each other. The patient's stance is characterized by decreased single limb stance time on the right and a foot flat initial contact. Knee flexion may not be present following contact, but the patient leans forward onto the left side during single limb support on the right so that the right hip remains flexed. Late stance is characterized by decreased or absent propulsion.

The kinematic data described are typical results of observational gait analysis. However, when taken alone, they merely reinforce the abnormality of the gait pattern. When put in the context of the specific tasks of stance and swing, these data will lead to a well focused, functional plan of care. The tasks of stance are first, support and second, propulsion. Present data do not include a review of the patient 's muscle strength, but for support, the patient requires adequate strength in hip and knee extension as well as in hip abduction. Strength in these areas should be assessed and facilitated as necessary. Propulsion is an important part of the stance phase requiring active plantarflexion. The patient has an AFO and continues to use the device. In the presence of a rigid ankle foot orthosis, active contraction of the plantarflexors for propulsion is precluded. However, a hinged AFO allows the tibia to advance over the foot. As control of the tibia is developed, facilitation of propulsion can occur. Propulsion also requires proper alignment of the trunk with the stance lower extremity. The role of plantarflexion in the stance phase is to provide a thrust in the forward direction which means that the trunk and pelvis must be in front of the stance foot. If the patient has weakness of the trunk and hip, particularly the hip extensors, the patient may be unable to advance the trunk and pelvis over the stance limb. If the hip is flexed, the patient will have difficulty in advancing the pelvis and lower extremity over the stance foot; and, consequently, the ankle will not be in a position to provide propulsion, even in the presence of contracting plantarflexors. This forward lean position may contribute to genu recurvatum and a plantarflexed ankle in late stance. Therefore, emphasis in treatment should be placed on pelvic advancement during weight bearing activities and use of plantarflexion for propulsion.

Swing requires limb clearance which means an ability to shorten the extremity adequately to avoid contacting the ground as well as the ability to transfer momentum through the extremity. The patient has active hip flexion, but actual strength of the hip is not reported. Therefore, the therapist must consider whether the patient has adequate strength to impart a forward thrust of the thigh which is the motive force for advancing the entire lower extremity. In addition, the knee joint must be swinging freely so that the forward momentum of the thigh can be translated into knee flexion, thus shortening the lower extremity. If this patient has increased extensor tone, then knee flexion and, consequently, limb shortening will be difficult. Treatment must also be directed toward facilitating thigh advancement with a freely swinging knee joint.

GOALS

Treatment goals are for the patient to:
1. increase strength in right lower extremity
2. increase endurance in ambulation skills
3. improve postural alignment during stance and during ambulation
4. improve gait pattern.

FUNCTIONAL OBJECTIVES

Following 3 months of treatment, Mrs. Smith will:
1. use active plantarflexion for propulsion during gait with verbal reminders
2. ambulate 100 feet independently with her walker
3. with verbal reminders, walk 10 feet with her walker without demonstrating genu recuravatum or forward lean
4. use pelvic advancement on the right side to equalize stride length while ambulating in the parallel bars.

TREATMENT RECOMMENDATIONS

Achieving these objectives requires a progressive training program which first considers the general strength of the patient. Although strength by itself does not predict a gait

pattern, certain threshold strengths do appear necessary for normal gait. The patient's pelvic and trunk strength must be assessed and enhanced to promote upright posture. Mat activities such as quadripedal and kneeling balance activities will promote proximal strength, as will activities on a therapy ball. Distal strength should be facilitated to enhance propulsion and to improve foot clearance.

Standing balance activities or activities on a rocker board will help facilitate distal strength. Progressive resistance exercises traditionally have been avoided in patients with increased tone. However, clinical experience has demonstrated significant improvement in gait and balance disorders with aggressive strengthening, even in the presence of increased tone. Movement patterns can be facilitated to disassociate trunk and pelvic rotations which will improve momentum transfer. Mat activities facilitating trunk or pelvic rotation in supine, sitting, and kneeling will help to disassociate trunk and pelvic movements, as will crawling activities. Manual facilitation during gait training in parallel bars also is useful in developing appropriate pelvic advancement over the stance limb, encouraging hip extension in stance, and promoting propulsion as well as preparing the limb for a more vigorous advance during swing. The patient should be encouraged to develop a two point gait pattern with the assistive device which will encourage upright trunk alignment during swing and stance.

In conclusion, the emphasis of the physical therapy program should be on developing adequate strength for support, propulsion, and limb advancement and on developing upright trunk alignment during stance. As momentum is transferred more readily, Mrs. Smith is likely to expend less energy with each gait cycle and, therefore, prolong her walking tolerance. This case demonstrates how kinematic data may be useful in developing an appropriate plan of care when the data are examined in light of the essential tasks of the gait cycle.

CASE STUDY #2
DANIEL JOHNSON

Age: 59 years
Diagnosis: Parkinson's Disease
Status: Four years post initial diagnosis

ASSESSMENT

The complete history for Mr. Johnson is presented elsewhere, but a brief review reveals a steady deterioration of ambulatory function over the four years since the diagnosis. The patient's symptoms began with general fatigue, but progressed to difficulty in rising from a seated position, a shuffling gait, a progressive forward lean, limited trunk rotation, and increasing rigidity of the upper and lower extremities. His present symptoms consist of constant bilateral tremors and increasing difficulty with balance, particularly with a tendency to fall during ambulation. Initiation of motion and transfers are becoming more difficult. Ambulation occurs without arm swing. Mr. Johnson also complains of a mild memory loss and demonstrates signs of depression. The patient's memory impairment and depression must be considered in developing goals and a treatment plan, keeping tasks simple and goals practical. All exercises should be written clearly so the patient has a record of his exercise regimen and does not have to depend on memory for completion of the program.

The patient's basic biomechanical limitations are increased rigidity and decreased isolated movements of the trunk on pelvis and the trunk and pelvis on the lower extremities. This absence of independent movement of the trunk and limbs precludes the ability to transfer momentum along one limb or from one limb to another. The patient's progressive forward lean increases the danger of forward falls, but also inhibits the patient's ability to impart forward propulsion. Thus, Mr. Johnson's treatment program should be directed toward increasing extension in the thoracic and lumbar regions to enhance upright posture and facilitating independent trunk and pelvic rotations. In promoting trunk extension, the therapist must consider the strength of the trunk and hip extensors and use exercises to promote adequate strength in these muscles.

GOALS

Treatment goals are for the patient to:
1. ambulate safely in a variety of environments
2. increase trunk and hip extension during stance
3. demonstrate improved transfer of momentum during gait.

FUNCTIONAL OBJECTIVES

Following 3 months of treatment, Mr. Johnson will:
1. ambulate independently within his house and with stand-by assistance in the community without falls
2. stand with shoulders in vertical alignment over the hips (no forward lean) with self monitoring through the use of a mirror
3. demonstrate a heel to toe pattern during ambulation for a distance of 30 feet.

TREATMENT RECOMMENDATIONS

PNF patterns are particularly useful in promoting extensor strength throughout the trunk and limbs, and exercises such as wall squats and quadripedal limb elevation will be helpful. Trunk rotation should be facilitated in a variety of positions from supine to kneeling and standing. Simple, slow rhythmic motions in hook-lying (supine with hips and knees flexed), sitting, and standing can be used initially, but should be progressed to larger arcs of varying speeds. Facilitation of arm swing can be used to enhance trunk rotation and to disassociate trunk from pelvic rotation. For example, Mr. Johnson can be instructed in golf swing movements of both upper extremities in kneeling which will enhance trunk control and facilitate rotation. Conversely, arm swing during

ambulation may be decreased because trunk rotation is limited; thus, the trunk is unable to impart rotational momentum to the upper extremities. Therefore, facilitation of trunk rotation may elicit more upper extremity movement. Trunk activities on a therapy ball also can be useful in promoting upright trunk responses.

This case study reinforces the concept that concentration on joint kinematics could mask the central problem in gait. It is undoubtedly true that this patient demonstrates decreased movements in all joint excursions, but the underlying problem is one of an absence of independent movement of trunk and limbs. Keeping this perspective allows the therapist to concentrate on the most promising areas of treatment during the limited treatment time, that is, those areas which are most likely to produce functional benefits.

CASE STUDY #3
SHIRLEY TEAL

Age: 21 years
Diagnosis: Post motor vehicle accident
Closed head injury
Status: Four months post accident

ASSESSMENT

Ms. Teal's complete history is presented elsewhere, but pertinent elements of her present status are reviewed below. The patient is alert and has understandable speech 80-90% of the time if she speaks slowly. She is extremely combative during physical therapy. The patient has active isolated movement of the right upper extremity with decreased strength and coordination. She has a 40° plantarflexion contracture at the right ankle. She has full active range of motion of the left upper and lower extremities, but with decreased coordination. She is able to perform pivot transfers and stands in the parallel bars for five minutes with minimal assistance. She has decreased weight bearing on the right lower extremity without cues and tends to lose her balance easily if she moves quickly. The patient's behavioral problems will influence dramatically her physical therapy program and require a team approach of behavior modification. The patient is scheduled for discharge in two months.

The patient demonstrates several problems which must be addressed, including behavioral problems; biomechanical problems, specifically a 40° plantarflexion contracture; and coordination problems. The behavioral problems will be addressed through a vigorous behavioral modification program involving the entire health care team. The biomechanical problem of the plantarflexion contracture is a severe one and most certainly influences her decreased balance and ambulation tolerance. The kinematic effects of such a contracture are anticipated easily and when Ms. Teal begins to ambulate include ground contact with the toes, absence of foot flat, inadequate knee extension in mid-stance, and unequal step lengths. A plantarflexion contracture results in a functional limb length discrepancy and interferes with limb advancement in swing as well as support and propulsion during the stance phase. Thus, the effects of the contracture on the specific tasks of stance and swing must be considered. Because the lower extremity on the involved side is functionally longer, safe clearance of the foot will be impaired. To ensure safe clearance, Ms. Teal would have to increase her hip and/or knee flexion in swing. This compensation would disturb the delicate timing between adjacent limb segments during swing and decrease the flow of momentum through the swing limb or between both lower extremities. The flow of momentum would be disturbed even further as she moves through single limb support in stance on the involved limb. Because the limb would be functionally much longer than the opposite limb, single limb support on the right would be characterized by an excessive rise of the patient's center of mass. Such a rise would interrupt the forward progression of the body over the stance limb and cause an interruption in energy flow, resulting in decreased efficiency.

In addition to the energy considerations of the contracture, the contracture itself decreases the available base of support on the involved side which, of course, decreases stability. The base of support is also asymmetrical. Anyone who has tried to walk with one high heel shoe on and with the other foot bare can appreciate the balance difficulties which arise. However, this patient reportedly has impaired balance. If these balance disturbances arise from vestibular abnormalities rather than the mechanical asymmetry alone, the patient may lack the necessary compensatory mechanisms to carry out the support function of stance, and she will appear quite unstable and may even fall.

The final task in gait, propulsion, will be influenced by the plantarflexion contracture. Propulsion normally is provided by a shortening contraction of the plantarflexors pushing the ankle from 5 or 10° of dorsiflexion to 20 or 30° of plantarflexion. However, this patient lacks dorsiflexion range of motion and does not have adequate range available to use a shortening contraction. She is incapable of imparting significant propulsive force. Therefore, an aggressive approach to resolving this contracture is required not only because of its impact on her overall function, but also because the patient is scheduled for discharge within two months.

GOALS

Treatment goals are for the patient to:

1. decrease plantarflexion contracture
2. increase strength in dorsiflexors and plantarflexors
3. ambulate in the parallel bars.

FUNCTIONAL OBJECTIVES

Following 2 months of treatment, Ms. Teal will:

1. increase passive right ankle dorsiflexion by 20°
2. in sitting, increase active dorsiflexion by 10° and in standing at the parallel bars, will actively rise to tip toe position

3. with verbal prompt, ambulate 20 feet in the parallel bars.

TREATMENT RECOMMENDATIONS

Serial casting of the right ankle or surgery should be considered to provide a rapid increase in dorsiflexion range of motion so the patient will have an enlarged base of support and symmetrical limb lengths. The patient's balance disturbances may be, in part, due to her plantarflexion contracture, but may also be the result of vestibular disturbances. As the patient is being treated for the ankle contracture, her balance reactions can be facilitated using tall kneeling positions and a therapy ball. Ms. Teal's coordination problems appear to be the result of difficulty in sequencing activities or planning motor activities as well as the result of flawed motor output. Multiple repetitions will be useful to improve motor output, and her ability to sequence tasks will be enhanced by keeping the tasks simple and using necessary cues. As the patient's ambulation ability improves, she can be trained using simple obstacle courses to facilitate motor planning.

This case study demonstrates the effect of a significant biomechanical lesion in the midst of more diffuse motor pathology. Improved coordination and motor planning will be of little use if the biomechanical effects of the plantarflexion contracture are not dealt with adequately.

CASE STUDY #4
SHAWNA WELLS

Age: 4 years
Diagnosis: Cerebral palsy; spastic quadriparesis;
mild mental retardation
Status: Onset at birth

ASSESSMENT

Shawna's history is presented elsewhere, but the most pertinent elements should be reviewed. The patient is approximately one year post right heel cord release. She ambulates with a posterior control walker. She reportedly has good head and trunk control, although she is most comfortable sitting in a "W" position. She also reportedly thrusts herself into extension when agitated. She rolls segmentally and creeps using a homologous pattern, but, with cues, can creep with a poorly coordinated cross diagonal pattern. She ambulates with minimal assistance with poor disassociation of the lower extremities and uses an ankle foot orthosis on the right. With the orthosis, she has a minimal heel strike. She demonstrates head righting in any direction, but has slow responses of protective extension. She demonstrates good responses to slow tilting in prone and supine, but inadequate responses in sitting. She is unable to maintain her posture in any position when moved quickly. Movement through space causes autonomic distress.

The patient's locomotor pathology is consistent with her basic problems of diminished postural responses and inadequate isolated movements of the lower extremities. These problems limit Shawna's ability to provide adequate support and propulsion during stance; and in the presence of poorly stabilized stance, contralateral swing is affected making safe limb clearance difficult. Further evidence of possible hip weakness is the poorly disassociated lower extremity movements in ambulation. The child may be using thigh contact between the limbs to provide additional stability during stance, thus compensating for gluteus maximus and gluteus medius weakness and generally reduced pelvic stability.

A complete review of the patient's strength throughout the trunk and extremities is essential for establishing appropriate goals and an effective treatment regimen. As indicated previously, adequate support during the stance phase depends on hip and knee extensor strength as well as hip abductor strength. In their absence, Shawna may be resorting to any form of stability that is available. While under the present circumstances this may be the best compensation available to her, the role of the physical therapist is to diminish the need for such compensation by increasing strength. In addition, the therapist must assess the patient's ability to contract muscles in isolated movements, that is, in the absence of compulsory activity of other muscle activity unrelated to the isolated task. If the pattern of muscle activity is synergistic in nature and not just a reflection of muscle weakness, the therapist must facilitate isolated muscle activity to provide Shawna with a broader repertoire of movements.

Decreased righting reactions and hyperactive autonomic responses to movement also limit Shawna's stability. Therefore, a variety of activities to promote balance should be used. Also, desensitization of Shawna to vestibular input will make her less susceptible to autonomic disturbances during movement.

To enhance appropriate momentum transfer, disassociation of the lower extremities during stance must be facilitated, although this goal is contingent upon Shawna's improved central control and her ability to maintain support on the stance limb.

GOALS

Treatment goals are for the patient to:

1. consistently right herself to midline when passive displacements are performed

2. increase hip extensor and hip abductor strength

3. ambulate independently with the posterior control walker.

FUNCTIONAL OBJECTIVES

Following 3 months of treatment, Shawna will:

1. in sitting, right herself to midline when quickly displaced 10° to the left or to the right, 1 of 3 trials

2. in the walker, stand on one leg without dropping the opposite hip for 10 seconds

3. ambulate independently from her class to the cafeteria (50 feet) using the posterior control walker.

TREATMENT RECOMMENDATIONS

A wide variety of activities to increase proximal strength are available to the physical therapist. Postural activities in prone, supine, quadriped, and kneeling can be used to facilitate activity of the trunk and pelvic girdle musculature. To promote trunk control and righting reactions, the patient can be exercised on a therapy ball to develop appropriate trunk shifts and to facilitate righting reactions. Activities in tall kneeling and half kneeling postures also can facilitate appropriate trunk responses as well as promote strength in the trunk and pelvis. Such activities may be used to desensitize the patient's vestibular system and facilitate isolated movements. As Shawna's central control improves, activities to promote disassociation of the lower extremities can be introduced such as creeping, side stepping, and walking backwards.

Shawna demonstrates the need for proximal and isolated control to meet the requirements of the stance and swing phases of gait: support, propulsion, and transfer of momentum. Such control depends on adequate strength because, although superior strength is not a direct requirement of normal gait, it remains an important ingredient in certain circumstances. ❑

REFERENCES

1. Krebs DE, Edelstein JE, Fishman S: Reliability of observational gait anaylsis. Phys Ther 65: 1027-1033, 1985
2. Eberhart HD, Inman VT, Saunders JB, et al: Fundamental studies of human locomotion and other information relating to design of artificial limbs. A report to the National Research Council, Committee on Artificial Limbs, University of California, Berkeley, 1947
3. Murray MP: Gait as a total pattern of movement including a bibliography on gait. Am J Phys Med 46: 290-330, 1967
4. Larsson LE, Oberg PA: Selspot recording of gait in normal and in patients with spasticity. Scand J Rehabil Med Suppl 6: 21-27, 1978
5. Simon SR, Deutsch SD, Nuzzo RM, et al: Genu recurvatum in spastic cerebral palsy: Report on findings in gait analysis. J Bone Joint Surg 60 A: 882-894, 1978
6. Winter DA, Patla AE, Frank JS, Walt SE: Biomechanical walking patterns in the fit and health elderly. Phys Ther 70: 340-347, 1990
7. Winter DA, Greenlaw RF, Hobson DA: Television-computer analysis of kinematics of human gait. Comput Biomed Res 5:498-504, 1972
8. Finely FR, Karpovich PV: Electrogoniometric analysis of normal and pathological gaits. Res Quart 35 Suppl: 379-384, 1964
9. Gyory AN, Chao EY, Stauffer RN: Functional evaluation of normal and pathological knees during gait. Arch Phys Med Rehabil 57: 571-577, 1976
10. Johnston RC, Smidt GL: Measurement of hip joint motion during walking: Evaluation of an electrogoniometric method. J. Bone Joint Surg 51 A: 1083, 1969
11. Inman VT, Ralston HJ, Todd F: Human Walking. Williams and Wilkins, Baltimore, MD, 1981
12. Murray MP, Kory RC, Clarkson BH: Walking patterns in healthy old men. J. Gerontol: 24:169, 1969
13. Murray MP, Kory RC, Sepic SB: Walking patterns of normal women. Arch Phys Med 51: 637, 1979
14. Murray MP, Frought AB, Kory RC: Walking patterns of normal men. J Bone Joint Surg 46: 335, 1964
15. Murray MP, Kory RC, Clarkson BH, Sepic SB: Comparison of free and fast speed walking patterns of normal men. Am J Phys Med 45: 8-24, 1966
16. Craik RL, Oatis CA: Gait assessment in the clinic: Issues and approaches. In Rothstein JM (ed): Measurement in Physical Therapy. New York, NY, Churchill Livingstone, 1985, pp 169-205
17. Himann JE, Cunningham DA, Rechnitzer PA, Paterson DH: Age-related changes in speed of walking. Med and Science in Sports and Exercise 20: 161-166, 1988
18. Craik R, Cook T, D' Orazio B: Variations in healthy gait with changes in velocity. Phys Ther 60: 575, 1980 (abstr)
19. Smidt GL: Hip motion and related factors in walking. Phys Ther 51: 9-21, 1971
20. Winter DA: The Biomechanics and Motor Control of Human Gait. Waterloo, Ontario, Canada, University of Waterloo Press, 1987
21. Jacobs NA, Skorecki J, Charnley J: Analysis of the vertical component of force in normal and pathological gait. J. Biomech 5: 11-34, 1972
22. Bresler B, Frankel SP: The forces and moments in the leg during level walking. Transactions of the ASME: 27-36, 1950
23. Paul JP: Forces transmitted by joint in the human body. Proc Inst Mech Eng 181:8, 1967
24. Seireg A, Arvikar R: The prediction of muscular load-sharing and joint forces in the lower extremities during walking. J Biomech 8: 89-102, 1975
25. Crowninshield RD, Brand RA, Johnston RC: The effects of walking velocity and age on hip kinematics and kinetics. Clin Orthop 132:140, 1978
26. Morrison JB: Bioengineering analysis of force actions transmitted by the knee joint. Biomed Eng. 3:164-170, 1968
27. Harrington IJ: A bioengineering analysis of force actions at the knee in normal and pathological gait. Biomed Eng. 167-172, 1976
28. Stauffer RN, Chao EYS, Brewster RC: Force and motion analysis of the normal, diseased, and prosthetic ankle joint. Clinical Orthopaedics and Related Res 127: 189-199, 1977
29. Winter DA: Overall principle of lower limb support during stance phase of gait. J Biomech 13: 923-927, 1980
30. Winter DA, Yack HJ: EMG profiles during normal human walking: stride-to-stride and inter-subject variability. Electroenceph and Clinical Neurophys 67:402-411, 1987
31. Milner M, Basmajian JV, Quanbury AO: Multifactorial analysis of walking by electromyography and computer. Am J Phys Med 50: 235 , 1971
32. Dubo HIC, Peat M, Winter, DA, et al: Electromyographic temporal analysis of gait: normal human locomotion. Arch Phys Med Rehabil 57: 415, 1976
33. Perry J, Fox JM, Boitano MA, et al: Functional evaluation of the pes anserinus transfer by electromyography and gait analysis. J Bone Joint Surg 62 A: 973-980, 1980
34. Hagy JL, Mann RA, Keller CW: Normal Electromyographic Data Gait Analysis Laboratory, Shriners Hospital for Crippled Children, San Francisco, CA, 1973
35. Mochon S, McMahon TA: Ballistic walking. J Biomech 13: 49, 1980
36. Winter DA, Quanbury AO, Reimer GD: Analysis of instantaneous energy of normal gait. J Biomech 9: 253-257, 1976
37. Robertson DGE, Winter DA: Mechanical energy generation, absorption and transfer amongst segments during walking. J Biomech 13: 845-854, 1980
38. Morrison JB: The mechanics of the knee in relation to normal walking. J Biomech 3: 51-61, 1970
39. Wells RP: Mechanical energy costs of human movement: An approach to evaluating the transfer possiblilites of two-joint muscles. J Biomech 21: 955, 1988
40. Winter DA: Biomechanics of Human Movement, John Wiley , New York, NY, 1979
41. Das P, McCollum G: Invariant structure in locomotion. Neuroscience 25 (3): 1023-1034,1988
42. Winter DA: Biomechanics of normal and pathological gait: Implications for understanding human locomotor control. J Motor Behavior, in publication
43. Olgiatti R, Burgunder JM, Mumenthaler M: Increased energy cost of walking in multiple sclerosis: Effect of spasticity, ataxia, and weakness. Arch Phys Med Rehabil 69: 846-849,1988
44. Cerny K, Waters R, Hislop H, Perry J: Walking and wheelchair energetics in persons with paraplegia. Phys Ther 60: 1133-1139, 1980
45. Bendersky E,Machold P, Rorh M: Assessment of community ambulation skill. Unpublished Masters Thesis, Beaver College, Glenside, PA, 1990
46. Krebs DE: Isokinetic, electrophysiologic, and clinical function relationships following tourniquet-aided knee arthrotomy. Phys Ther 69: 803-815, 1989
47. Stauffer RN, Chao EYS, Gyory AN: Biomechanical gait analysis of the diseased knee joint. Clin Orthop Rel Res. 126: 246-255, 1977
48. Tardieu C, Lespargot A, Tabary C, et al: Toe-walking in children with cerebral palsy: Contributions of contracture and excessive contraction of triceps surae muscle. Phys Ther 69: 656-662, 1989
49. Oatis CA: The use of a mechanical model to predict the motion of the knee in normal locomotion: A study of healthy younger and older adult males. Unpublished Doctoral dissertation, University of Pennsylvania, Philadelphia, PA, 1982
50. Brinkman JR, Perry J: Rate and range of knee motion during ambulation in health and arthritic subjects, Phys Ther 65: 1055-1060, 1985

ACKNOWLEDGMENTS

I would like to thank Erica M. Fletcher, PT and Patricia G. Morris, PT, M.S. for their clinical insight and assistance in preparing these case studies.

Chapter 12
The Patients In Treatment

Patricia C. Montgomery, Ph.D., PT
Barbara H. Connolly, Ed.D., PT

INTRODUCTION

Patients with neurologic deficits seldom have isolated problems, but rather multiple problems as identified in the preceding chapters. For teaching purposes, assessment and treatment of each problem area have been presented separately. However, in the clinic, we must deal with the whole person, not problems in isolation. The purpose of this chapter is to provide examples of comprehensive treatment sessions for the patients used in the case studies. In each of the cases, the goals and functional objectives are written for a 2 - 3 month period.

CASE STUDY #1
MRS. JANE SMITH

Age: 74 years
Diagnosis: Right hemiplegia,
secondary to left cerebrovascular accident
Status: Six months post onset

GOALS

Quarterly goals of physical therapy are for Mrs. Smith to:

1. demonstrate improved awareness and use of the right side of the body as well as the right side of visual space

2. perform transfers with increased speed and safety

3. increase strength and coordination in right extremities

4. improve gait pattern and functional ambulation skills with walker.

FUNCTIONAL OBJECTIVES

Following 3 months of treatment, Mrs. Smith will:

1. be able to perform 3 sets of 10 repetitions of resistive exercises to the right dorsiflexors and knee extensors with green thera-band (sitting in wheelchair)

2. be able to maintain a midline posture in standing for 30 seconds with vision and 10 seconds without vision (standing with walker)

3. transfer independently in and out of her wheelchair to the walker and mat table, 100% of the time

4. identify with 75% accuracy small, familiar objects with the right hand without having explored them with the left hand

5. orient spontaneously to visual stimuli on the right, 2 of 3 times

6. demonstrate less circumduction and retraction with the right hip during gait, using increased knee flexion and ankle dorsiflexion

7. use full active range of motion when reaching forward or to the right and reaching across the midline with the right arm.

SAMPLE TREATMENT SESSION

Mrs. Smith comes to the rehabilitation department as an out-patient. She receives 45 minutes of speech therapy, followed by a 15 minute break, then 45 minutes of physical therapy. Following physical therapy and another 15 minute rest, she receives 45 minutes of occupational therapy.

Mrs. Smith's physical therapy program involves numerous changes of position to allow practice of transfers and to increase concentration. However, the sequence from session to session is similar so she has a consistent routine to follow. This helps her anticipate activities and decreases her frustration when practicing more difficult elements of her therapy program.

Mrs. Smith comes to the physical therapy department in a wheelchair. Her shoes, AFO, and socks are removed and she begins her therapy program with a series of "warm-up" exercises. These consist of resistive exercises using theraband to right ankle dorsiflexors and knee extensors. A few repetitions first are performed on the left side before performing exercises on the right side. She also performs bilateral activities of the upper extremities, including hand-to-mouth patterns, holding the arms in forward flexion with elbow extension, and raising and lowering the arms with elbow extension.

While still barefoot, Mrs. Smith transfers from her wheelchair to standing in a corner of the therapy gym. She practices maintaining a midline, upright posture using a mirror with her eyes open, and for brief periods (3-5 seconds) with her eyes closed. A number of textured surfaces are used (carpeting, tile, doormats) to increase tactile input and increase awareness of the right foot and lower extremity. Mrs. Smith then transfers back into her wheelchair and her socks, AFO, and shoes are put on.

Mrs. Smith transfers from her wheelchair to a stationary bicycle. She pedals the bicycle at a low resistance using a metronome to improve timing and reciprocation. She takes rest breaks whenever she becomes fatigued or loses her timing. She also is encouraged to maintain her grasp bilaterally on the handlebars to increase upper extremity sensory input and to maintain a symmetrical position on the bicycle. The bicycle is placed with the left side against the therapy wall, so that Mrs. Smith has to orient to her right and look into right space to observe the therapy room and other objects and people in the environment.

Following work on the bicycle, Mrs. Smith uses her walker to walk to the parallel bars. While in the bars, Mrs. Smith performs semi-deep knee bends, with emphasis on symmetry to increase strength in the hip and knee extensors. She practices standing with her weight on the left and swinging her right leg with her knee flexing and extending. She also practices standing on the right leg without knee hyperextension and lifting the left leg. PNF resistive exercises to increase pelvic rotation and hip extension are done. Mrs. Smith walks in the bars trying to rotate her right hip forward and increase knee flexion during gait. She then attempts to use this same pattern with her walker.

Following gait training, Mrs. Smith walks to the mat table and transfers onto it. She then works on upper extremity patterns and control. Prior to working on movement patterns the therapist rubs Mrs. Smith's upper extremities (first the left, then the right) with various textured materials, such as velvet, corduroy, cotton, and wool, asking her to identify if the material is smooth or rough. Active-assistive and active exercises are then performed. For example, with Mrs. Smith supine, the therapist positions the right arm at 90 degrees of flexion with the elbow extended and asks Mrs. Smith to hold this position, then to lower the extremity against gravity. Mrs. Smith holds her shoulder in 90 degrees of forward flexion, then attempts to flex and extend her elbow.

Mrs. Smith transfers from the mat table back into her wheelchair. Transfers stress using the correct sequence of weight-shifting with smoothness to maintain momentum, as well as safety factors, such as locking the wheelchair, positioning it optimally for the transfer, and requesting assistance for more difficult transfers. Once she is sitting in her wheelchair, a number of sequenced upper and lower extremity tasks are attempted. She is asked to imitate the therapist to perform tapping movements first of the left hand and foot, then the right hand and foot. Eventually, she is progressed to more complicated combinations of left hand, right foot and right hand, left foot movements. She practices manipulating and identifying objects (without vision), such as a key, pencil, shoelace, and block, first with the left hand, then with the right hand. At the end of the session she is given a functional task to complete while she rests before occupational therapy. These tasks have been devised in consultation with the occupational therapist and represent tasks of interest to Mrs. Smith. Today, she is asked to place and arrange artificial flowers in a large vase. The flowers are placed on her right side and she is instructed to reach and obtain them with the right hand before transferring them to the left to be placed in the vase. The vase is made of plastic, for safety purposes, and is tall and cylindrical, requiring that Mrs. Smith stabilize it with her right hand while she places the flowers inside.

Mrs. Smith has a home program of exercises to perform each week. These are outlined in writing with stick figures to illustrate the specific exercises. Exercises include theraband strengthening exercises for the right ankle dorsiflexors and knee extensors, as well as bilateral upper extremity exercises in forward flexion with elbow extension and maintained forward flexion with isolated elbow flexion and extension. She has been instructed to suspend a ball on a string from the ceiling and to practice visual tracking left and right as it swings. Trunk symmetry exercises in sitting, consisting of leaning left and right, then to the middle, using a mirror for feedback are also part of her home program.

CASE STUDY #2
MR. DANIEL JOHNSON

Age: 59 years
Diagnosis: Parkinson's Disease
Status: Four years post initial diagnosis

GOALS

Quarterly goals of physical therapy are for Mr. Johnson to:
1. demonstrate improved short term memory

2. increase trunk mobility, especially active extension and rotation

3. initiate voluntary movements more quickly and with improved coordination

4. perform transfers safely

5. maintain independence in gait

6. participate in a Parkinson's support group.

FUNCTIONAL OBJECTIVES

Following 3 months of therapy, Mr. Johnson will:

1. remember and repeat the initial activity during therapy sessions, 3 of 3 times

2. perform 10 repetitions of trunk rotation exercises in kneeling

3. place 10 colored pegs in a cribbage board when given a command for each color (within 5 seconds for each peg)

4. maintain standing balance on a 2" piece of foam for 60 seconds

5. walk a 100 foot obstacle course with 10 obstacles to negotiate within 2 minutes

6. perform three sit to stand to sit exercises independently from a bench or chair without armrests

7. participate in group exercise program and support group with a minimum of 75% attendance.

SAMPLE TREATMENT SESSION

Mr. Johnson comes to physical therapy as an outpatient once each week. He is asked at each session to remember the initial activity and to demonstrate it again at the end of the session. During this session, he initially practices kicking a soccer ball across the treatment room several times. Mr. Johnson then performs a number of mat exercises, including rolling to both sides, first leading with the arms, then with the hips, to improve trunk mobility. He also works on prone extension of the trunk by pushing up on extended arms and also by assuming a pivot prone position. In kneeling, he practices a "golf swing" and trunk twisting (rotation) to both sides. In this position, he also performs lateral trunk flexion to each side. In all fours, he works on isolating extension of one hip with his knee flexed and performs repetitive exercises to increase strength of hip extensors.

While sitting on a chair without armrests, he does reciprocal pulley exercises (non-resistive) on verbal commands emphasizing initiating and stopping movement as well as different rates of movements (i.e., start, stop, fast, slow). He practices active trunk rotation while seated on a bench and sit to stand to sit exercises to practice rising from a chair as well as to increase strength in knee and hip extensors.

After resting for a brief period, he works on upper extremity tasks. He is given three step commands, i.e., place a red peg in the cribbage board, throw the ball to me, then place a blue peg in the cribbage board.

Mr. Johnson works on standing posture by standing with his back against a wall. He is asked to stand as erect as possible with his upper back touching the wall. He practices rocking back on his heels and attempts to maintain his balance on his whole foot, rather than on the balls of his feet. Working barefoot increases his awareness of weight-shifting in standing. He also practices standing on foam surfaces of different compliances. With his shoes back on, Mr. Johnson practices walking and attempts to march to music of different speeds. He also practices stepping over obstacles of different heights with stand by assistance of the therapist as necessary for safety.

At the end of the session, Mr. Johnson is asked to demonstrate the initial activity (i.e., kicking the soccer ball). He and the therapist review the written home program established for him at the group sessions. The therapist provides encouragement for Mr. Johnson's continued participation in the support group.

CASE STUDY #3
SHIRLEY TEAL

Age: 21 years
Diagnosis: Post motor vehicle accident
Closed head injury
Status: Four months post accident

GOALS

The goals for Ms. Teal to attain in two months are to:

1. increase strength and coordination patterns in the right upper extremity

2. increase range of motion in right lower extremity

3. improve stimulus identification ability in both hands

4. become more symmetrical with equal weight through both sides of her body in sitting and standing

5. improve balance and stability in the upright position without vision

6. begin assisted ambulation.

FUNCTIONAL OBJECTIVES

Following two months of therapy, Ms. Teal will:

1. reach and grasp an object placed at shoulder height, using shoulder flexion and elbow extension for 15 trials

2. increase passive right ankle dorsiflexion by 20 degrees

3. match 3 dimensional circle and square forms using tactile and proprioceptive cues (without vision), with 75% accuracy

4. match a vertical taped line in midline of her shirt with a taped vertical line in mirror, while standing in the parallel bars, 4 of 5 trials

5. stand in the parallel bars with neutral alignment of hips and knees and with both feet flat on the floor for 30 seconds with the eyes closed

6. ambulate length of parallel bars with minimal verbal prompting.

SAMPLE TREATMENT SESSION

Ms. Teal comes to physical therapy three times a week at the extended care facility. Usually, she comes to therapy in the mornings when she appears to be less easily agitated. Each of her therapy sessions lasts approximately 45 minutes.

Her physical therapy program begins with Ms. Teal in supine on the therapy mat after she has transferred independently from her wheelchair. Active-assisted exercises using PNF patterns for the right upper and lower extremities are performed with the therapist specifically emphasizing active right ankle dorsiflexion and hip and knee extension.

Because of her difficulties with benign paroxysmal positional nystagmus and vertigo, activities in the therapy department initially are focusing on habituation for this problem. These activities consist of 5 repetitions to the left side in a modified Hallpike position. She begins in a sitting position on the side of the bed and tilts rapidly to her left side to recline on pillows placed on that side, allowing her head to tilt slightly upward. After waiting for the dizziness to subside, or 30 seconds, she sits back up. After waiting for the dizziness to subside in an upright position, or 30 seconds, she repeats the exercise. Ms. Teal performs these exercises two times per day with the assistance of the nursing staff as a part of her habituation program.

Ms. Teal remains in a sitting position and practices maintaining a midline position. Using verbal and visual (mirror) cues to establish midline, Ms. Teal is asked to practice weight shifting in all directions, returning to midline after each of the tilts. She then is asked to practice without vision by closing her eyes. Once she feels that she is in midline, the therapist asks her to open her eyes and to correct her posture as needed by using the mirror.

Ms. Teal transfers to a chair with arms. She begins working on strengthening and coordination of the right arm by reaching out for a hairbrush and then brushing her hair. Other activities for the upper extremity include having her reach for objects that are held in various positions (i.e., over head, out to her side) and then placing the objects onto a table or shelf. To help her with response selection, simple one part commands are used initially in executing movements with the upper extremity and then progressed to two choice commands using the terminology "left" or "right" to indicate which hand she is to use in reaching.

While sitting at a table, Ms. Teal works on palpating an object with her eyes closed. The object is then removed from her hand and she opens her eyes. She states the name of the object or locates a matching object in a box of objects. She also is asked to palpate common objects while she has her eyes closed and then demonstrate their usage.

At the end of the session, Ms. Teal is asked to stand in the parallel bars. The following activities are done while she is standing to help improve her balance, weight shifting, and mobility of her right ankle:

1. turning her head and trunk to look behind her in both directions

2. standing, reaching forward, backward, and laterally to reach objects held by the therapist while she maintains her feet as flat on the floor as possible

3. standing on her right foot, without leaning to the side and holding for a count of five with her eyes open and then with her eyes closed

4. standing on her right foot, placing her left foot to the front, and holding for a count of 5 with her eyes open and then with her eyes closed

5. walking forward in the parallel bars with minimal prompting from the therapist to move her legs forward.

Ms. Teal completes her exercise program by practicing standing and walking short distances (5 feet) with a rolling walker with maximal assistance from the therapist.

CASE STUDY #4
SHAWNA WELLS

Age: 4 years

Diagnosis: Cerebral palsy; spastic quadriparesis; mild mental retardation

Status: Onset at birth

GOALS

Quarterly goals of physical therapy are for Shawna to:

1. decrease avoidance responses

2. increase variety of trunk movements

3. improve active glenohumeral movement

4. increase lower extremity reciprocation

5. improve balance and protective reactions during a variety of motor tasks

6. increase hip extensor and hip abductor strength

7. ambulate independently with the posterior control walker

8. improve selective attention.

FUNCTIONAL OBJECTIVES

Following three months of physical therapy, Shawna will:

1. tolerate being swaddled in a blanket for 5 minutes without fretting

2. use a segmental trunk pattern when rolling on the floor and maintain a stable pelvis in tailor sitting on the floor while rotating to reach an object behind her

3. reach for an object with 90 degrees of forward flexion at the glenohumeral joint without elevating her shoulder, 2 of 3 trials

4. creep 25 feet with a reciprocal pattern with verbal reminders and demonstrate longer distances between knee placement as measured by chalk prints on the floor

5. independently fall forward out of her walker onto a 3" thick mat, catching herself effectively with extended arms, 3 of 5 times

6. in the walker, stand on one leg without dropping the opposite hip for 10 seconds

7. ambulate independently from her class to the cafeteria (50 feet) using the posterior control walker

8. attend to a table activity for 5 minutes without being distracted by two other children working at the same table.

SAMPLE TREATMENT SESSION

Shawna is seen in physical therapy on a twice weekly basis through her preschool program. She is in a classroom with 9 other children that is located approximately 30 feet from the therapy room. In addition to the direct physical therapy that she receives twice weekly, the physical therapist consults with the classroom teacher and offers suggestions on how many of the activities from the treatment session can be incorporated into the classroom.

Shawna walks to the physical therapy room using her walker and with stand by assistance from a classroom aide. Therapy begins by wrapping a cotton blanket around Shawna and then requesting Shawna to remove the blanket. She then wraps her own arms with a towel and unwraps the towel with guidance and assistance. This treatment is followed by having Shawna search for toys that are hidden in containers of sand, rice, or beans. After doing this searching, Shawna does fingerpainting with pudding or whipped cream so that she gradually has to experience more aversive sensory input to her hands during the session.

Shawna's aversion to fast movement is dealt with in a variety of activities. First, she is asked to roll up an inclined wedge independently. Then, she is allowed to roll quickly down the wedge with the therapist helping to increase the speed by propelling Shawna at the pelvis. Next, Shawna is placed in sitting on a mat and then pushed forward and sideways by the therapist to get Shawna to place her hands to the front or sides. The speed of the displacement is gradually increased by the therapist. The therapist then moves in front of Shawna and grasps her legs. With Shawna lightly placing her hands on her thighs, the therapist then lifts either both of Shawna's legs upward or one leg in a diagonal movement across midline. Either displacement moves Shawna's center of gravity backwards or to the sides. This will cause Shawna to place her hands appropriately for support. This activity is presented as a game to Shawna and the therapist counts as Shawna is waiting to be lifted. Each lift occurs at different times during the counting. Shawna moves to a kneeling position and is pushed forward by the therapist at differing times to get her to place her hands out to catch herself.

To further work on Shawna's fear of movement and on her lack of lower extremity dissociation, Shawna rides a small tricycle. Her feet are in cuffs that are attached to the pedals of the tricycle so that her feet do not slide off the pedals during movement. The therapist ties a rope to the handle bars of the tricycle and then begins to pull Shawna forward. Shawna is encouraged to push the pedals on her own and the therapist moves the tricycle over both flat and slightly inclined surfaces (ramps) so that Shawna varies the degree of propulsion that is needed.

After riding the tricycle, Shawna stands in her posterior control walker. The therapist rolls a medium sized ball to Shawna and asks her to kick the ball with her right foot. This allows Shawna to shift her weight to her left leg and causes her to maintain her pelvis in alignment as she stands momentarily on the left foot. Next, she kicks with her left leg and shifts her weight to the right leg. This alternation of kicking is done for about 5 minutes.

At the end of the session, Shawna sits at a small table with the therapist. She works on a number of puzzles with pieces that have either small or large knobs attached. The puzzle pieces are held at different heights and positions so that Shawna has to use a variety of reaching strategies to obtain the puzzle piece with either her right or left hand. Small 1/4 pound weights are placed on each of Shawna's wrists during the activity to increase proprioceptive input and to increase the strength in her upper extremities. The length of time that she sits at the table and works on the puzzle increases in 1/2 minute increments per week from one minute to five minutes.

After completing the session in the therapy room, Shawna walks back to her classroom in the posterior walker with her classroom aide. However, a piece of carpet and a 4'x4' piece of thin foam rubber are placed in the hallway so that Shawna walks over a variety of textures and surfaces while using her walker.

CONCLUSION

Not all goals, objectives, or therapeutic techniques for each of the patients were addressed in this chapter. Setting goals and objectives provides a framework for administering treatment. A variety of techniques can be used to meet the same objective or several objectives simultaneously. Although repetition is important in treatment, a variety of activities makes the sessions enjoyable and motivating for the patient and the therapist. Creativity, therefore, is the art of physical therapy. ❑

Index